The Implementer's Guide To Primary Care Behavioral Health

A Publication of the Collaborative Family Healthcare Association in partnership with Access Community Health Centers (Madison, WI).

Edited By Neftali Serrano

E-book ISBN: 979-8-218-36773-2
Print ISBN: 978-0-615-96751-6

All proceeds from sales of this book will go to the Collaborative Family Healthcare Association (CFHA). CFHA is a not-for-profit member association promoting the integration of physical and behavioral health in the US health system.

℅ Neftali Serrano
Collaborative Family Healthcare Association
11312 US 15-501 N., Suite 107-154
Chapel Hill NC 27517
United States

http://cfha.net

Cover artwork by Leiana Edwards

A Note On Web Links In This Book:

This book was designed as e-book first where all links are active. For the physical edition of the book go to this site for the links by page number:

https://www.cfha.net/resources/the-implementers-guide-to-primary-care-behavioral-health-link-page/

Note that links posted more than once in the text are only listed once in the link page. Our apologies for broken links as web page addresses may change over time.

This book is a tribute to those who tirelessly strive to improve healthcare and to the patients who have taught us valuable lessons about what truly works.

Foreword

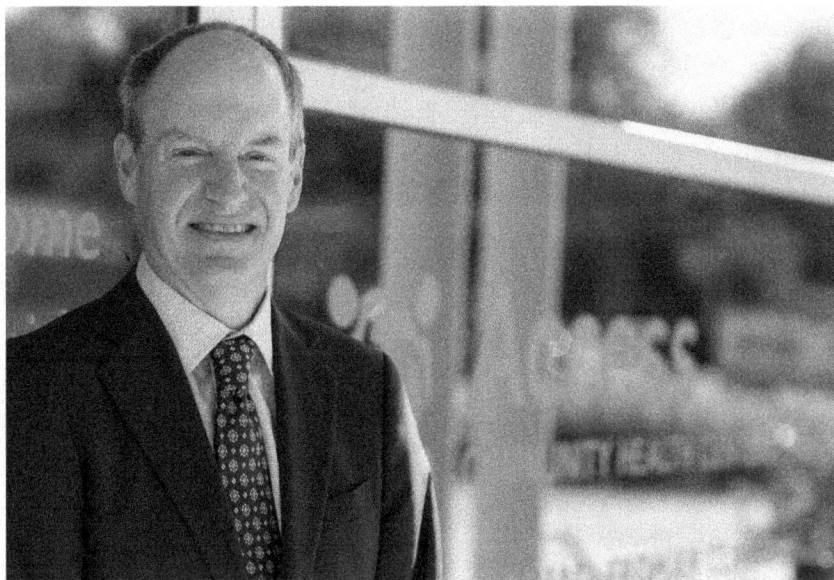

I am honored and grateful to be reprising my forward for the second edition of this groundbreaking text. I wrote in the first edition that "the best thing to come along in primary care medicine in my career is the integrated behavioral health model." That sentiment has grown as I've watched our behavioral health team expand and flourish and help our organization do the same.

The provision of health care is in a constant state of flux. We always strive to strengthen the care we provide, improve the patient experience, and grow to serve more community members who need a trusted healthcare home. What has been especially notable over the past several years is how behavioral health integration has grown deep roots in our organization and helped us adapt to our changing environment. We've built a more inclusive culture, created mechanisms to appreciate our employees actively, practiced resiliency in the face of the COVID-19 pandemic, and recruited, retained, and promoted a committed and diverse staff. When we recently struggled to recruit dental assistants, we successfully adopted the "train your own" mentality of the behavioral health practice, where they have a longstanding training program that has been the primary recruiting source of our workforce from the program's inception.

Behavioral health integration has also solidified critical components of our clinical care. As the opioid epidemic continues, we have significantly expanded our substance use disorder services, including medication-assisted treatment. There was widespread support for the effort from the medical providers because they knew they would be working with the support and expertise of the behavioral health consultants.

Our Chief Behavioral Health Officer, Dr. Beth Zeidler Schreiter, has been instrumental in advocacy to support the integrated model. She has built relationships throughout the state and successfully advocated for more practical payment models that align with the integrated model and pay us for the additional services our patients need. We have recently augmented our model with the Collaborative Care model to effectively manage our population of patients with behavioral and mental health needs and receive reimbursement for that essential work.

The integrated behavioral health model at Access Community Health Centers encompasses all aspects of our organization. As a result, our employees experience a more inclusive and functional workplace, and our patients receive better care.

This book is cosponsored by Access and CFHA and is a testament to the power of integrated care. It is written by the people doing the work in the clinics daily and highlights the necessity of sharing this model more widely across the primary care landscape. I'm grateful to be an advocate who knows firsthand that the model has made our organization a better place to work for employees and a better place for our patients to receive care.

Ken Loving, MD
Chief Executive Officer,
Access Community Health Centers
Madison, WI

Prologue

Nearly a decade ago, we wrote the first edition of this text nearly on a whim. We knew we had a story to tell, and we wanted to tell that story in a way that differentiated the text from other manuals and scholarly articles. Much has changed since we first published the inaugural edition, including many positive developments in the field of integrated care, but the need for this kind of book has yet to. This book remains the only narrative-based text on implementing the Primary Care Behavioral Health (PCBH) service delivery model in real-world settings. We write again to update our story and add more wisdom and learning we have discovered in the ensuing years.

Much has changed including the "we" referenced above and throughout the book. The editor, then the Chief Behavioral Health Officer at Access Community Health Centers, became the Chief Executive Officer of a national nonprofit, the Collaborative Family Healthcare Association. That association is now a co-sponsor of the text with Access. The book's authorship has expanded with new voices and stories, including stories from other exemplary clinics.

We invited authors from other organizations to tell their stories to highlight that Access' story is not the only one out there and to underline the point that what we have learned at Access is shared elsewhere as well.

Where applicable, we have included sections or segments from the first edition to provide a sense of the progression from a clinic seven years into program development to one that had reached maturity at nearly 17 years of growth by 2024. The interested reader can refer to the first edition to fully scope the changes.

Our true north in writing is to encourage the emerging workforce and the program developers in the world still fighting for a vision of healthcare that prioritizes the whole person. Integrated care is a core piece of restoring the lifeblood of primary care and revisioning the work of healthcare teams. We write because telling stories is one of the critical ways we learn and one of the best ways we remind ourselves of what is good in the world. We hope you are reminded and equipped by our stories in the following pages.

Neftali Serrano, PsyD
Chief Executive Officer, Collaborative Family Healthcare Association
Editor

Chapter 1: Did We Make A Dent In The Universe?

By Neftali Serrano, PsyD

What We Were Trying To Achieve

PCBH, like any service delivery model, has evolved. While there is no formal history of the model in print, see here for a good overview. The initial aims of the model were to address a fundamental problem: what to do with the large number of individuals accessing primary care for behavioral health support. So, did we solve that dilemma? Did we make a dent in the universe after over 20 years?

Like most things in life, an authentic assessment incorporates much grey in the answer; this is true of the PCBH model since we learned that the actual need in primary care was more complex than we initially thought. It is important to remember that when PCBH was developed, the notion of care teams, the patient-centered medical home, and even basic concepts like registries for chronic disease conditions were still in their infancy. We assumed that PCBH had a role in working with all of the primary care functions, but those functions have evolved, and, with it, the role of the Behavioral Health Consultant (BHC). A good example is Medication Assisted Treatment (MAT) which did not exist in its current form at the outset of the PCBH model. What we can say is that PCBH has shown itself to be adaptable. These developments have been matched by PCBH adherents and incorporated into clinical workflows, process improvements, and other program development efforts over the last two decades. So that has been a definite win.

As to the initial goal of PCBH (the need to embed a behavioral health provider into a care team effectively), the last two decades have shown that this is the best way to embed a clinician. There have yet to be any demonstrations of alternative methods (that have the same goals as PCBH) that have been successful. In other words, if you aim for improved access to the population, improved integration with the care team, and a generalized impact across mental and behavioral conditions, there has yet to come along a PCBH alternative. (Note, for adherents of other models, which we love as well and which PCBH plays nicely with, those other models have different goals.) So, the co-located clinician running a specialty model in a primary care clinic is not an adequate PCBH model replacement. After 20 years, this is a well-defined finding bolstered by the proliferation of the model.

Did We Solve The Workforce Issue?

The main outstanding concern with the model is how to staff it; this was a problem at the outset and continues to be a significant issue for most programs, especially in rural and smaller states. While more resources and training are available for prospective BHCs in general, the lack of defined pathways for professional development limit the available supply of BHCs. Most BHCs receive on-the-job training, which is an expensive and far-too-often unsuccessful process, and data on this phenomenon needs to be published. Still, the consensus among technical assistance providers is that the rate of successful onboarding of BHCs, meaning the rate at which they stick around long enough and get what working in PCBH means, needs to be higher. Most professionals do not enter the profession with socialization for primary care - they only receive this after their training in specialty mental health. Again, there are certificate programs, internships, post-docs, and even a doctoral program that caters to future PCBH'ers, but most new hires still are retro-fit professionals. So, no, we have not solved the workforce issue.

Clinical Outcomes Research: How are we doing?

Another grey area in evaluating the impact of the PCBH model is the issue of clinical efficacy. Here we get into an oft-cited and often misguided critique of the model. Does the PCBH model improve clinical outcomes? As is often the case, the problem is with formulating the question. There are several considerations we need to investigate here.

First, to what should we compare the PCBH model? Given that the goal of the model is providing access to behavioral health support, should we use patients receiving no care at all as the comparison group (which is a problematic control group to access)? Most critics are really asking, "Do 15-30 minute interventions, spaced farther apart, work just as well as specialty therapy which takes 45 minutes and many sessions of often weekly meetings?" Remember that PCBH does not introduce any new interventions per se but repackages them for a unique setting and distributes them differently than specialty psychotherapy. So, the real question is not whether the tools work themselves (same tools used in psychotherapy), but whether the delivery and packaging work well (again, in comparison to what?).

This brings up yet another conundrum the field still needs to work out: understanding and measuring the role of context and the care team as a unit of care delivery. The PCBH model is not intended to add a BHC that delivers care independent of the context or team. The effective BHC leverages the primary care context and the care team to broaden their impact on the population and enhance intervention efficacy with individuals. So, should we study clinical efficacy in the same way for specialty psychotherapy as we do with the work of a care team running the PCBH model? To add to the puzzle, which disorder should we study? Primary care, as a context, deals with all manner of human conditions, and PCBH is designed to support the care team's work across all of those conditions. So, would we be justifying the existence of PCBH if we found that depression scores decrease compared to controls? We need to define PCBH according to its own goals.

Another critical consideration still needing to be settled by the field is the issue of effective functional outcomes measurement. Since the model is philosophically predicated on improving patient function across many domains, most PCBH'ers chafe at purely symptom-oriented outcome measures. However, a functional outcome measure has yet to rise to the level of wide-scale use as the PHQ-9. A tool like the Outcome Rating Scale may point to a brighter future in this regard.

So, the last twenty years have yet to settle whether PCBH improves clinical outcomes, although there are studies with varying degrees of methodological rigor that point to positive effects. And if you agree with our argument that this is perhaps the wrong query formulation, we can still see that a research enterprise that fits the PCBH model has yet to be clearly defined. However, intelligent people are working on it, including researchers interested in core PCBH model characteristics like warm handoffs. We are especially heartened by the work of some to provide a research framework to guide future research in PCBH.

Where To Now?

The future of PCBH must include three core elements:
- The development of functional outcome measures administered in an automated fashion as part of routine care
- A direct, planned pipeline for workforce capacity building

- A more sustainable set of community standards for BHC job requirements

Let's take a look at these briefly as part of our evaluation of the promise of PCBH.

Outcomes Measurement

While PCBH can rightly claim that measurement in the style of specialty care, SBIRT, or the collaborative care model does not fit PCBH's goals, PCBH cannot declare independence from the notion of measurement. Measurement is essential to modern primary care, from blood pressure and temperature to A1Cs and other laboratory tests. PCBH needs to mirror this ethos not so much to justify its existence but rather to exert the quality control that comes with measurement. For example, in primary care, it is theoretically possible for a primary care provider to treat diabetes without A1Cs, perhaps focusing just on the patient's reports of symptoms and regular blood glucose monitoring. However, the overall quality of care, especially across a population, would be noticeable. You would have some patients suffering from the long-term consequences of the illness because of faulty assumptions on the part of the patient-provider dyad. You would also have a more challenging time tracking portions of the population who need enhanced care and may get lost in follow-up.

Similarly, PCBH must develop a standard panel of behavioral health "labs" to serve similar functions for BHCs and their care teams. In truth, a series of commonly used tools could already be considered standard, although unofficially. These might include the PHQ-9 for depression, the Vanderbilt ADHD scales, the GAD-7 for anxiety, and the AUDIT/DAST for substance abuse. These are fine and have some utility. However, most of these tools are screeners repurposed in many settings for routine measurement; this is an important distinction to consider, so let's spend a little more time on this.

Screening tools are the equivalent of the TB test in primary care. They have a focused utility of case finding in a population. In other words, a screener like the PHQ-9 is designed to identify people who struggle with symptoms of depression. It may seem logical that repeating the screener would automatically help determine a patient's clinical needs. However, that is only sometimes the case. The TB test is a good analogy in this regard. One could screen positive for TB, having previously had TB, after receiving treatment for TB (with certain tests), without any clinical need for intervention. In the same way, a patient with a screen score of 13 on the PHQ-9 and a later score of 13 on the PHQ-9 may not need current clinical intervention based on the "lack of progress." Clinical intervention depends on several variables and is usually driven by the patient's subjective sense of their functionality. In other words, the patient came into care having depressive symptoms, improved functionally, and is content with their progress (and thus often discontinues care) and, if measured again, may still show some symptoms but does not require treatment adjustment or ongoing care. In PCBH parlance, we might state in a note that the patient only requires as-needed maintenance care, for example. So this is why screening tools are not always helpful for outcome measurement. The other key detail is that many of these tools were never normed for formal outcome measurement.

So, what do we do? Well, the PCBH approach has always been to focus on functioning. Functioning sounds like a dry way of describing something quite rich: living. In other words, the PCBH model focuses on helping patients live better, and that, of course, is heavily defined by the patient encounter versus an objective symptom count. So, PCBH must use tools that measure how the patient feels they are improving. There are tools, like the Outcome Rating Scale, and many others with different emphases. Some focus on the alliance between the patient and the consultant (because we know from research that alliance is related to improved outcomes overall), some focus on the quality of life, some focus on domains of living, and some focus on specific aspects of coping with stress or chronic illness. In truth, like primary care, BHCs will likely need to use various tools flexibly to get the job done. In other words, no one tool is expected to dominate the market. We need our own "lab" panel.

However, BHCs need the same ease and convenience that PCPs have with their labs to do this effectively. In other words, the process of outcomes measurement needs to be automated. Remember, a PCP usually makes a few clicks, and then the labs are drawn by other professionals, and the results are populated in the EHR. BHCs need that kind of ease, not the struggle of administering in person at each visit in the chaos of primary care. Technological tools like surveys sent via text to patient phones or surveys sent to the front desk check-out tablet are much better solutions that can foster the consistency needed to maintain the number of tools necessary for population outcomes management. Fortunately, various technology companies are emerging to offer these services, but challenges still must be overcome with EHR integration and clinical flow features. We are getting there, however.

The Workforce Pipeline

The second thing we need to promote the promise of PCBH is to build the workforce pipeline; this starts with a radical notion. We need to re-conceive mental health care delivery in a stepped-care model which envisions the creation of a primary care level of care. A wholesale re-conceptualization would include other levels as well, including public health and re-imagined tertiary care. For our purposes here, we will focus on the primary care level of care. If the power structures in the current healthcare marketplace conceive of the need for a primary care level that complements the specialty level of care (and below it, the public health level), then a concerted effort to build the workforce from the ground up would ensue.

What would this mean practically? It would likely mean introducing the concept in Bachelor's level introductory social work and psychology courses. At the graduate level, it would mean tracks or dedicated Master's and Doctoral level programs for primary care clinicians and researchers; this would require significant changes in accreditation guidelines to ensure curricular consistency and approved standards for primary care practitioners; and this would involve a substantial re-training program to prepare current academics to develop and train the primary care workforce. This is no small feat, but it is achievable with government incentives/signaling, accreditation body task force work, and marketplace forces. The ingredients are there, especially current marketplace forces, namely the scarcity of trained workers and the increasing number of positions available. We have consensus and even exemplar curricula that could be used by accrediting bodies to implement guidelines. And we have some experience with governmental incentives in the form of Behavioral Health Workforce Education and Training (BHWET) grants of the early 2020s.

Workforce Standards

Current standards for the BHC workforce need to be defined and should be influenced by the existing primary care workforce. Considering the current workforce is under duress, there may be better ways to create a sustainable BHC role on the primary care team. As we advance, one of our primary concerns for the BHC workforce is that it will fall prey to some of the same stresses faced by primary care providers, namely unreasonable productivity demands, poor administrative support for problem-solving, and high expectations for quality outcomes with little support for reaching those outcomes. It makes sense to address these pitfalls now while the workforce norms are still in their infancy.

Here are some of the critical questions around the standardization of workforce norms that are yet to be addressed:
A. What are reasonable productivity expectations, and how do we measure that productivity to encompass the fullness of the BHC role?

- Currently, most sites expect BHCs to see between 8 and 12 patient consults per day, but there is significant variability. Furthermore, patient consults are not the entirety of the BHC role. BHCs provide curbside consultation, EHR in-basket support, and other team functions such as liaison roles to an MAT service. Additionally, some BHCs may have higher numbers of patients that challenge the 15-30 minute standard approach, such as patients necessitating interpreter services.

B. What is the appropriate organizational structure to support a PCBH service?
  - Far too many PCBH services are not appropriately homed in their organizational structure. In other words, the service needs to report to the correct power centers in the organization. As a result, the PCBH service needs to improve its ability to solve problems and is often isolated from critical organizational decision-making. Access is an excellent example of how an appropriately homed PCBH service with a Chief Behavioral Health Officer reporting directly to the CEO works well.

C. Quality outcomes are the future (often already the present) of reimbursement in value-based payment arrangements. What expectations will PCBH services share with their primary care colleagues, and will there be enough support to reach these expectations?
  - Quality expectations often overburden primary care providers through metrics like HEDIS measures. Achieving these can be burdensome, especially without organizational support in the form of data

support tools and staffing support. Will the same happen to BHCs as quality expectations increase for metrics like emergency department utilization, depression score decreases, and medication adherence measures?

So, we have some work to do in building the vision of PCBH. However, the following pages should serve as an encouragement to you. We have come a long way. We have made a dent in the universe, and the world of healthcare will never be the same. Integrated care and PCBH are here to stay. The story of Access and some of the other clinics represented in this text are stories of possibility, and they demonstrate that this vision is achievable and, in fact, necessary. While we cannot claim that these stories are the norm everywhere for PCBH programs, we can claim that these stories represent success stories that you can emulate with confidence in your setting because these are programs that have stood the test of time. And that is the most exciting thing about this second edition: the notion that what we wrote nearly a decade ago has not only persisted but thrived and evolved. We hope that our stories become your stories.

About the Author

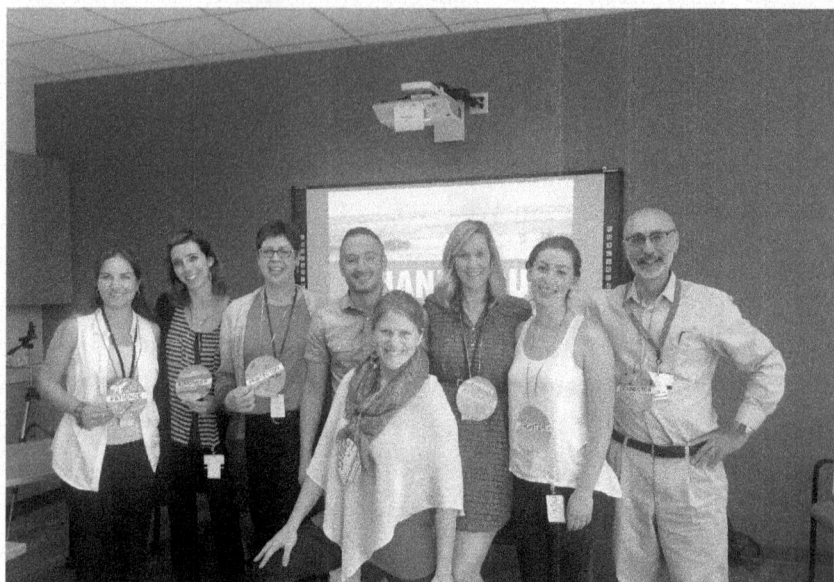

Neftali Serrano (center) is a primary care psychologist who has spent his entire career in primary care. Currently, he is the Chief Executive Officer of the Collaborative Family Healthcare Association a national non-profit dedicated to promoting integrated care. Other than integrated care, he loves soccer, spending time with his wife and three teenagers, and reading history. The picture above was a tearful team goodbye as Dr. Serrano left Access in 2015.

Chapter 2: The Making Of A Professional Identity

By Neftali Serrano, PsyD

My journey into primary care began after my doctoral studies in clinical psychology. I assumed that my professional identity was complete and that I had arrived, and I was now a grown-up. The problem was that even before falling into my postdoctoral year at the Lawndale Christian Health Center (Lawndale) on the west side of Chicago (IL), I had already experienced what psychologists term "cognitive dissonance" related to my identity as a psychologist. My bi-cultural identity as an American-born Hispanic descendant of immigrant parents from Puerto Rico and Colombia was a critical factor in creating this dissonance. During my graduate training, I felt uneasy about the care models taught to me.

Psychodynamic theory struck me as pathology driven and impractical in the face of the day-to-day lives of the Hispanic immigrants I grew up with in Queens, NY. Cognitive-behavioral approaches seemed artificial, dry, and disconnected from contextual realities. And in the end, I felt that none of the systems solved the fundamental dilemma of getting patients to the front door. Which of the people I grew up with would ever want to sit with a stranger in an office and talk about their problems (let alone have the means or insurance to pay for it)?

It wasn't that the theories were wrong or unscientific. Indeed the part of me acculturated into Western thinking understood their genesis in dualism, the scientific method, and Western medicine. The problem was that the part of me acculturated as a New York Latino also saw the cultural baggage of the models and their associated service delivery models. I knew intuitively that the healing technologies that people in my community of origin looked to were different than the professional therapist of Western culture.

Another critical factor in creating this dissonance for me was a book I encountered early in my training by a psychotherapist, Philip Cushman. Cushman's thesis (Constructing the Self, Constructing America: A Cultural History of Psychotherapy, 1996) planted an even more dangerous thought than the poor psychotherapy match issue with ethnic minorities. His cultural history of psychotherapy in America posited that the West's healing technologies essentially helped sustain the fundamental individualism and consumerism that was at the root of many of the psychological ills of the culture. In short,

Cushman was suspicious that there was a symbiotic relationship between this 'therapy' that took people out of their contexts individually and inadvertently reinforced their ability to surmount intrapsychic difficulties to become 'better' individualists and consumers. Cushman called the result "the empty self."

Aside from the general challenge that his book issues to any reader, it caused and allowed me to question whether the traditions of Western psychotherapy and psychological science, in general, were the best we could come up with. Is there a better way to conceive of life's challenges and deliver or make care available than the requisite intake appointment, treatment plan, and series of 50-minute visits?

The third factor influencing my identity issues was my rooting in a religious tradition. As a devout Christian, I had grown into an understanding of health and healing that was inherently integrationist in nature. In other words, psychological healing was always connected with other aspects of healing in the worldview I grew up with, whether physical, spiritual, or even communal. This multidimensional view of healing was at odds with the specialist and reductionist approach to psychology I was taught. In essence, it made less sense to me to read research on the impact of affective states on test-taking than to conceive of studies looking at the impact of faith communities on health outcomes (physical and psychological).

And so it was that I was a confused and frustrated young man coming out of graduate school. But I needed this confusion or creative helplessness to borrow a term from Acceptance and Commitment Therapy (ACT) when I fell into a job as the Director of Mental Health Services (technically called Director of Clinical Pastoral Care) at the Lawndale Christian Health Center. I fell in because I initially rejected applying for the job. First, I was right out of graduate training and felt overwhelmed by the idea of directing anything, especially in my confused state.

Secondly, Lawndale was a big, intimidating place. The clinic was one of several sister organizations that served the community - each of which was tied together by the founding church, Lawndale Community Church. The clinic served a population of Mexican immigrants to the south and African-Americans to the north, numbering about 20-30,000 (60,000 annual visits). Of course, after investigating a bit further, my interest was piqued, intuitively at least. I was not conscious of it then, but Lawndale was the perfect place to consolidate the pieces of my personal and professional life. It was to be my Rosetta Stone.

I will always remember my first meeting with Bruce Miller, the Chief Operating Officer at the time. I would come to truly love Bruce and learn a great deal from him, but looking back, I am astounded that he even gave me the job. My initial presentation of what I would do if hired reeked of inefficiency and inexperience. I proposed (as the lone mental health professional) to work intensively with 4-6 families and work on developing the program from there (there were also administrative responsibilities associated with two pastoral staff I was to supervise). My thinking was that a. I was afraid to become overwhelmed with the needs in this underserved community, and b. I had developed a poorly thought-out philosophy that 'true' psychological healing could only result from intensive family-based work. He must have seen something in me.

I quickly became utterly irrelevant to the clinic's work, which was mostly my fault. I asked to have an exam room refitted to look more like a therapy room; this meant replacing the exam table with couches from IKEA and the sink with some nice decorative touches like an accent lamp and some art pieces. The room was located at the end of the pediatric hallway, so in that sense, it was 'integrated,' but in no other way was it substantially a part of the clinic's life. The 50% show rate further cemented that divide. It was frustrating to see providers working busily while I sat around seeing 1-2 patients per day, and it was even more frustrating to them when they saw the need in their exam rooms every day.

It soon became apparent that something had to change, but there was a lot of internal resistance to making those changes. As loosely as I held my professional identity as a psychologist, it was all I had. I was used to segregated charts (I even made up my chart note form with fancy graphics and sections), clinical interviews, and 50-minute visits. For some reason, stepping in on patients already in the clinic was tough to swallow. Indeed, some of me even blamed the patients for their non-compliance with my obviously stellar service. If they would only come, they would reap the great benefits of the intensive psychotherapy I had planned for them!

With time I began hanging out in provider areas and making myself available to see patients. Looking back, I think my idea was to see patients for a first visit and then see if I could get them to come back to see me - a sort of advertising for the 'real thing.' What I discovered was the genesis of a paradigm shift. I would walk into an exam room, and within seconds, the patient would cry and tell me something they had not told anyone in their entire life. That blew my first preconceived idea that a therapist must build rapport over sessions to achieve meaningful relationship work. I also began to see the great benefit and relief many patients received from either these one-time visits or a shorter series of visits. I had something of value to offer, and it didn't take an intake to figure out what that was. At times it was simply the collective benefit of the common factors associated with therapy; at others, it was reframing the situation; and at others, it was an education about the best approaches to resolving specific conditions or symptoms. Patients found me relevant and helpful, and providers found me accessible and comforting.

I also discovered a shocking reality. I knew a bit more about psychopharmacology than many of the providers did. I learned why as my wife made it through medical school. Training in psychiatry is several months at best for the typical primary care provider. So, I would see many patients with panic attacks placed on benzodiazepines instead of selective serotonin reuptake inhibitors (SSRI). And I would see many patients on sub-therapeutic doses of medication. I tentatively began to point these things out to providers; remarkably, they listened and changed their habits.

I was more exhilarated, exhausted, and intellectually stimulated than ever. Most nights, I wanted to sleep by 6 PM, and the pace and quantity of visits had my head spinning. Things were beginning to make sense for the first time in my life.

In these exam room encounters and in the clinic spaces where I would naturally interact with my primary care colleagues, I saw a glimpse of what could be the landscape of truly modern psychology. I also saw how the pieces of my life fit so well with this new vision.

The bicultural part of me (and much of that sound training in communication) helped me to connect with patients quickly and effectively while also being able to facilitate communication between provider and patient. That part of me also felt great satisfaction at being able to see patients, which reminded me of the people I grew up with. Their acceptance of this model of care confirmed to me that there was a way to reach these people. Integrating the medical, psychological, and spiritual in the exam room made sense to these patient groups. The patient who cried after 30 seconds of my entering the room, I realized, was establishing rapport with me because she was extending the trust she had in her provider to me. I learned I had been granted a superpower that emerges when a patient trusts someone with their body and naturally extends that trust to their mind and heart (especially when somatic concerns tie all three together).

Cushman's critique also found at least a partial solution at Lawndale. The setting of a clinic, especially this clinic with its history, creates a community. Part of the power of integrated care, I learned, is that the experience of going to see the doctor is, for many patients, a communal experience. You may meet community members in the waiting room, get to know the nurses and medical assistants, hobnob with registrars, and yet find a safe place to deal with medical and other concerns. The healing seemed to have a context I could not find in the sterile therapist's office. In many ways, the recovery tied that individual to this community. Of course, not all clinics and doctor's offices have this component - but Lawndale did.

My longing for an integrated approach also found its place at Lawndale. It made much more sense to be working with a patient concurrently on their diabetes, their conflictual relationship with a family member, and the panic attacks related to all of the above. We could address how faith could be utilized as a coping resource to deal with ongoing conflict while we started an antidepressant and worked on medication adherence, all in one visit and one place. Stuff was making sense to me.

Of course, this growth, particularly early on, was difficult. As I already mentioned, I was exhausted and drained much of the time. Not only was I clinically overloaded, but I was also responsible for growing a program and supervising the pastoral care workers. I also had a steep learning curve in the first few years as I reconfigured my identity and learned brand-new content daily. Everything from psychopharmacology to health-related conditions had nuances I needed to be on top of. And it seemed as if I saw some new presentation of some illness or situation every day. I will never forget the odd week when I saw two patients with a variant of obsessive-compulsive disorder called olfactory reference syndrome. In short, I was stretched to the max.

Of course, it was in the midst of this that I had one of my worst moments in primary care. After a year or so of doing this work on pure intuition alone, Lawndale received a grant for technical assistance from the Bureau of Primary Health Care to do this kind of integration. I had the privilege of meeting Kirk Strosahl, Ph.D., one of the founders of the Behavioral Health Consultant model, who arrived to shadow me for a day. Our lone patient on that busy clinic day was what primary care folks call a train wreck. This young woman was referred to me because she was depressed and diagnosed with bipolar disorder. She had a prior referral to see a psychiatrist at a local hospital but, for whatever reason, had not made the appointment. She was not taking any medication and looked vacant that morning. I was intimidated by being shadowed by Kirk and way out of my league with the case itself. I spent the better part of the visit assessing symptoms and figuring out how to get the patient to see the psychiatrist. As there often are, there were many barriers, not the least of which was the illness she bore.

After briefly debriefing with the usual candor that characterizes Kirk, he asked me if I really knew this person. He explained that the psychiatric side was the easiest part of this case presentation. She could be placed on a mood stabilizer trial while waiting for a referral, but what had yet to be addressed in this visit was who she was and what was important to her. I remember him saying, "She made it here today, correct? So, what got her here? What is truly important to her?" It was my first exposure to the ACT model (Acceptance and Commitment Therapy), which Kirk would later school me on, but even more so, it was the first time I realized that this kind of integrated work had also created its own perspective. Call it an orientation, perspective, approach, or whatever – but I realized that the functional approach to care was a means to integrating various perspectives, including psychological theories, evidence-based therapies, and pharmacological therapy. I have found that almost anyone doing this kind of work ends up with this functional approach which ties together the vast knowledge base of psychology and reduces it to the patient's main goals, hopes, dreams, and opportunities. Kirk's question that day hit me in some deep places of my soul. I was embarrassed, and I felt ineffective. I use that moment to anchor my experiences today with patients. Whenever I feel lost in a patient consult or overwhelmed by the breadth of data to digest, I remind myself to know the patient, wonder what makes them tick, and then get at how they live and breathe each day effectively, despite severe symptoms and difficult circumstances.

Kirk met with me a few times after that and was gracious in his approach. As a New Yorker, I appreciated his sometimes brash and direct style. I also understood the toll it must have taken on him professionally and perhaps personally to travel and help people like me. Kirk was one of the first-generation psychologists to make any headway in integrated care, which most certainly came at a cost. As I have often found in my presentations and discussions with other mental health providers, the paradigm shift that I have described here is both simple and monumental at the same time. I often describe this model of care as the simplest solution to the problem, given that you define the problem correctly. And yet it is a leap of faith for many in mental health who are tied to the aging paradigm of traditional specialty mental health services. And as we know in counseling, introducing paradigm shifts often engenders resistance, sometimes ugly opposition. For that, we must be grateful for persons like Kirk, his wife Patricia Robinson, and others who braved the initial onslaught of critics.

Now I consider myself a primary care psychologist, a member of the modern care team, and I have become acculturated to the thinking and practice of primary care. In fact, generally speaking, I feel more of a kinship with my primary care brethren than with other mental health professionals. It is a unique culture and one which fits me personally. But more so, it is the one place where I have seen mental health work for all. As Steve Jobs would say, it is a place to make our dent in the universe.

Chapter 3: What A Mature Program Looks Like

By Neftali Serrano, PsyD

The movement that is primary care behavioral health is now entering into a mature phase, or at least what could be termed an adolescent phase. There is significant clarity about what works, a growing body of research, more fellowships, jobs, and interested parties. There is, of course, still a great deal of growth needed, particularly in the evidence base specific to the components of prevailing models and in the payment systems required to undergird these models. However, without a doubt, the landscape of integrated care feels vastly different than it did all those years ago when I stumbled onto the BHC model at Lawndale. Back then, I had no counterparts to bounce ideas off of, and most anyone I spoke with had no fundamental knowledge of the model, which is why the visits from Kirk were essential. Today there are robust conferences (for example, the Collaborative Family Healthcare Association), books, and amazingly a PubMed search brings up relevant articles! It is a different world that cannot revert to when integrated care did not exist.

After five years at Lawndale, I began working at another community health center in Madison, WI, called Access Community Health Centers (Access). At Access, I found fertile ground to develop the BHC model in ways I had not even imagined, and this is the story I want to tell in this section: the story of a mature program. First, it will be helpful to understand why Access was fertile ground. Hint: compare this to your current organizational setting.

Lawndale was a wonderful and rich learning environment for me. As I wrote in the previous section, it was a place that neatly tied my life's personal and professional aspects, especially in my identification with the community. However, the clinic itself was a behemoth. It was large physically and in capacity and grew exponentially. When I left in 2005, the clinic saw nearly 100,000 annual patient visits in three sites. Two BHCs (including myself) and a postdoctoral fellow were theoretically responsible for this patient population. As a result, there were a great many inefficiencies that developed, which made it difficult to grow the BHC program. Some of those lessons are covered in future chapters. What is important for now is not what Lawndale needed to have but the qualities specific to Access that made it as successful as it was. To my great satisfaction, Lawndale's BHC program is doing well today with an expanded staff who saw over 10,000 visits in 2022.

I arrived at Access in late 2005, almost on a whim. At the time, I was only interested in volunteering some time at the clinic since I was a stay-at-home dad for my then-one-year-old daughter, Emma. (Emma was driving me up a wall, thus the need for some time out of the home.) In his wisdom, the medical director at the time, Ken Loving, MD, instead offered me a part-time position and indicated excitement at the possibilities, given that the organization had decided in its strategic planning process that integration of mental health treatment was a key goal. Like Lawndale, Access had no mental health services besides a volunteer psychiatric nurse practitioner, and I was back to square one.

There is excitement associated with developing these programs, but there is also often a sense of dread or, at the very least, anxiety. I could already anticipate having to convince that one negative clinician about the value of my services and, even more so, what we could do together. The effort needed to work with the resistant medical assistant whose only desire was to ensure she got out on time. Worse yet, I could feel the dread of convincing administrators that we needed to scale the program to achieve the desired efficiencies. I had learned these lessons at Lawndale, and I was prepared, but by and large, I did not have to face any of these issues at Access.

The CEO at Access, Barb Snell, was a former social worker who together with the CFO, Joanne Holland, and Communications staff, Tammy Quall and Paul Harrison, quickly picked up why the model worked and what it needed to grow successfully. For the first time, an entire administrative staff could explain to visitors how the BHC model worked and why it was crucial for our patients and clinicians. Access was fertile ground because the organization 'got it.' It was also fertile because the organization, in general, ran efficiently. Medical teams worked well together, patient waiting times were within reason, the clinic was financially solid, and communication was functional throughout the organization. I learned through Access how important the general efficiencies of an organization impact the efficiency of an integrated care program; this is what led to the truism noted throughout this text: "No program can exceed the efficiency of the clinic at large."

As I began to work at the clinic, which I always reduce to the most straightforward approach possible, namely starting to 'hang out,' I learned that Access clinicians were also ripe for the model. As with Lawndale clinicians, these healthcare workers cared deeply about their patients and disliked how hampered they felt in caring for patients with mental health concerns. In most cases, they told me they were stuck trying to treat patients since access to mental health services was virtually non-existent in the community for uninsured and underinsured patients. Relationships developed smoothly by and large, although, as is to be expected, some clinicians wanted to test whether I was cut out for their patient panels. Several years removed from the debacle with the patient Kirk shadowed me, I had learned my lessons and was ready for the test. What ensued were terrific, rich relationships with the Access clinicians. We grew together in the model (cross-pollination), another truism found throughout this text.

What initially struck me in my work at Access - which originally was only two half days a week - was the prevalence of severe and persistent mental illness. Ironically my work at Lawndale, an impoverished urban community, had consisted of much more garden-variety depression and anxiety alongside the stresses of inner-city decay. In Madison, a more resource-rich environment with less social decay, I found that some patients were bipolar-disordered or had some variant of a psychotic disorder. Many of these patients were under-identified and thus under-treated, perhaps with an antidepressant. My growth curve began again as I became more adept at working with patients in this area. Through me, the clinicians became more adept at identifying illnesses more readily and treating them according to evidence-based algorithms. After all, I soon learned there weren't other alternatives for these patients. It was us or nothing. And that nothing was often costly, as in trips to the emergency room or any other variant of the eventual decompensation of the patient, such as domestic violence or incarceration.

I also learned another truism: treatment intensity must match patient motivation and capacity. I had initially believed, as many still do, that more severely mentally ill patients need more severe and intensive services. I learned that patients need services that match what they can handle. For the few patients who had some resources we attempted to refer out, we found ourselves frustrated by the barriers to completing the referrals; more often than not, patients would no-show to external referrals. We learned that patients were no-showing because of their illnesses and social conditions. And yet, due to their no-shows, patients were losing access to those specialty clinics.

Rules were often in place that kicked people out of the specialty systems as a result of multiple no-shows. Furthermore, patients were often frustrated by the prolonged intake processes. Delayed treatment initiation, when the patient feels like the treatment has started, is a crucial barrier to completed care. Indeed, the time to treat mania is when one is manic, not in two weeks when it may have dissipated on its own.

So, we learned to use the functional and step-wise approach to intervene quickly with these patients, increasing function as soon as possible and then continuing to match treatment intensity (including visit strategies) to patient goals and motivation. I learned from our patients that this worked well for many of them. Over time, even when patients stabilized, many chose to keep their care with their primary care team since they often had good relationships with their primary care clinicians. The lessons learned from that patient I saw with Kirk were in full bloom.

Understand me; it was stressful. Many times I and our clinicians went home wondering if we had handled a suicidal or floridly psychotic patient appropriately. Most of the time, we could console ourselves with the notion that some treatment was better than no treatment. But that did not resolve our desire to do our best for this vulnerable population. Over time, this drive to provide the best care led to our efforts to increase our competencies and develop systems that fit the BHC model to deal specifically with severely ill patients. Over time, this dread dissipated, though there will always be those patients that fall through all the societal safety nets, exceed our professional competencies, and challenge us to do something or face the prospect of a dangerous nothing. It is, in fact, that challenge that should drive us to make our dent in the universe.

Serendipity and Growth

One of the critical lessons in developing programs is knowing when to jump on opportunities and when to avoid them. I worked independently in the initial program development stage, covering the first year and a half of my time at Access. However, I quickly began planning for a training program, which based on my experience at Lawndale, was the best way to grow a program. These efforts led me to contact local schools, which resulted in a serendipitous sequence of events that propelled the growth of our staff and training program. A health psychologist at the University of Wisconsin Hospital sent me an e-mail wondering if I would be interested in co-sponsoring a postdoctoral fellow that would rotate between the hospital and our primary care clinics; this was nowhere on my radar, nor was it on our organization's radar, but I decided to pass the suggestion along to our medical director. Within a few weeks, we approved the position and hired Dr. Meghan Fondow, who would later become a staff member. This postdoctoral fellowship has been responsible for more than 50% of our staff hires since then. I mentioned this because opportunities are often not explicitly planned for, but if you are developing relationships, ideas and partnerships can germinate; this doesn't mean that all opportunities are equal, as we will discuss later on, but it does mean that relationships are at the center of opportunities.

Access' BHC model, at the time of the edition of this text, is 15 years mature and stands as one of the nation's most fully developed PCBH integration models. Approximately 20% of medical patients are served annually at the clinic (by the BHC team). That is integration. Although there will be much more in the chapters that follow on each of these aspects, reviewing the components of Access' BHC program will be instructive as a starting point. It will also serve as an endpoint to the narrative of my personal story (although there's a twist at the end!).

Core Model Components

The core of the BHC model (for more on the general model, see our Wikipedia article) at Access is the relationship between the primary care clinician and the BHC. Everything else hinges on that relationship; if primary care clinicians are not engaged and directly supported, then you don't have an integrated care program - you have a program.

BHCs see, on average, ten patients per day, with some variability pushing that daily figure to 14 or more on the busiest days; this is accomplished by staggering follow-up visits at 9 AM, 9:30 AM, and 10:30 AM in the mornings and 1 PM, 1:30 PM, and 2:30 PM (we also have some evening clinics staggered similarly). Since consults are typically between 15 and 30 minutes, this allows for warm hand-offs throughout the day. These warm hand-offs replace 'referrals,' a word that no longer exists in our language, which involves the primary care clinician briefing the BHC on the nature of the patient situation and then often inviting the BHC to see the patient (sometimes only a curbside conversation is what is needed). After the visit, the BHC briefs the primary care clinician and suggests a course of action. This sequence, multiplied over time year after year, creates a unique symbiotic relationship between BHC and clinician and their patients. The entire team morphs into something greater than the sum of its parts as each part learns from the other. Access clinicians readily admit they cannot conceive of practicing without a BHC. BHCs, of course, would not even exist without our clinicians.

Consulting Psychiatry

The need for consulting psychiatry arose when the severity of patients became prevalent enough (and without other options) that the dyads of BHCs and primary care clinicians became concerned about competence to treat. Garden variety depression and anxiety are well within reach of most clinicians regarding competence to treat (though comfort certainly varies based on experience). However, two factors complicate the treatment of more severe patients: a. lack of confidence in treating the condition and b. the prevalence of the severity of this type of patient in the clinician panel. In other words, most clinicians are willing to go out on a limb with some help in isolated situations - this happens even in other medical areas where a clinician will consult a specialist who may give them a treatment algorithm to follow. The problem arises when a critical mass of these patients develops, making clinicians very uneasy; this led to our development of the consulting psychiatry model, reviewed in detail in an upcoming chapter. The consulting psychiatry model is not unique to us, but we will discuss some of the nuances of the model as implemented at Access.

At the time of the writing of this text, Access has a 75% FTE consulting psychiatrist supporting the work of our 12 BHCs and about 45 medical clinicians with varying FTE levels. By providing recommendations directly to our medical teams, our consulting psychiatrist provides the confidence boost and sense of security that our clinicians need to manage very ill patients; this is not to say that clinicians still wish our patients had better access to specialty psychiatry (or that they would go if access were provided), but rather that it allows for a way where there once was none (or the one that was there felt like a rickety bridge).

The success of this program reinforced my belief that our nationwide access problem for patients with mental illness is solvable if we adequately support our primary care clinicians. In other words, some combination of consulting psychiatrists or prescribing-consultant psychologists/psychiatric nurse practitioners embedded in primary care practices could enable our existing primary care clinicians to expand the prescribing provider base in the United States dramatically.

The consulting psychiatry approach is a more reasonable solution than simply trying to grow enough specialty psychiatrists or prescribing psychologists to meet the need. Of course, there is a great deal of human politics that stands in the way of this occurring, including, not surprisingly, plenty of economic self-interest. But in the end, it is better for patients, particularly those with severe and persistent mental illness, to have expanded and facilitated access (along with integrated access) to prescribers; this is the kind of dent in the universe we need.

Care Management

One of the other things that became apparent as we began to reach scale in our program at Access was that the sheer volume of patients made tracking the consistency of care difficult. BHC work mimics primary care, focusing on today's work. A mantra in primary care open-access scheduling systems says, "Do today's work today." That works fine for issues that can be resolved in one day, like a sore throat, but for many mental health and primary care conditions, some form of consistent follow-up is needed, often as determined by evidence-based algorithms. This is where care management becomes helpful. Again we will go into this in more detail later on, but for now, it is instructive to note the basic outlines of the service. This aspect of the program involves targeting specific populations, registering them in a database, and tracking key indicators that tell you whether the care you provide is adhering to evidence-based algorithms and whether patients seem to be getting better and accessing care appropriately.

At Access, we follow patients with mood disorders and ADHD in this way. One of our BHCs serves as the part-time point person for managing the databases; more recently, dedicated staff has been added to give increased focus to the work (see later chapter on "care management"). Those familiar with diabetes care management will note the similarities here. The future of primary care is in these registries, hopefully better embedded in electronic health records, which will ease tracking patients with various disease conditions. The trick is that no one has entirely developed a great tool embedded in an EHR like this, although Access has used the reporting workbench tools in EPIC as of late to mimic this function.

Furthermore, no one has figured out how to make it flexible enough to cut across disease categories versus the current models, which results in separate databases for different problem areas. And, of course, we have yet to figure out how to pay for this kind of extra-office visit work, although the Collaborative Care model codes provide an option for clinics as long as they adhere to the parameters of the billing model. Again, more on this later.

Training

Scaling a BHC program made the problem of developing a workforce a pressing reality. As the demand for BHC time increased, it became apparent that Access would need a proactive solution to staffing its team. This was one of the Lawndale lessons. At Lawndale, the program suffered because demand far outstripped our staffing, which caused all sorts of inefficiencies. By making some impulsive hires, I also learned the hard way that finding the right fit was more important than finding a warm body. And I learned the right fit was often easier to create/train first and then hire. In other words, the adage is usually true; it seems: "You can't teach an old dog new tricks."

Students are often more open, malleable, and less attached to aspects of professional identity that don't work in primary care. As such, we began our training program in 2006 with a Marriage and Family Therapy student with little direct care mental health experience. We soon followed with a postdoctoral fellow in health psychology that also rotated through the local hospital. By 2023 Access had a robust training program, including an average of 10 annual psychiatry residents, two postdoctoral fellows, 2-4 intern or practicum trainees, and one social work fellow. This training program was responsible for nearly all staff hires.

Training programs need to be scaled for integrated care to take off. We need more students exposed to primary care in their training and more opportunities for clinical practice.

Research

It is uncommon for community programs to engage in research, but Access is uniquely positioned to work in this area. As the program grew, I realized that there were a couple of persistent threats to its sustainability, no matter how popular the program was internally. These threats included: a. fee for service payment model and b. no community ecosystem supporting it. With the former, the threat revolves around the inadequate nature of paying for integrated care by paying for office visits. The primary end product of integrated care is not an office visit. The primary end product is seamless, continuous, and collaborative care that results in an improved medical team (home) and an empowered patient who utilizes care efficiently and effectively. Insurance companies should pay for that, not an office visit. So, research is needed to show that integrated care achieves this end product to stimulate payers to adopt alternative payment systems, such as bundled care. More on that later, but for now, the point is that it is incumbent on practitioners to work to integrate research into their practices to get ahead of changes in healthcare reimbursement.

With the latter threat, the lack of a community ecosystem, the workforce development issue is but one of the threats I identified. In reality, integrated care must be the de facto community standard of care for it to thrive. As long as most practices eschew integrated care, our approach faces potential changes in things like regulations, which can threaten our program's viability. Again, research and the advocacy it can promote, are essential ways to ensure we influence the standard of care in the community. We started our research initiative in 2011 and, to date, have published several peer-reviewed articles describing various aspects of our program. Our approach has been to tie quality improvement evaluations to these research endeavors, which keeps us from working on esoteric projects of no value to our clinic. We hope that we can influence our region, Dane County, and perhaps the state of Wisconsin to recognize integrated care as the standard of care such that all practices in the state either have or are on the path to integrating. Due in part to our efforts, one local HMO and one large health system have developed their integrated care programs with Access alumni. Being unique is fun for a while, but we prefer to be bland and typical.

So, it is time for me to be honest. Thus far, I have used the terms "we" and "our" to describe the work, mainly because I still feel so connected to Access. However, the truth is that I left my post as Chief Behavioral Health Officer at Access in the summer of 2015; this makes the longevity and quality of the program even more special. Dr. Elizabeth Zeidler Schreiter, a pre-existing Access BHC, took over as the CBHO and continued to grow and sustain the program using the same core principles covered in this book. Her story of handling that transition is reviewed later in this text and is a testament to her leadership and the overall health of an outstanding organization. Access is a medical home to emulate.

This is our vision for making a dent in the universe. We are not content with the status quo, and we are not satisfied with incremental improvements on the status quo. As Steve Jobs implored his staff at Apple, our goal is to be "insanely great." Hopefully, this text inspires its readers to do and be just that.

Before we adjourn this chapter on what a mature program looks like, I want to meander before you enter the very pragmatic portions of this book. The reason for this meandering is that there are significant implications to the work of integrating care for patients. One might even say, dangerous implications. Understanding this will help you identify and hold firm to your true north as you face resistance in program building. So, here is me on my soapbox.

The Way Forward

Like any large-scale change, there are likely elements here that are off the mark (meaning I could be wrong) and others that are simply offensive to individuals who currently have a stake in existing parts of the system; this is understandable. However, it is still crucial that we develop a vision that seeks to solve the problems of our day. Too often, the solutions have more to do with protecting our futures or our respective guilds. There should be no more room for that kind of thinking. But make no mistake about it: when engaging in program development, this is often behind the headwinds you feel.

Primary Care Is The DeFacto Mental Health Provider

You will find this statement at the beginning of many articles on integrated care. However, it is often cited as a lament - as if we must mourn the centrality of primary care. In the sense that it marks a failure of the mental health system, it should be lamented, but otherwise, it is simply a statement of patient preference. The way forward is for the healthcare system to recognize this.

Most patients in the community (note I'm not addressing the minority of patients that self-select to participate in specialty care) do not tolerate our day's expensive, time-consuming, and siloed mental health practices. They prefer their care to be efficiently integrated with primary care. A redesigned system considers this and builds capacity within primary care to handle the entire population's mental and behavioral health concerns; this means that most group primary care practices should have BHCs and access to psychiatric consultation. Ideally, these medical home practices would have additional supports typically found in community mental health practices, such as social work support.

For rural or solo practices where a Behavioral Health Consultant or consulting psychiatry may not be sustainable, these practices should make arrangements for telehealth services. Insurers could even make such services available to practices on demand.

The design of such a system should mimic the medical system, which seeks to manage as much as possible within the primary care environment, where most issues can be handled efficiently and at a lower cost. In other words, this new primary care behavioral health system can become the center of mental health provision in the United States; this challenges individual practitioners of mental health who run their own businesses. Does this mean that jobs will be lost? Not likely, though the long-term trend would be that new psychologists-in-training would likely enter the field with less of an expectation of working in their practices, which over time could diminish the number of individual specialty practitioners.

The analogy to the current medical home movement may be helpful here. When the argument is made that more patients should be managed in medical homes and that specialty care should be de-emphasized, no one argues that we need fewer surgeons or endocrine specialists. We assume that we have plenty of work to keep those folks busy. It is being said that those resources need to be utilized more efficiently within the system and that those services should not be the center of the system since they are costly and often inappropriately used. In the same way, specialists in mental health providing therapy, assessment, and psychiatric services will always be needed - they should not be the center of a system because, as we have already discussed, they are not designed to provide population-based care.

However, it would be unreasonable to sugar-coat the changes needed in this system transformation. There are very dysfunctional aspects of the current system that would need to adapt or become extinct. Our current crop of educators would need to gain skills in primary care training. Psychiatry residency, long in need of more considerable systemic changes, would need to center the training experience in primary care versus inpatient and specialty settings. Community mental health centers need to develop strong ties to primary care and reshape their practices to become more efficient and available to neighboring primary care practices than they have been. And the ailing substance abuse treatment system will need to consolidate and integrate more deeply with primary care and ensure that the access problems that plague it are solved.

Each of these aspects of the system does mean changes in the job market and the nature of the work done, but I don't believe they mean fewer jobs. If mental health professionals can prove their worth to the medical system over the long haul, I imagine it may imply more positions. The mental health and substance abuse sectors often battle for funds and attention mainly because their worth is too esoteric for the larger health system. "We help people get better!" we cry out to the health system, and the larger system cries back to us, "Too few people and too expensive!"

In some instances, consolidation may occur. That is, not all practices will survive. Again, our approach should not be to protect territory that is not worth saving. I know from a personal standpoint that individuals have poured their time and effort into building these institutions, and the thought of seeing their demise is personally painful. That makes sense. What does not make sense is ignoring what is best for the population. Often we defend our practices based on our limited personal knowledge of the patients we see, not understanding that those populations are not representative of the more significant needs of the masses. What is worse is when we defend interests for the sake of our guilds and attempt to defend such practices by stating that it is in the best interest of patients. At the very least, we should be honest about our motivations. As they say, money makes the world go around. Those who defend the status quo or mistakenly believe it can be reformed usually end up on the wrong side of history.

Specialty Care In Service To The Primary Care Medical Home

As stated, centering mental health on primary care does not mean eliminating specialty mental health. So what is its role? The best approach is for specialty care to see itself as an extension of primary care. As with the Behavioral Health Consultant mantra, primary care should be a primary customer of specialty services. What this means is operating under the assumption that patients seeking mental health care should be directed to the primary care medical home as a first contact (if it has yet to happen naturally) and work through the primary care system to elicit appropriate referrals. This flow is essential because it introduces logic into the system. This logic would help determine which patients genuinely need specialty care and which should be managed in primary care (and introduce an open loop where patients could be shuttled back and forth based on various factors). At present, there is no logic as to where patients receive care and what intensity of care is provided.

In addition, specialty mental health practices must adapt their practices to be more efficient. One of the most frustrating aspects of community mental health programs are the programs that confuse patients and referrers alike. They divide resources and make it difficult to know where to send patients (and if patients qualify for specific programs). The best-case scenario is for specialists to operate as generalists and take all comers (no convoluted intake practices); this means fewer therapists and psychiatrists who only work with specific populations and more that have skills across the range of human problems.

The substance abuse treatment paradigm has not been wildly successful and suffers from the same inefficiencies of the mental health system. Due to political realities, substance abuse is paid for and treated as separate from the rest of the health system. It is time to re-integrate substance abuse care into the health system. Aside from the roles played by detoxification programs and inpatient centers, there is nothing unique to the treatment of substance abuse that should preclude a mental health provider from being capable of providing care, whether in a specialty setting or an integrated primary care setting. There is a good deal of research supporting brief interventions for substance abuse in emergency rooms and primary care clinics. In addition, most community practitioners realize the lack of logic in separating substance abuse treatment due to the high prevalence of medical and psychological comorbidities. Why send someone to another clinic to work on their alcohol abuse when you are working with them on their bipolar disorder and diabetes? In short, the money and effort would be better spent making substance abuse just one of the other aspects that patients are cared for in an integrated environment.

Such an approach has a variety of ramifications and is bound to ruffle some feathers. A lot of money and politics would stand in the way of such wholesale changes. Still, this kind of dent in the universe is possible, given our collective will to recognize the problem, see beyond our guild survival, and act in the best interest of patients.

Ok, now I'm off my soapbox. I hope you can see that building a program like Access' is doable, but I also hope you can see that it will not come without friction.

Chapter 4: Advocacy Skills

By Neftali Serrano, PsyD

One of the unique historical realities of PCBH implementers of the current generation is that many will be called upon to provide care in this model *and* develop programs from scratch. The primary purpose of this text is to provide skills in program development to this generation of self-starters. Thus the power of persuasion, not one of the ordinary skills instilled in mental health professionals, is one of the primary skills needed to be effective.

Mental health professionals are trained to see all sides of an issue and to be tentative in their conclusions and collaborative in their work style. Generally speaking, these are admirable traits and one of the strengths we bring to the other health professions. We would make horrible salespeople; many of us could be better businesspeople. This chapter focuses on the messages and strategies that help communicate what and why we do what we do in ways that can move the field and individual programs along.

Know Your Audience

Surprisingly, especially for professionals trained in approaches like motivational interviewing, mental health professionals often do a poor job of anticipating how administrators and business managers will receive them; this is due to a poor understanding of how these individuals operate and a subsequent misinterpretation of the professional/cultural cues. Let's take the typical gripe of mental health professionals when dealing with practice managers. "All they care about is money and numbers." If we were dealing with a patient, we would likely take more time to test this hypothesis or at least provide some greater context to such a loaded assumption - but often, when dealing with other professionals, we don't.

My dealings with those on the administrative side of things have been typical of any cross-cultural encounter. These individuals are trained differently, socialized differently, operate from different assumptions, and have professional strengths and weaknesses. It's my job to understand that background and work within their frame of reference to arrive at a mutually agreeable approach to our work. If this sounds like what happens in a patient consult, you are starting to get it; this does not mean that we need to be demeaning or treat these individuals as patients, but simply that we need to apply some of those same skills we use to enter their worlds before we demand they see the logic of ours.

It would be too simplistic to detail a set of recommendations for speaking with professionals of all kinds, but it can be helpful to remember a few things. The culture of business training values hard work, responsibility, and achievement; this means that when you propose a solution that involves, for example, no financial accountability, you are striking at the core values of that professional's training. Far too often, mental health professionals want to do the "right" thing without a detailed evaluation of the financial cost or, at the very least, a rationale for the business. As a result, administrators are offended and lose respect for the mental health professional. A typical battle is that of "numbers" or the workload of the mental health professional. Again, if we remember that a core value of the business professional is work, grumbling about needing to meet "numbers" sends a message that you don't care about the organization.

Recommendation:
1. Learn about your administrators' cultural frameworks.
2. Take their perspective.
3. Figure out what motivates them.
4. Find common ground and the right frame for your concerns and requests.

For example, if you are concerned about workload, prepare a plan that focuses on working efficiently and has a good work environment and sustainable organizational practice as its goal. And never whine.

The two measures that typically drive administrators are productivity and income; this is not bad - this is what their jobs revolve around. So, why would you start a presentation with clinical data? Their gauge of success is whether they can make their organization profitable, so expecting them to listen to your measure of success is a poor cross-cultural strategy; this is not to say that tying in a mission focus or clinical focus can't be done, but to state that is not usually a good starting point.

Recommendation: Any argument you make should be justified with data that speaks to their concerns.

And while on the subject of data: get some. Justifying your practice on the notion that you are helping many people does not fly in a world that demands that you prove it; this does not mean you need to justify your work with a double-blind, randomized study. Business people always use broad trend data, so be creative about the data you gather. It could be as simple as keeping a tally of the number of times providers curbside consult you as a measure of the number of patients who indirectly benefit from consultation services.

Show energy, initiative, and focus. Business people are trained to have drive and value individuals that show these traits. The training of mental health professionals values contemplation, which often can feel slow and lifeless to business people. One CEO I worked for remarked that he always felt suspicious about mental health professionals' need for so many "meetings." In his view, they talked too much and did too little. Recommendation: Walk fast, speak briefly and cogently, and display good organizational skills.

Administrators are not trained in people skills like mental health professionals; this might seem like an obvious statement, but it is important nonetheless. Because they are in positions of power, mental health professionals and others often assume that administrators are immune from being caught in interpersonal dynamics of their own and others' doing; this could not be further from the truth. You will often see aspects of their interpersonal functioning that could be more desirable. The key is to not lose respect for the individual because of these flaws but to learn how to work effectively despite them. I have worked with many administrators with blind spots in areas such as managing conflict or regulating anxiety. It was not my job to fix these things, but I logged those things in my mental databank and worked with those individuals respectfully and productively.

Recommendation: Understand your administrators and their strengths and weaknesses.

Get to know the medical culture and the sub-cultures. Since programs always need medical champions, it becomes imperative to convince primary care clinicians of the value of behavioral health consultation. To do so, you must know the culture of medicine and its varied sub-cultures and interests. For example, if you have primarily academic clinicians (such as at a university-affiliated center), you would probably want to have an elevator speech that cited critical research and the benefits of resident training. If you are addressing pediatricians in community practice, you would emphasize the assistance they would receive in managing ADHD referrals from local schools. If you were addressing a family practitioner, you might notice that they are reasonably open to an argument based on whole-person care (a softer sell) versus an internal medicine provider who might respond more to what academic clinicians will respond to (data, facts, assistance with specific disease categories such as diabetes). These are all based on the socialization experiences of these professions. There is significant variability in training, especially regionally in the United States, but I have found the general assumptions helpful as starting points in working with clinicians of all kinds. The point is not to be disingenuous or manipulative but rather to speak the language of your audience and tailor what you say to their needs. They are, after all, our first customers. Recommendation: Hang out with your providers as much as possible and learn their styles and cultural frameworks. You need to know what is essential to them.

What To Say

In case you haven't guessed, I am a big fan of the late Steve Jobs (at least his better attributes). One of the things he did well was convince people that what he was selling was not only a great product but a transformative product that would change how you looked at that aspect of your life. Most of the time, he seemed to be correct. In the same way, we have to inspire that sense of confidence in others that what we are proposing is fundamentally transformative of how we think about healthcare. So, not only is the content of your message crucial, but the energy and inspiration that goes along with it must be as well. Here are some sample elevator speeches (you can try to guess which groups they are addressed to):

Highlighting Efficiency:

"The biggest thing we are shooting for with this behavioral health consultant approach is increased efficiency. We can make great use of times when clinicians are not in the exam room and even, at times, intervene with a patient before a clinician has seen them, which helps move the process of care along quicker. Ultimately, we hope that the patient's needs are met and that the primary care clinician feels supported and free to focus on other aspects of care; this also means we see a lot more patients than in a traditional model, where we are sitting back waiting for referrals to show."

Detailing A Specific Benefit In A Typically Difficult Area:

"One of the areas this program is going to be helpful with is chronic pain. All patients who push the clinician's buttons (because they feel manipulated to prescribe narcotics) are possible warm handoffs to behavioral health consultants who can go in before or after the clinician visit and engage the patient in motivational interviewing while helping the medical team set reasonable boundaries. Clinicians find this support extremely helpful in diminishing or working through conflict."

Displaying Grounding In Evidence-Based Practice:

"Integrated care models have been extensively studied in large-scale clinical trials in areas such as depression, smoke cessation, and substance abuse, and the results show conclusively that they are as effective as specialty care in terms of clinical outcomes and superior in engaging patients when compared to specialty care referral approaches. In addition, clinician satisfaction is especially high because of the support provided to clinicians who are typically overburdened by patients with mental health concerns."

Highlighting Interest To A Particular Sub-Group:

"There are many residency training programs across the country that see the addition of behavioral health consultants as a great way to train clinicians in the medical home model of the future. By exposing residents to BHCs, we are training them on installing these programs in their future practices and enhancing their knowledge of how to treat mental health concerns."

Displaying Interest In Sustainability:

"Ultimately, our success in integrating care will depend on our payer mix, productivity, and provider satisfaction. Moving forward, we need to develop a plan to track these markers to ensure that what we do is sustainable for the clinic."

Highlighting A Particular Benefit:

"Behavioral health consultants would be very helpful when a parent is overwhelmed with a challenging child, and you might be concerned about possible delays or disorders. You could hand off the patient to the consultant and then have another set of eyes and ears to ensure the child is screened properly and the parent is well supported. And, of course, it would save you some time too."

Highlighting The Systemic Impact of The Model:

"One of the intended benefits of the model is that everyone on the medical team gets better at each others' jobs. That means that the primary care clinician gets better at identifying and treating mental health concerns, and the behavioral health consultants get better at co-managing physical health conditions such as diabetes. Medical assistants benefit and often learn how to use the BHC to enhance clinic flow, triage, and refer patients with specific concerns to the BHC."

Detailing A Plan For Addressing Sustainability:

"There are various ways to make an integrated care program sustainable, as many clinics nationwide have found. To determine how we will make it work, we should identify key data, such as what our payor mix looks like and what kind of reimbursement we can expect/estimate while we also continue looking for grant funding. Beyond that, we should also consider the impact the BHC program could have on improving cycle times, which could improve our customer experience while also reducing some strain on the primary care clinicians, which is key for retention over the long term."

Highlighting The Data-Driven Approach of the Model:

"Our data, collected over the last month, shows that primary care clinicians consulted behavioral health consultants more than 25 times per day, resulting in an average of 8 warm handoffs per day in addition to scheduled patient consults. A provider survey showed 95% satisfaction with the service, and the main complaint was that there were times when a consultant was unavailable. Based on these figures, we should be on track for sustainability, assuming our standard payor mix doesn't shift."

Of course, many other variations exist, but hopefully, you get the point. You speak to your audience's needs; you are brief and display confidence, passion, and purpose. Easy right? Of course not, this is challenging. But we hope that the rest of this book provides tools for growth so that your program development skills grow to become as good as your consultation skills over time.

Chapter 5: Nuts & Bolts Of Getting Started: Year 1

By Neftali Serrano, PsyD

Nothing is more critical in developing your primary care behavioral health program than starting with a laser-like focus. If you are a clinic and want to create a program, your first step is simple: find the right talent. If you are the talent selected and looking to develop the program, your first step is simple: build those provider relationships.

Don't Make It More Complicated Than It Is

One of the common errors or misunderstandings that clinics have about primary care behavioral health integration is that it is complicated. As a result, clinics get stuck on many details and ignore the singularly most essential element: talent; this is true of all hires, especially the first hire. Your first hire will likely be a clinician who sees patients and is your service line leader or director of the growing program. Therefore, the program's development will hinge on the skills this person brings to bear on your patients, leading a team, working collaboratively with other clinic teams, and tolerating the organization's growing pains. In fact, given that reimbursement issues and other logistics are usually quite solvable, finding the right talent is the most challenging element of the puzzle. The harsh reality is that there are not a lot of mental health professionals either trained for this work or with the right combination of temperament and skills to make it work.

Unfortunately, many clinics desperate for help choose someone with a good reputation as a clinician and then are disappointed one year into the program development because the person is not performing adequately. They have then lost a year and set the program back even further in the jilted minds of the medical providers. It would have been better if they had waited six months to find the right person; this means don't hire someone because they are a family friend or because someone you know says they are a good therapist. This job demands a lot more than that. You can review the chapter in this book for more on hiring and maintaining your staff. For now, the thing to focus on is the simplicity of hiring a talented individual who fits the following makeup:

- Leadership skills
- Confidence
- Good communication skills
- Flexible
- Passion for the vision of primary care behavioral health
- Buys into the idea of developing a program
- Enjoys working with others, even tricky people

- Solid clinical skills that are adaptable to primary care consultation
- Cares about quality and productivity
- Interpersonal maturity (sets good boundaries, even keel, balanced perspective)

Working on other details related to program development is OK while looking for the right person. What does not make sense is waiting until you get these details right to begin looking. It often takes a long time to find this person, and often, this person can be the one to work out the details in a much more efficient fashion. Organizations should also prepare to wait for total productivity from the program until as much as a year or more after its inception. Often, organizations want to get their ducks in a row because they wish to begin making money from Day 1; this is highly unrealistic no matter how much pre-work is done due to the nature of integrating a new program and team member. There is a steep learning and growing curve which must be accounted for. So, yes, patience is required. But patience often saves money in the long run because it is much more costly for an organization to make the wrong hire than to wait, make the right hire, and then grow the program.

In case I haven't clarified enough, hiring the right talent is the crucial focus of starting a primary care behavioral health program. Nothing else matters if this does not occur. The same applies if you are a first hire and are charged with growing the program further. Who you hire for the following Behavioral Health Consultant positions is the most critical thing you will do. And as discussed later on in the text, treating your talent well is just as key.

Build Provider Relationships

A truism immutable in PCBH is that everything rides on the relationship between the primary care provider and behavioral health consultant. Nothing else matters if this is not solid, and this should be the primary focus, period. This relationship is facilitated through the daily interactions between primary care clinicians and behavioral health consultants. Once primary care clinicians find the behavioral health consultants helpful in a variety of situations, the bedrock of the model is set; this means being present and visible and constantly working on the minutia of good patient flow and individual provider preferences for how to work things.

First-time directors or lone BHCs often take time to work on newsletters, protocols, or meetings - some of which might be fine but account for so little of the overall success of a program that it is not worth doing to the exclusion of the day-to-day relational stuff. I have learned that many of these activities I engaged in early on were about anxiety management (my own). Preparation makes more sense after you have some live data (data in the general sense as in relational data). So all the protocols and clinic flow pathways will develop organically in an integrated care setting where providers trust each other and understand how each other works.

One of the challenging aspects of this non-specific work in building relationships is that it takes time, and that it means it might feel like you are not being productive. I spent a lot of time early on sitting with and hanging around providers, listening to their conversations and, at times jumping in with either a helpful suggestion or a snide comment. The steady accumulation of presence, helpfulness, and specific cases worked between provider and behavioral health consultant create a bedrock for your program. It is that simple. If you get this part right, you can solve other issues. If you don't, the other issues won't matter anyway.

At their core, integrated care programs are about organizing how human beings work; this is one of the weaknesses of protocol-based programs - they ignore that non-specific relational factors impact how people work.

The nurse who is excellent at organizing patient requests and triaging issues gets a lot more done with her providers than the care manager who hides in his office and keeps his door closed. The primary care provider who communicates well with front desk staff can implement micro-system changes, whereas the medical assistant with poor communication skills is chronically slow and ineffective. Relationships mediate the goals of systems, and the Behavioral Health Consultants in a system become key relational cogs that can significantly improve the systems around the medical team. So, working with primary care clinicians is the most effective way to build a program.

What To Watch For

When working with primary care clinicians, you want to watch for elements of their work that will inform your work with them. These include watching for how they communicate with staff and patients, what they value most (speed/efficiency vs. relational connections), their specific flow as they move from patient to patient, and their baseline understanding of your role.

For example, in provider curbside consults, I often asked flow questions such as, "Are you done with this patient, and if not, what is next?"; this gives me an idea of what the provider's day is like as well as how they work flow with their patients. Suppose the provider hurriedly indicates that there is still much work to do and that they are backed up. In that case, I will quickly state that I will make the visit as brief as possible and alert the medical assistant as soon as I am done to make sure the next step occurs; this helps the provider feel like their needs are met along with the patient's needs. This can do much more for stimulating referrals than any paper-based protocol.

Start A PCBH Champion Committee

We didn't start our BHC program at Access this way but it has since become more common and helpful to start with a committee of champion representatives from throughout the organization. For example, you could invite medical, nursing, medical assistant, billing and front-desk champions to join a regularly scheduled meeting (usually more frequent early on and less after year 1) to discuss and help form the PCBH program. This creates buy-in across the organization from the get-go and provides a forum to troubleshoot key issues.

Key to making these groups work are tightly run meetings with a pre-made agenda, the right meeting cadence (not too often, not too infrequent), and the right participants. The group should not be large (anywhere from 4 to 8 participants for a standard clinic) so as to water down the investment of each participant. Remember that a key goal of the committee is to champion PCBH across the organization, so participant connection to the group will be key.

Measure Progress

We recommend starting with tools to help you measure progress with implementation. These can be administered to your champion committee or more broadly to the organization. Plan for a pre-, mid-, and post-evaluation, usually spaced around 6 to 12 months in-between administrations. The goal here is to feedback information to the organization about how implementation is proceeding. I have found it particularly useful to plan a meeting with champion committees to discuss the evaluation's findings, which then elicits conversation on shoring up lacking areas.

Two tools we recommend are the Practice Integration Profile out of the University of Massachusetts and the MeHAF out of the Maine Health Foundation. The best way to use these is to send them out to representatives of different parts of the organization, compile the results and then meet to discuss the results. In particular, it is helpful to identify the items where the group members differed the most in their perspectives and spur a conversation as to why the perceived discrepancy exists. This then can lead to either adjusted perspectives or real-world changes in the implementation that the team can agree to. Access did not start with such a process but we wish we had to involve more people in the process and to have more information about where we were in our process.

Keep It Simple

So, in sum, in year one, you keep it simple. Build these relationships by being in the clinic as much as possible and learning about the day-to-day life and habits of your primary care teams. And don't go it alone. Find your champions and have them invest in the program along with you. It is exhausting and relationally tiring but, in the long run, a rich and rewarding process as you see the teams grow into a sum that is much greater than its parts.

We start with this focus because it is so easy to get lost in the details of the work that you lose this fundamental aspect. Forget control early on, get in the clinic, and work things out that way as much as possible. Next, we move on to the fundamentals of your program, starting with the BHC schedule.

Chapter 6: Nuts & Bolts Of Getting Started: The Schedule

By Neftali Serrano, PsyD

O ne of the most fundamental aspects of behavioral health consultation, yet one of the ones new BHCs seem to make unnecessarily complicated, is the schedule. The reason why it feels complicated is that the schedule is reflective of the transition behavioral health consultants are making professionally. So naturally, there is some reluctance to implement the simplicity of the new schedule. As human beings and mental health professionals, we have control issues.

Indeed, this chapter ought to be obscenely short because scheduling in the behavioral health consultant model is simple - but I have seen enough new BHCs struggle with it to know to spend some time on it. Let's start with the primary goals of the schedule and then move to the nuts and bolts.

The Basic Goals of A Behavioral Health Consultant Schedule

Perhaps it is best if we start with the goals of a mental health specialist's schedule. The schedule's purpose is to alert patients regarding the times the specialist has made available for hour-long appointments for the panel of patients the specialist has agreed to see. There might be a few other nuances to the schedule in some settings, such as the type of appointment - intake or follow-up - which might impact the schedule, but generally speaking, this is the purpose.

By contrast, the behavioral health consultant schedule has multiple purposes. The schedule communicates to receptionists the follow-up slots the behavioral health consultant has made available for clinic patients that have already been seen in warm handoffs. These are 15-30 minutes long, but only theoretically since they are not bound by time precisely like the specialist schedule. More on this in a moment. The schedule also is a holding environment for the open spaces, which allow for the curbside consultations, which are the heart and soul of behavioral health consultation. The behavioral health consultant's schedule emphasizes immediacy and open access, whereas the specialist's schedule is on boundaries and structure.

The behavioral health consultant schedule's goal is to provide as much access to the clinic population as possible at the time of need. More specifically, on a day-to-day basis, the schedule should allow for the needs of all patients and providers in the building to access the behavioral health consultant(s) (in-person or via curbside consultation). So, one way to look at the behavioral health consultant's schedule is that it does not belong to the behavioral health consultant but to the medical team. Thus it makes sense why new behavioral health consultants have difficulty throwing themselves in wholeheartedly: the BHC schedule gives them less control over their day. So, my advice to new behavioral health consultants is simple: let go.

Of course, both schedules have pros and cons, and the point here is to draw a contrast and understand the goal of the schedule.

While there may be room for variation, be mindful of that pull for control; it sneaks in and creates barriers for providers and patients to access the behavioral health consultant. So, keep it simple and follow what has worked for many other clinics.

Logistics

Here are some rules which work well:

1. The only thing you seek to limit is the follow-up slots. Too many follow-up slots, and you don't have enough time for same-day work (curbside consults and warm handoffs). Access has three follow-up slots per half day. Registrars have access to schedule in just these slots. Simple.

2. Slots are typically front-loaded in a half-day or clinic session because the expectation is that there will be

fewer warm handoffs in the early part of the session and more later on. Access' slots are at 9 AM, 9:30 AM, and 10:30 AM for the morning session and 1 PM, 1:30 PM, and 2:30 PM.

2.1. A nuance you will need to navigate here is how to manage the slot access by staff. Some electronic health records (EHR) will make it easier to lock down access to specific team members (e.g., not allowing registrars to book in the warm handoff slots), while others do not. In the EPIC EHR, Access chose to color code the slots red and green and train registrars not to schedule in the red slots; this provides flexibility for circumstances where a BHC may ask a registrar to overbook a red slot, for example.

3. The scheduling strategy should allow the behavioral health consultant to add the warm handoffs they see throughout the day. So, often this means having the same kind of software security access as registrars. As the behavioral health consultant sees patients, they add the patient they have just seen for billing and record-keeping purposes (e.g., to enable a note to be associated with a visit). Note that there may be better workflows for some clinics, but having the flexibility to schedule helps.

4. Time outside the slots can be spent on various activities, including warm handoffs, curbside consultations, phone-based patient follow-up, and even same-day patient access (e.g., a suicidal patient who calls in and would benefit from being seen right away). Occasionally we might overbook the schedule with such a patient in

need a day or so in advance, but you can't make a habit out of this since it will clog up access.

5. Patients rarely need weekly follow-ups in primary care as they might in specialty care. Typical follow-up occurs in 2-6 week chunks. If follow-ups are scheduled too closely, access problems develop, and the schedule gets clogged; this is where your program metrics can help you (see the chapter on data). In an ideal circumstance, follow-up slots should be available two weeks in advance.

6. When you have multiple behavioral health consultants on a team, it works well to have a generic schedule by site versus one based on the particular behavioral health consultant provider. For example, there would be a schedule for "BHC South Clinic" instead of a schedule specific to "Neftali Serrano"; this fits the behavioral health consultant model where various members can see a patient of the BHC team (the patient would schedule with behavioral health generally versus scheduling with a specific behavioral health consultant). The advantage is that you avoid having behavioral health consultants develop patient panels that follow them around, creating access problems. For example, a popular behavioral health consultant might begin to attract a following and then have patients upset because they cannot access a follow-up appointment for just that provider. This scheme also reinforces the team-based mindset of the behavioral health consultant model.

What Does Not Work

Just in case you feel tempted to try interesting variations on the scheduling scheme presented here, here are some things that do not work:

1. Random follow-up slots. The lack of structure to follow-up slots presents a challenge to registrars and behavioral health consultants. It typically leads to overbooking and booking of patients at inopportune times of the day.

2. Half-day traditional schedule and half-day warm-handoffs; this is the proverbial compromise situation made by clinicians who are having difficulty transitioning their identities and have yet to fully buy into the idea that consultation can be just as effective as traditional specialty therapy. Schedule-wise, this pulls the behavioral health consultant out of the clinic for a half-day which is problematic for provider awareness (they need the behavioral health consultant at all times, not just designated times). However, even if there were another behavioral health consultant to cover while the other consultant is engaged in specialty therapy, the practice sends mixed signals to primary care clinicians and patients alike. In this scheme, the behavioral health consultant practice becomes a mere bridge to specialty care versus an actual place of collaborative care for the medical team. Remember that the model intends to retain most patients in primary care and only refer those who fit and need specialty therapy. One other side-effect, and perhaps the most damaging, is that behavioral health consultants tend to have stunted professional growth in their identities as participants in the medical home. They don't seem to make the

transition wholeheartedly. The final result is that these scheduling schemes are never as productive as full-throttle behavioral health consultant programs.

3. The behavioral health consultant has a different schedule which only they manage. A good rule of thumb when doing integrated care is to use existing processes when possible. There is no reason a behavioral health consultant needs to manage their schedule when you have people paid to do that for medical providers. All the same systems, including call centers, registrars, etc., should apply to the behavioral health consultant's work. What happens when the behavioral health consultant manages their schedule is that no one else learns about the practice habits of the behavioral health consultant. Furthermore, managing the schedule adds more time and complexity to the behavioral health consultant's work with patients (answering phone calls and negotiating dates and times in consults).

4. Forget warm handoffs and see patients for 15-minute visits all day. It might sound absurd but trust me, some places have tried this. First, while the intent might sound population-based (see lots of people), the result is not since there is little interaction with and cross-pollination with primary care clinicians in this model. It is not integrated care and does little for productivity since no-show rates are still obscenely high. Additionally, many clinicians will adapt to this "high productivity" scheme by creating a panel of patients they see regularly, meeting their productivity goals but having a decreased population penetrance as compared to a true BHC. Cramming in more slots is a tried and

true recipe for failure. The heart and soul of behavioral health consultation is the warm handoff. Given either follow-ups or warm handoffs, the good behavioral health consultant will always prefer the latter. Many behavioral health consultants will tell you that these are often the most productive visits from an activity standpoint. Plus, you will burn out your BHC quickly with this schedule type.

So, keep it simple. The schedule is the cornerstone of the behavioral health consultant's work, and once it is set, it rarely needs tinkering. Get this done within the first month of practice, and you are good to go.

Chapter 7: Nuts & Bolts Of Getting Started: Charting

By Neftali Serrano, PsyD

So far, we have suggested that you start with identifying the right talent and setting up a proper behavioral health consultation schedule. So, suppose you are struggling with finding ways to fix the schedule to make it more familiar to specialty mental health. In that case, you know you are struggling with fundamental identity issues. I have seen it happen many times. What is simple is made to be obtuse and complex, but underlying it all is a simple struggle for identity. And if that is the case with the preceding section topics, it is all the more true of this one. Few issues cause as much identity conflict as the simple act of charting. My directive here is similar to the other section topics: keep it simple.

Once again, let's review and contrast the goals of charting in specialty mental health and compare it to medical record charting.

Charting In Specialty Mental Health

Generally speaking, specialty mental health providers have distinguished between two forms of note-taking: process notes and progress notes. Process notes are usually described as notes with a great deal of personal detail related to the patient and factors associated with the content of sessions, even in some therapeutic traditions, down to the transferential issues the therapist observes in session. They can be thought of as reflecting the process of therapy itself.

Progress notes are the more official version of details related to patient care, often including the facts necessary to track patient care over time, the goals of that care, the diagnosis associated with these sessions, and other essential information which insurers may require. The purpose of progress notes is to document the work done and to serve as a historical record of treatment progress. Progress notes also usually include aspects of the patient history, often reported initially in a clinical interview.
In the case of process notes, the audience for these notes is the therapist themselves, though legally, this may not be the case (courts can subpoena any documentation). In the case of progress notes, the audience is the therapist, the insurer, and possibly the patient themselves since they officially own their records. In some cases, progress notes can be released to other providers with the patient's permission, so future providers should also be considered an audience for these notes.

Charting In The Medical Record

Charting in the behavioral health consultant model mirrors charting that primary care clinicians engage in. A good rule of thumb is that if primary care clinicians chart something regularly, behavioral health consultants should also. If they do not, then behavioral health consultants should not.

The goal of charting in the medical record is similar to the progress note goals of specialty mental health in that it serves as a record of treatment provided and the associated diagnoses. So a chart note typically includes a procedure code (also called a CPT code), an associated diagnosis code(s), and a narrative, often in the SOAP note format. Since the consultant is just one person working with the patient in the medical home team, the consultant is not responsible for documenting a comprehensive psychological history often appearing in the specialty mental health record. The behavioral health consultant often adds a note related to their visit that day. They might put some relevant information into the history sections of a chart. Still, they are just a contributor, not the main author (the primary care clinician is the leading actor here).

The behavioral health consultant SOAP note differs from progress notes primarily in its intended audience. The note is written for the medical team, often primarily the primary care clinician since the consultant's role is to consult. More broadly, since the note exists in the general medical record, it also documents treatment progress and billable activity for insurers. In addition, since the medical record belongs to the patient, the patient is part of the audience as well. Mental health providers' main difficulty with charting in the medical record is related to historical factors around the development of charting and privacy concerns within the profession. Historically, therapists have often confabulated the distinction between process notes and progress notes. So some therapists come from traditions that did not do a good job of distinguishing the type of content in each. Also, since mental health issues carry a stigma in most societies, mental health professionals have developed traditions around strict confidentiality. These traditions are codified in ethical statements and instilled from the start of a mental health professional's training.

Notice that I use the term "traditions." Traditions are culture-bound phenomena, not absolutes. In many cases, the struggles of therapists with writing in a medical record have to do with traditions, not absolutes, and certainly not legal requirements. They have to do with what we were told is good for patients and our profession.

The reality is that primary care clinicians have been documenting mental health treatment in the medical record for decades, including documentation of suicidality, substance abuse, trauma, domestic violence, and treatment for all primary psychiatric diagnoses. They have done this just as they have documented treatment for sexually-transmitted diseases, HIV, sexual dysfunction, obesity, neurologic conditions, and everything else under the sun. In light of this reality, the concern that mental health professionals often profess at writing "confidential" information in the medical record strikes primary care clinicians as absurd.

Federal law also does not distinguish between aspects of the medical record. In other words, HIPAA does not have requirements for an über-protected part of the record that deserves more protection than other parts that deserve less. All aspects of a medical record are to be kept equally confidential, and HIPAA provides patient-directed rights to release parts of the medical record. So, patients have a right not to release aspects of the medical record related to HIV status or mental health concerns - this would include a note for depression written by a primary care clinician.

So, process notes have no place in a medical record since they are more akin to the private thoughts of the therapist. A SOAP note should be written with the audience of the note in mind, not the least of which is the patient; in fact, some clinicians write their notes with their patients. We as mental health professionals have to give up ownership of mental health issues as our own domain and realize that, in reality, it is and always has been the domain of the patient-doctor relationship (medical). So when we become a part of the medical home, we do not own any part of the record. The team does, and ultimately the patient does as part of that team.

So, as you can imagine, I am not an advocate for "break-the-glass" features in electronic health records, separate charts, or even separate mental health tabs in paper charts. No legal or ethical mandate requires these (though lamentably, some state regulations often require this of state-certified agencies), and in the end, it is a bad practice for the medical home and the patient.

Why is it a bad practice for the medical home? To begin, it creates an arbitrary line of demarcation between the team members, which goes against the integration goals. Primary care clinicians resent that they cannot access mental health records when they know their patients in some of the most privileged ways imaginable. Practically, separating mental health notes also creates barriers that encourage primary care providers to ignore mental health data. Thus, the exchange of information crucial to integrated care does not occur.

Why is it a bad practice for patients? This is perhaps where we must be the most self-reflective as a profession. We have spent so much time and energy working to protect mental health information that we have reinforced that mental health concerns should remain hidden, dark parts of our lives. Yet, in a strange form of double-speak, we encourage people to talk about their mental illness and seek to reduce the stigma associated with it in public ad campaigns.

There is nothing that does more to reduce stigma, in my professional experience, than integrated care. The patient begins to experience the aspects of their mental functioning in the context of their life's physical and even spiritual elements because they are treated as one person with interrelated concerns. The medical record should reflect this reality. The patient will always retain the right to release aspects of their medical record as they wish, and organizations should ensure that release of record procedures are sound in this respect. That is the only protection patients need. The "protection" we have afforded the patient record in specialty settings has done more harm than good, leading to disintegrated and disjointed care, increased stigma, and professional isolation. Nothing good has historically come of it.

So, please keep it simple. Unless you can argue that the information you gather is more confidential or critical than what primary care clinicians discuss with their patients, you cannot justify not charting in the medical record. Of course, the key is knowing how to chart so that your notes omit process note content and extraneous content or details irrelevant to the consult or identified problem. The key is simply writing well with the audience(s) in mind.

Here are some keys to getting started with charting:

1. **Chart in the medical record**. If your clinic uses paper charts, use the same paper and format. If your clinic uses an electronic health record, use the same sections primary care clinicians use. Separate mental health modules are typically irrelevant and expensive.

2. **Mirror standards at the clinic.** If providers use a SOAP note format, then use that format. If there is an alternative version, use something similar. I prefer using the SOAP note format but in an APSO order; this places the assessment and plan sections at the top of the note, which is very helpful for readers (for whom these are the salient parts of the note) and also trains the behavioral health consultant to think more efficiently in their consults. (More on this latter aspect in the section on training.) All BHCs should use the same template.

3. **Make charting quality one of the goals for the first year.** Notes should be brief, specific, relevant to the concerns of the medical team, effective at moving patient care along, and easy to read (formatting, consistency). For more specifics on the content of the SOAP note or, as we use, the APSO note, see the section

on training. We make charting the first competency we teach our new behavioral health consultants because it teaches the logic behind the model and is a foundational element of the work.

4. **Start with a minimalistic design, and then build on that as needed.** Too often, the tendency is to want to gather more information, probably due to the same anxiety we discussed in previous sections. Adding elements is often easier than removing them, so start with a basic process and basic note structure and stick with it for a while. After some time, it will become clear what pieces of the note process need amplifying based on feedback from primary care clinicians and others (e.g., the billing department).

5. **Ensure that your clinic has a suitable HIPAA-compliant release of records process and consent form.** If done correctly, it should already have the check-off boxes needed to cue patients on what aspects of their record should be released. Don't tinker with it unless it is not HIPAA compliant. Get one from another clinic if you want to compare versions. (In most cases, these forms are standardized, and you should not alter them in any way.)

6. **If you have had poor exposure to SOAP note training** or your training needs to be improved for note writing in particular (not much attention is given to this formally in academic settings), seek some consultation from someone in the primary care behavioral health community. There are tried and true methods. You don't have to reinvent the wheel. CFHA has some excellent training materials online.

7. **Do not chart in a separate record** in addition to the medical record. It is unnecessary and only opens up more liability concerns. The behavioral health consultant is a consultant to the medical team and, as such, does not have a special relationship with the patient. Therefore having a separate record is only potentially harmful and not helpful.

8. **Informed consent regarding charting**, that is, alerting the patient to the fact that all members of the healthcare team place data relevant to the patient's care in the medical record, is an emerging but not uniform practice. For example, not all clinics even have patients sign an informed consent to treatment. All clinics provide the patient with a copy of their HIPAA rights and other clinic-related information, which is considered informed consent. Some clinics with integrated behavioral health provide a statement or separate documentation. In the end, we all know that patients rarely read the information provided upon registration, so most of this comes down to providing legal coverage for your clinic or what is commonly referred to as CYA (cover your ass). The best practice would be integrating a statement related to the integrated chart in a general informed consent procedure for all new patients at the front desk. I would not recommend having behavioral health consultants ask all patients to sign a consent before each visit; this is cumbersome, introduces differences between the medical and behavioral health consultation services, and is rarely in the patient's interest. Patients should be informed of the practice but cannot be provided with an alternative. In other words, if they sign, they are

assenting to the fact that they have been informed, not because they have a choice. The behavioral health consultant cannot see or work with the patient without the ability to document the medical record.

9. **Train the care team,** including registrars and others with access to the record, in best practices related to confidential patient information. An explicit component of the training should include a mention of the importance of protecting sensitive data. Fortunately, all modern HIPAA training already has these elements.

10. **Use documentation as a training tool**, especially for case conceptualization. I train students to use this equation when writing their note: S+O= A, therefore P. The subjective data a patient provides (S), plus the objective data you collect (O), should equal/ inform the assessment you create, which should result in a plan (P) that flows from this assessment. If this logic is not self-evident in the note, then it should be re-written or perhaps the consult was ineffective.

11. **Teach case conceptualization skills** using your documentation. I teach students to write an assessment using this formula: PT with XX (symptoms, issues, presenting concern), as a result of (or mitigated by) XX who would benefit from XX (intervention approach). For more see here.

12. **Initial and follow-up note templates** are not necessary. Some places have them but if you understand primary care you realize how unhelpful the distinction between a first visit and a follow-up visit is. The step-wise care model has you always assessing and intervening at each visit so every visit is a mix of a first

and follow-up visit. Furthermore, nearly 50% of visits are one-time visits in any given year in PCBH. Teach your staff to write subsequent notes using the same template.

13. **Feel free to copy and paste.** Below is a sample APSO note template, an example of the note filled in, and a form to assess documentation standards in your practice.

APSO TEMPLATE EXEMPLAR (EPIC EHR)

ASSESSMENT:
PT with (1***), related to (2***), in the context of (3***). Patient would benefit from (4***).
Stage of change: {Stage of change: 5}
Intervention Type: {BHCintervention: 6}
Diagnosis: {Current visit dx: 7}

PLAN:
1. F/U with behavioral health consultant {Time Interval:8}.
2. Medications: {Medication: 9}.
3. Behavioral recommendation(s):
      A. 10 ***
      B. ***

SUBJECTIVE:
Pt here for {11 INITIAL CONSULTATION/ REFERRAL/ FOLLOW-UP/ OTHER:} regarding 12. {13 Gender/Parent:} reported the following symptoms/concerns: 14 ***
    Progress towards prior plan: {15 BHCprogress:}
    Duration of problem: {16: "1-2 Weeks","2-4 Weeks","1-3

Months","3-6 Months","6-12 Months","Several Years","Lifelong Course","Lifelong Course With Waxing & Waning","Lifelong Course With Recent Exacerbation"}
Severity: {17 BHCSeverity:}

OBJECTIVE:
Referred by: {18 PCP:}.
Orientation & Cognition: Oriented x3. Associations logical, no gross signs of thought disorder.
Mood, Affect: {19}.
Appearance: Appropriately dressed and groomed.
Harm to self or others: {20}
Substance use: {21}
Psychiatric medication use: {22}
Health risk behaviors: {23}
Completion of screening measures: 24 Yes/ No; {25}

Time spent face-to-face with patient: *** minutes

@Name of clinician@

{BLANK:19884::"The patient was informed of the following characteristics of their care within the primary care medical home at XXX Community Health Centers: a. Behavorial health providers operate as consultants to the medical team and not as stand-alone providers of care, b. All information discussed with team members as applicable/appropriate will be documented in the shared electronic health record and visible by all care team members, c. The Behavioral Health Team works as a group providing care to all Access patients and as such a patient is likely to work with multiple Behavioral Health providers. Patient consented to meet with BHC."}

----

*Note that the elements in {brackets} would be drop down or list elements in EPIC that are unique to your build. In other words, you can't copy this into EPIC and have the lists work, but you can easily replace the lists with similar lists in your iteration of EPIC.

DROPDOWNS:

1 to 4: -Every time you see *** it means, free for providers to document as much information as needed.

5:
Precontemplation
Contemplation
Preparation
Action
Maintenance
**** (For providers to add any additional information)
6:
 Acceptance/Commitment Approach, Problem Solving
 Behavior Modification, Psychoeducation, Behavioral
Activation, Relaxation Skills Training, Cognitive-Behavioral,
Stress Management, Crisis Management, Supportive
Interventions, Insight Development, Systemic Intervention,
Interpersonal Skills Training, Health and Behavioral
Interventions, Mindfulness Training, SBIRT, Motivational
Interviewing Assessment, Parent-Child Interaction
Other ***

7. Should pull up the diagnosis inserted in the Diagnosis field in Epic.

8.
2 weeks
1 month
at the next PCP visit
as needed
other ***

9.
None
Per PCP
NA
Other ***

10. Free for providers to document as much information as needed.

11.
initial consultation
follow up
health and behavioral consultation
referral
other ***

12. Free for providers to document as much information as needed.

13.
He
She

They
Parent
Other ***

14. Free for providers to document as much information as needed.

15.
Ongoing
N/A- First time seeing BHC
***

16.
1-2 Weeks
2-4 Weeks
1-3 Months
3-6 Months
6-12 Months
Several Years
Lifelong Course
Lifelong Course With Waxing & Waning
Lifelong Course With Recent Exacerbation

17.
None
Mild
Mild to Moderate
Moderate
Moderate to Severe
Severe
Other

18.

PCP
BHC follow-up appointment
Self
Other ***

19.
 Dysphoric, Irritable, Blunted, Euthymic, Flat, Agitated,
Depressed, Distressed, Tearful, Anxious, Labile, Other ***

20.
Pt denies
Morbid ideation only
Passive suicidal ideation. Denies intent or plan.
Active suicidal ideation
History of
Non-suicidal self-injurious behaviors
Non-assessed
Other

21.
Pt denies current substance use/abuse
Problem or risky substance use
Current use of
Not assessed

22.
Unchanged from prior contact
Stopped medication on her own on
Intermittent use of
Adherence
N/A
Other ***

23.
Problem or risky alcohol use
Problem or risky substance use
Current tobacco use
Other health behavior concern
None
Not assessed
***

24.
Yes
No
PHQ-9, GAD-7, SLUMS, AUDIT, DAST, SBIRT
Other ***

25. Free for providers to document the amount of minutes spent with patient.

APSO TEMPLATE EXEMPLAR FILLED IN

ASSESSMENT:
Pt with persistent depressive disorder, alcohol use disorder, in sustained remission presenting with recent increase in depressive sx, anxiety and sub-optimal sleep hygiene in the context of psychosocial stressors. Pt with good self-awareness and motivation for values based living and as such would benefit from returning to use of values-based coping strategies that have helped before as well as implementing sleep hygiene strategies.
Intervention Type: Cognitive-Behavioral, Motivational Interviewing

PLAN:

1. F/U with behavioral health consultant in 2 week(s).
2. Changes to psychotropic medication regimen: None.
3. Behavioral recommendation(s):
    A. Reinforced on-going medication adherence.
    B. Sleep hygiene behaviors. Limit screens before bedtime. Develop nighttime ritual.
    C. Goals: 1. Re-engage with regular church attendance; 2. Re-engaging with daily prayer (morning and evening).
4. Referred to nursing triage to address physical health concerns.

SUBJECTIVE:
Pt here for follow-up regarding mood. Pt last seen by BHC in May 2019. Pt verbally consented to meet with BHC. She reported the following symptoms/concerns: increased periods of depressed mood, low energy, lack of engagement with value based living (has stopped going to church, no longer engaging in morning prayer/meditation). Pt discussed recent falling out of close friendship and sadness/feelings of rejection along with many negative automatic thoughts. She has remained active in the recovery community (12 years in recovery from alcohol use). Pt discussed grief from death of father and value of taking FMLA to be with him and assist with care. Sleep issues persist with poor sleep hygiene. Difficulty falling and staying asleep with noted anxiety/worry. Frequently watches screens before bed. Falls asleep around 1 am and is up at 6 am for work. Pt discussed recent physical illness and negative and catastrophic thinking associated with her health. States desire to met with nursing today to listen to her lungs and discuss medical concerns. We discussed personal goals, barriers, and behavioral action plan.

Progress towards prior plan: Ongoing
Duration of problem: Several Years
Severity: Moderate

OBJECTIVE:
Referred by: PCP Name
Orientation & Cognition: Oriented x3. Associations logical, no gross signs of thought disorder.
Mood, Affect: Dysphoric.
Appearance: Appropriately dressed and groomed.
Harm to self or others: Pt denies.
Substance use: Pt denies current substance use/abuse. H/o alcohol use disorder. In sustained remission.
Current psychotropic medication use: Unchanged from prior contact. Pt taking both fluoxetine and Effexor.
Health risk behaviors: None.
Completion of screening measures: PHQ=17

Other(s) present in the room: None.

Time spent face-to-face with patient: 30 minutes

Dr. Neftali Serrano

The patient was informed of the following characteristics of their care within the primary care medical home at Access Community Health Centers: a. Behavioral health providers operate as consultants to the medical team and not as stand-alone providers of care, b. All information discussed with team members as applicable/appropriate will be documented in the shared electronic health record and visible by all care team members, c. The Behavioral Health Team works as a group providing care to all Access patients and as such a patient is likely to work with multiple Behavioral Health providers. Patient consented to meet with BHC.

APSO NOTE AUDIT TOOL

Behavioral Health Consultant Documentation Audit

1. Goal is to complete a review of Behavioral Health notes within the EHR annually or as indicated by agency needs.
2. Focus is on the Behavioral Health notes, not the overall chart.
3. Assumption that larger medical team is taking care of their responsibilities including documentation of insurance, guardianship if applicable, organizational consent for treatment, etc.

Person Being Audited:

Auditor: Date:

Elements					
	APSO/SOAP Overall Note Elements	Yes	No	N/A	Reviewer Comments
1.	Are there clear sections for subjective, objective, assessment, and plan?				
2.	Are required elements as dictated by coders included in the template? Can include modality of treatment, verbal consent to treatment, presenting concern, progress since last visit or others.				
3.	If first visit with Behavioral Health or visit after gap in care, is informed consent documented at end of note?				
4.	Is there enough information included in the note to assist in moving care forward?				

Use this tool to give BHCs feedback on documentation proficiency (developed by Meghan Fondow, PhD)

Chapter 8: Nuts & Bolts Of Getting Started: Hiring

By Neftali Serrano, PsyD

I f the adage in real estate is location, location, location, then the saying for behavioral health consultation is talent, talent, talent. I have seen far too many organizations get excited about integration, select the first mental health provider, and then see their integration efforts fall short of their expectations. Finding the right talent to build or expand your primary care behavioral health program is an organization's most significant decision; this is true of most programs, but even more so of primary care behavioral health.

Consider what we have identified as the cornerstone of primary care behavioral health: the relationship between primary care clinician and behavioral health consultant. Since this relationship, not a protocol, is the centerpiece of the model, the fit and relational skills of the behavioral health consultant are paramount. You can have a great set of protocols for depression, but if you have a slow, traditionally-minded behavioral health consultant, your program is dead on arrival. So, the questions for us in this section are how to find the right person and who to select from the applicant pool you create.

Outer Parameters

There will be some baseline criteria for the candidate you select, some of which are dictated by your setting. These are things like Spanish-speaking only or a specific type of degree such as an LCSW or PsyD. These form the outer boundaries of your search. Unfortunately, many organizations assume they are done looking once they find someone who interviews well within these parameters. The truth is that these parameters tell you very little about the ability of the individual to fit primary care behavioral health. However, they can be critical rule-out variables for organizations, so they are starting points for your search. Many organizations ask about terminal degrees that fit the primary care behavioral health model. You can't make solid assumptions based on degrees; these only establish the outer parameters, which should only be a starting point for your search. There are some generalities I have found to be helpful concerning degrees, and each has strong caveats, however.

1. Clinical psychologists (PsyD or Ph.D.) can have better initial credibility/buy-in from primary care clinicians; this has to do with three factors: a. the doctoral degree status brings some credibility; b. there is some affinity between the socialization experience of psychologists and physicians; c. compared to LCSWs, psychologists do not carry the baggage of "social work" in their title,

which to primary care clinicians often means case management. However, this initial credibility wears off quickly if the person is unhelpful. In other words, a social worker can build up this credibility over time, and a psychologist can lose it soon if they are a poor fit.

2. Clinical psychologists can be more prepared for program development. The training of a psychologist includes program evaluation and research experience (though to varying degrees and for varying situations); this can be particularly helpful for initial hires where program development is critical. However, some social workers have better program development experience and can have better innate skills in this area, depending on their work experience.

3. Clinical psychologists typically have broader experience in dealing with the full range of psychopathology and psychopharmacology. In other words, they may be better at discussing medications more comfortably with primary care clinicians and diagnosing a variety of patient presentations. Then again, there are social workers who, due to their years of experience, can trump some psychologists.

4. Clinical psychologists can have better medical experience, particularly health psychologists (a sub-field of clinical psychology); this means they have specific training in working with comorbid medical conditions such as diabetes. However, based on experience, some social workers might have more expertise if they have worked in a medical setting than a comparable psychologist.

5. Social workers tend to be more flexible than psychologists. Temperamentally, the field of social work draws candidates who are often more adaptable than psychologists. Psychology tends to attract and then train for specialization. The result is that psychologists can hold more strongly to their personal and professional space. In contrast, social workers who are used to adapting to different settings exhibit more willingness to be flexible. Of course, again, this varies wildly by person and training program.

6. Other master's trained mental health professionals, such as marriage and family therapists (LMFT) and licensed professional counselors (LPC) or licensed mental health professionals (LMHC), fall under the same pros and cons of social workers above. Experience can trump training, but training can be an edge. Since these professions are newer than social work or psychology, there tends to be more variability in skill level and fit between candidates with these other degrees. A popular terminal degree for BHCs are LMFTs due to their training in systems thinking and exposure to Medical Family Therapy. LMFT training also tends to be rigorous, especially compared to LPC, where there is more variability in quality. A critical factor in hiring non-psychologist or non-social work candidates is whether they are eligible for reimbursement from your clinic's primary payers. Fortunately, more major payers recognize a broader swath of license types making this less of an issue. Typically state Medicaid departments are the key holdouts, so make sure to obtain

confirmation related to which degree types they recognize.

So, in sum, I believe that a great-fit psychologist and a great-fit social worker will have equivalent effectiveness in the primary care setting clinically and programmatically. However, when searching for top candidates, I have found that the pool of candidates is typically consistently more robust on the psychologist side. In other words, let's assume we have ten psychologist candidates and ten social work candidates. My experience has been that the skills in the psychologist group are consistently better than those in the social work group (for primary care). However, one of those ten social workers may be better than all the psychologist candidates based on their skill and temperament. This should be obvious since the scope of practice for social workers is much greater than for psychologists, thus the increased variability of specific fit for primary care. Therefore, it is worth it to search for all types of mental health professionals while aware of the central skills and temperamental qualities you seek.

One other delimiting factor for many organizations is how much these degrees cost. Psychologists command higher salaries than all the other mental health disciplines (aside from psychiatry). For example, for primary care behavioral health jobs (in a low-end market), if a social worker might command $65,000, a psychologist would make around $80,000. We will discuss compensation more specifically later on in this chapter. An organization should pay for what it is getting or expecting. So, if you are expecting a CEO-type program developer who will build your program into something special, you need to set a salary to attract that kind of individual. I have seen many organizations ineffectively promote a robust job description for a BHC and not obtain candidates with the requisite skills because they need to pay more in salary. The adage applies here: "You get what you pay for"; this is true regardless of terminal degree.

Core Parameters Of The Ideal Candidate

The qualities that make an excellent behavioral health consultant are relatively easy to spot, though they are not especially easy to find in one individual. The main issue in hiring is divorcing oneself from the anxiety of hiring somebody. If you can tamp down this anxiety, you will more clearly see and assess the qualities you need in a behavioral health consultant. Generally, you are looking for an individual with three levels of skills: clinical, team-based, and program development. Undergirding these skills are temperamentally-related skills or attributes.

Clinical Skills

These skills are the baseline skills that define the ability of the hire to engage patients effectively across various concerns. Specific to primary care behavioral health, the behavioral health consultant should exhibit the ability to:

1. establish rapport quickly
2. think efficiently around diagnostic issues and yet adopt a more functional, recovery-based approach
3. cope with conflict well
4. have an excellent orientation to psychopharmacology (or be excited to learn)

5. work as a generalist - the ability to work with all primary care presentations
6. some exposure to medically-related issues

Team-Based Skills

These skills are the baseline skills a behavioral consultant exhibits when working in teams:

1. exhibit concern over others' workflow and roles
2. desire to be helpful and interactive
3. open, honest, frequent, and direct communication
4. fairly thick skin with a humble demeanor and not easily offended
5. confident in own abilities and yet collaborative in style

Program Development Skills

These are the skills that a hire should have, especially if they are a first hire, to help develop a program:

1. essential leadership skills, including mobilizing others with specific strategies such as delegation, planning, task creation, etc.
2. basic awareness of program development cycles
3. some awareness of the use of data
4. employee management skills
5. skilled computer utilization
6. problem-solving skills

Typically hires with a good combination of these attributes will have the temperamental qualities I list below, but better to be specific since temperament is vital. Character often trumps missing skills in my hiring practice because I assume I can always teach a skill but can't teach temperament.

1. Flexibility: this quality relates to the ability to work with different personalities and situations without demanding a great deal from those around them
2. Even-tempered: the ability to maintain a steady, consistent presence and affective state despite rapidly changing circumstances
3. Engaging: typically quiet, demure individuals do not thrive in a primary care environment
4. Socially skilled: the ability to communicate confidently with a variety of personality types and avoid unhelpful interpersonal entanglements
5. Passion: this kind of work requires commitment and excitement - lukewarm candidates do not do well

How To Find The Ideal Candidate

Now to the challenging part. Once you have a solid idea of who and what you are looking for, you must find them. There are no magic strategies for finding the right talent, but some methods have yielded better results.

Train your own: starting a training program is the most helpful strategy I have tried because it avoids retraining individuals upon hiring and allows for an extensive assessment of their skills. There are also many training programs looking for sites to train their students. Of course, this requires a first hire to make this happen; this is an excellent second step in program development activity for the first hire or program director.

Connect with others in the field and advertise via word of mouth: there are listserves, schools, and individuals you can connect with who can alert their networks about your job opening. Nothing is more helpful than working these networks and sensitizing them to precisely what you seek. This strategy usually requires multiple contacts and communication strategies. For example, the CFHA listserve is a common place for organizations to post their openings.

Advertising: The top job websites are typically good places to advertise, including the <u>Collaborative Family Healthcare Association</u>, Indeed.com, Monster.com, and others. When you advertise your organization, emphasize the specific traits you are looking for and the developmental aspect of the job to cue the right individual. Use terminology such as "excited individual," "leader for our clinic in behavioral health," "passion for population-based care," and other attributes which can help communicate what you are looking for. Do not assume that your human resource department is particularly adept at creating language for posts. Far too often, posts are regurgitations of job descriptions. Job posts are advertising pieces that should engage the relevant audience with inviting language, communicating a sense of mission and purpose, and clarifying the benefits of working in PCBH. Job posts should also always have salary ranges.

Here is sample language to include in a post:

> "Come work with one of the best healthcare employers in Chatham County, NC! This exciting opportunity to lead and develop a new integrated

care program is perfect for a self-starter behavioral health professional passionate about providing care to underserved populations while supporting our primary care mission. The optimal candidate will know of or be willing to learn the Primary Care Behavioral Health model, an exciting, fast-paced model of care. Want to grow your skills and challenge yourself? This position is an outstanding opportunity for the applicant who can demonstrate flexibility and a willingness to collaborate in real-time as part of the medical care team."

centered and may include different visit types (e.g., warm handoffs, curb side consult, individual, groups, co-visits) and different interventions (e.g., CBT, ACT, psychoeducation, self-management of chronic health conditions, care management) based on patient needs.

Essential Duties and Responsibilities:
1. Provide consultation and co-management of patient physical and behavioral health needs in collaboration with the interdisciplinary team and provide feedback to care team about patient encounters.
2. Provide brief, targeted, evidence-based interventions to help patients better manage their physical, behavioral and psychosocial risk factors and improve daily functioning.
3. Demonstrate practical application of a variety of therapeutic approaches tailored to individual patient needs.
4. Demonstrate cultural competency in serving diverse populations across the lifespan.
5. Actively engage providers and patients and maintain a visible presence for same day visits and curb side consults.
6. Adhere to clinical protocols (e.g., screening, assessment, patient volumes, outcomes measurement, referrals, follow-up)
7. Assist patients in identifying and engaging with out of clinic resources and/or a higher level of care as needed
8. Complete clinical documentation that is concise, accurate, timely and in compliance with all regulations and organizational requirements.
9. Other duties as assigned.

Competencies:
1. 1Treats people with respect, establishes and maintains good relationships, works with integrity and follows policies and procedures.
2. Communicates clearly, listens and asks for clarification, and diffuses difficult or emotional situations.
3. Demonstrates good clinical judgement, maintains clinical licensure and participates in professional development opportunities

Qualifications:
1. Master's degree or higher from an accredited college or university
2. Current independent license in STATE as Social Worker, Psychologist, Counselor or

This is the basic language in a BHC job description.

When you have identified some potential interviews, we have found that a shadowing experience is the most helpful way of gauging an individual's fit. Have them come to the clinic and shadow a primary care clinician, preferably one interested in behavioral health, or shadow an existing behavioral health consultant if there is one already. We then follow that with a sit-down interview and debrief, asking candidates about their impressions of the morning and areas they would find exciting or challenging.

I generally see whether the candidate is genuinely excited or thrown off by the pace and environment. I also look to see if they interact comfortably with staff and exhibit good relational skills. And finally, I look to see if they ask the right questions. Good candidates start brainstorming how they would work in the setting and will ask questions about how certain situations are handled and how flow is managed. If you get the sense that they can think along with the model as you explain it to them, you've got a potential keeper.

In the worst-case scenario, where your organization feels they need more confidence in selecting a candidate, look for help from another clinic that does and see if someone there would be willing to do some interviewing. I'm often surprised that clinics don't put resources behind getting help for hiring, considering the financial risk of making a bad hire. Let's say, for example, that you want to make an $80,000 purchase. Wouldn't it make sense to pay someone a few hundred dollars to ensure the purchase is good? Typically paying now means paying less later.

To this end, here are a few ways to ensure that your investment in a candidate selection process is a fruitful one:

Get technical assistance: Many individuals and organizations now offer consultation support. It is well worth the investment, especially when ready to hire. CFHA, for example, provides consultation services, including assistance with developing your job posts and job descriptions, and can even interview your candidates for you. I promise I'm not just selling CFHAs services here. There are plenty of options out there. The key is getting support so that you make a hire that will stick, especially for the first hire.

Set a competitive salary: I've made this mistake plenty of times. If you tend to be cheap, like me, you will lowball a salary, waste time in the hiring process, and miss out on candidates who will not even apply due to the posted salary. For help selecting an appropriate salary range, refer to CFHAs biannual salary survey. Other tools with larger data sets can be helpful, including sites like Indeed.com or Zippia.com. I recommend that sites use the upper regional pay ranges for behavioral health professionals, given that you are looking for a combination of skills and attributes at the top of the license for these professionals. Data from the CFHA survey bears this out.

Chapter 9: Nuts & Bolts Of Getting Started: Staff Development

By Neftali Serrano, PsyD

Once you have the talent in place, you have to treat that talent accordingly. Here we can learn a great deal from successful large corporations like Google, Apple, and the Dallas Mavericks. These corporations understand that their success hinges on the talent of the individuals they recruit. So they seek to hire the best and treat their employees as if they are the best in their respective businesses. Mark Cuban, the owner of the Mavericks, provides the best food and environment possible for his players, who in turn have demonstrated consistent performance and loyalty during his tenure. Google boasts on its webpage the following about the benefits they provide:

"The goal is to strip away everything that gets in our employees' way. We provide a standard package of fringe benefits. On top of that are first-class dining facilities, gyms, laundry rooms, massage rooms, haircuts, carwashes, dry cleaning, commuting buses - about anything a hardworking employee might want. Let's face it: programmers want to program; they don't want to do their laundry. So we make it easy for them to do both."

Old-school management gurus might consider such employee treatment a waste of money or effort and focus more on incentive-based or productivity-based motivational tools. But few could argue with the success these organizations have had. Apple, at the time of this writing, was the most valuable company in the world based on stock valuation - it got there because of the talent it hired and its high expectations of that talent. However, they have also worked diligently to keep that talent, as evidenced by the stability of its senior leadership team that has been kept primarily intact for years. Aside from good benefits, Apple's secret hinges on the solid creative mission of the organization. Apple keeps its staff invested in its mission by creating an environment where creativity and innovation flourish and where good ideas can rise to the top. The idea is that it would be hard to leave Apple because where else could you innovate as quickly and effectively in the industry?

Too often in healthcare, the mission of primary care clinics becomes so reductionistic (see as many patients as you can in a given day) that these organizations begin to burn their talent out and then lose that talent either physically or spiritually. By physically, I mean that the talent leaves. Spiritually, the talent loses their passion for the work and then underperforms. Organizations rarely account for spiritual loss when they take stock of their productivity, and it can be the most damaging loss. At least when a person leaves an organization, they can no longer affect the morale of others on the team. But a person who is spiritually dead concerning their vocation is a cancer that will impact many others. The best clinics understand how valuable their staff is and do not view them as widget-makers but as creative forces and leaders. And these clinics understand what Google gets: that your talent is people, and people have needs, desires, and dreams. If you can tap into these dreams with a strong sense of mission and purpose, and if you can remove barriers or address needs, then you will have that strong creative force to propel your organization and create a culture that sustains the organization for many years.

So, a clinic or manager's underlying approach must focus on enabling your talent to achieve their best. Productivity should not be the focus; it should be a side-effect of employees' freedom to perform excellently. I've often reminded myself that if a staff member is underperforming, it is either because I have failed to remove an obstacle, present the proper challenge to the individual, or select the wrong person for the job. The answer is never that the person is lazy and needs me to set a productivity goal and consequences if they do not achieve that goal. Sometimes a precursor to this is an organizational review of priorities. In other words, to treat employees well, you must have a clear mission and set of goals into which you bring your talent. Many organizations need more clear priorities or clear missions.

So let's get to some specifics on how to treat your behavioral health consultants.

1. **Create a sense of mission and purpose on your team that ties into the individual staff's roles**. The Access team has a strong sense of mission towards the underserved and population-based care and to serving their primary care clinicians. Everything Access does serves the end of providing greater access and timely services to their patients and innovating wherever they can to enhance their reach into the clinic population while supporting their primary care clinicians. All staff buys into this; culturally, these facets are so ingrained that an employee would feel relatively isolated if they did not. Beyond this, when I hired each individual, I considered the individual's particular role or leadership area that they could take ownership of within this larger mission (more on this in the next chapter); this ties them into a place of ownership, and within this, they have great freedom to innovate – for example, to develop a well-child protocol or an addictions clinic strategy. However, at the same time, the mission and focus of the team provide boundaries so that we never lose focus of the core of our work: consultation with providers and accessibility to all comers. So, a necessary skill in this vein is to be a good evaluator of talents and abilities; this entails getting to know your talent and then sitting down with them and providing leadership responsibilities in areas that fit their best skill set.

2. **Communicate frequently and creatively.** I'm not a big fan of meetings, so I created a series of communication strategies to stay in touch with my staff. These include online video conferencing, monthly training seminars, individual meetings every three weeks, texting, group email, regular email, shared documents, to-do apps, and more. The point is that

staying in touch is essential. If I feel like I don't have the pulse for what turns my staff on and keeps them excited, then I don't feel like we have something sustainable. What I have learned to pay attention to within this communication as well is the reality that people change over time, and their interests and foci change. When staff has children, their focus will vary, so you must accommodate these life changes while keeping them engaged. You can work with these life changes if you respect your talent enough. Of course, without communication, you won't be able to adapt along with your staff.

3. **Identify barriers and troubleshoot collaboratively.** This involves trusting your talent. If you don't trust your talent to perform well given the right circumstances, the problem is yours, not theirs. You selected the wrong staff. So, if you feel like you chose the right team, trust them. If they are underperforming, then troubleshoot collaboratively. Think of anything that gets in the way, and work to remove those barriers to whatever degree possible. I worked hard over the years to reduce paperwork and unnecessary documentation. I also made sure to monitor fatigue and burnout in my staff. These barriers keep talent from doing what they do best: interacting with primary care clinicians and helping patients in exam rooms. I try to limit anything else that gets in the way of these fundamental activities.

4. **Understand that there will be variations in productivity.** Some staff are workhorses and will be much more efficient than other staff. What you want is to have each staff achieve their best. Once you identify their ceiling, don't push them to do what others are doing - instead, identify challenges in other areas that

they are best at that can serve the overall mission; this goes back to their leadership responsibilities.

5. **Set high expectations in essential areas, and don't sweat the small stuff, primarily by example.** A good leader mostly leads through modeling. Access has high expectations as a team regarding how well they treat their patients and primary care clinicians. They take it personally if they have a slow day in clinic, not because someone is forcing them to meet a number, but because they feel responsible to their primary care clinicians. They also have a healthy sense of competition and will often see how others on the team are performing and want to keep pace.

6. **Be honest and transparent, but be mindful of what and how you communicate.** Staff needs to connect to their leader personally; this requires you to be yourself. However, good boundaries help retain the roles and respect between team members; this is especially true at the outset of a program where you are trying to establish norms for your team. It is also essential over time to communicate what needs to be shared with your team without allowing communication to be distracting. For example, there were times when decisions regarding our clinic were in progress at higher administrative levels. I waited to communicate specifics around the communications until the leadership team decided. Why distract the team?; this also avoids gossip or undue speculation.

7. **How you communicate is also important.** It is shocking how some leaders use the wrong venue to communicate. An email is not a good communication tool for handling conflict. A face-to-face meeting is better for that. There may be better venues than an

informational team meeting to brainstorm ideas for program development. A shared document or group email would be better at the outset. You need to be mindful of the tool you are using to communicate just as much as the actual communication. One final tidbit: if you feel upset or emotionally agitated while writing an email, write it, save it, and come back to it in a day or so and see if it still makes sense to send it.

Pay Well

You get what you pay for. If you seek to underpay, you will attract talent commensurate with that pay, or you will lose good talent with better opportunities elsewhere. Staff should be considered a long-term investment, not a short-term commodity. We discussed salary in a previous chapter, but some additional direction here is appropriate. The following factors should influence your assessment of the value of a behavioral health consultant:

1. The role requirements of a behavioral health consultant are pretty expansive. A behavioral health consultant must have a generalist knowledge of every mental health condition and a working understanding of medically-related comorbid behavioral health issues.

2. The behavioral health consultant is responsible for seeing a higher volume of patients than a specialist would and engaging in a proportionally greater number of overall tasks (e.g., management of triaged messages from nurses for extra-office patient concerns, managing consulting psychiatry relationships, assisting PCPs with relevant patient paperwork).

3. The behavioral health consultant often has leadership roles. Every behavioral health consultant has a significant role within the specific care team and is responsible to their patients and teammates. Often the behavioral health consultant has other leadership roles in the clinic, such as helping the clinic develop patient management strategies for suicidal patients and working on other quality improvement protocols.

These factors, which also exist in other medical settings, are why psychologists and social workers who work in those settings tend to have higher salaries. In the same way, a suitably paid workforce in primary care will reflect this trend. It is a very complex thing to do to establish wages for a nation as large as the United States since factors as varied as setting, geography, and market forces (supply, demand) vary wildly, however here we hope to set a baseline from which you can make specific judgments. Of course, using the aforementioned CFHA salary tool is also essential.

A good general rule of thumb is to ascertain the local market salary trends specific to degree status (e.g., LPC, LCSW, PsyD, Ph.D.) and then set a baseline salary between $5,000 - $20,000 above the median. The broad salary range here is that you must consider various factors, including what you are hoping from the person you are hiring and aspects related to how difficult hiring is in your community (supply/ demand). If you expect someone to fill a director role, for example, that will require a more expansive skill set than someone who will be primarily a clinician (remember, your first hire is almost always your director by default). If your market is not well saturated with mental health professionals, a higher salary may be necessary to inspire someone to move to your area.

As an example, assuming a midwest market at the time of this writing, if we were to hire an LCSW in the first five years of professional licensed practice to an existing group of behavioral health consultants where a good deal of the program development was already well developed, we would identify a salary range of $65,000 to $80,000 (not including benefits).

A clinical psychologist (Ph.D./PsyD) in the same situation would command a salary between $75,000 and $90,000. The salary difference between LCSW and psychologists is justified simply by supply/demand factors (fewer psychologists) and the relatively more expansive training psychologists receive, particularly in psychopharmacology, psychopathology, and behavioral medicine. Additionally, psychologists often have program development skills as part of their repertoire; if you find a superstar LCSW (I know several) who is a great fit and has an expanded skill set by virtue of training or experience, then pay them accordingly. The issue should be the person's value to your organization, not the degree.

To add to the scenarios, let's assume you are adding the above individuals to your new primary care behavioral health program, which will require a director-level type individual. In that case, you want to start with a higher salary within those ranges to ensure you attract the highest quality candidates. If you add someone with more than five years of experience, you will likely need to pay more than the salary ranges described. For a psychologist, $80,000 to $100,000, and for an LCSW, $70,000 to $90,000.

These are at least some starting points for determining salary. The point is, particularly at the outset, you don't want to skimp on pay when it could cost you more later on. The value of your hires to your organization is much greater at the outset of program development, and as such good upfront investment is protective. Once you have a well-developed program, you can be more conservative, if needed, regarding how you hire and add to your team. For example, at Access, LCSW and other master's level clinicians are more likely future hires because the program development needs are well cared for by their team of psychologists. So they will expect slightly less from their prospective behavioral health consultants than they did from their first batch. This approach mirrors the 'mid-level' approach in medicine, where physician assistants work in teams with doctoral-level practitioners; this should not imply a lesser or demeaned status - it simply relates to the phase of development of your program.

Ultimately what you pay staff in any business has a relationship with what your business can sustain financially. The take-home point here is that if you expect the kinds of results we are discussing in this text, you have to have the talent to make that happen - and skill requires adequate payment; this is especially true as you make your first hires, who are the most talented individuals you are likely to need. That said, salary is just one component of hiring and retaining staff, and job design is the other. Let's turn our attention there.

Making Primary Care An Attractive Place To Work

Primary care is a fantastic place to work for the right person. Unfortunately, primary care clinics can also quickly burn out their providers. Primary care clinicians are famously overworked and stressed by the tasks they are expected to accomplish. The primary care behavioral health model is a critical way to improve clinician satisfaction with their work. Let's consider that primary care clinicians and behavioral health consultants are valuable assets. It behooves us to design their jobs and work environment so that they enjoy their work and remain productive.

The most important aspect of a job design is how staff are engaged. If you choose a behavioral health consultant, it should be because you believe that an individual possesses the core temperament and skills we discuss in this text and because you think that person has a commitment to primary care, and because you see innate talents that person has that match needs in your program. A well-developed organization will seek to nurture those skills and talents and provide opportunities for that development.

One of the ways that can occur in primary care is the creation of leadership roles and the provision of administrative time. Administrative time is the wrong word to use for what we are discussing here because it encompasses a variety of functions. The staff is given a day per week of administrative time for the Access team, but this is more than just time for paperwork. This time is used for program development activities such as writing, meetings, and planning. It is also used for clinic leadership activities such as working with other teams to manage complex patients and connecting with external agencies to create seamless patient transitions to specialty care services. It is also used for flex time, a valuable commodity for the modern worker. This flex time is used to manage home life with work life so that childcare responsibilities and appointments can be flexed with work responsibilities. It is a recognition that only some of our work must occur between 9 AM and 5 PM. Another function of this time is simply time away from clinical activity, which can be strenuous in the primary care behavioral health model. This strain is also why primary care clinicians often do not work 5-day weeks, either by design or by choice. Finally, this time also serves as a catch-up time for charting and other patient care activities. Staff can work from home during this flex time, a bonus. Some clinics are also designing work-from-home clinical work roles to allow staff to see patients from home for a portion of their FTE.

Ask our staff; this time is invaluable to making the model work. It has been my experience that clinics that expect their behavioral health consultants (or primary care clinicians, for that matter) to work 5-day clinical weeks reach a point of diminishing returns with productivity. Behavioral health consultants in these clinics see fewer patients and are more strained. Behavioral health consultants in these situations will naturally find ways, some conscious and some unconscious, to avoid seeing more patients out of a desire for self-preservation. No amount of incentivizing or threats can overcome that desire. I would rather have fresh, energetic, and engaged behavioral health consultants who work fewer hours than tired, stressed behavioral health consultants who work more. The former are the ones who will keep the reputation of the program intact with primary care staff who depend on them.

Some clinics may not have the luxury of providing this much administrative time. In that case, consider paying a behavioral health consultant for a 4-day work week and building your program that way. We should be mindful of learning the lessons of the rest of the primary care world, which needs to do better in caring for primary care clinicians. Although a different industry, CFHA staff operate on a 4-day work week and have replicated findings in various sectors showing <u>productivity and well-being advantages</u>.

Remote work was accelerated during the coronavirus pandemic and remains a portion of what BHCs do. Providing part-time remote work can be an attractive part of a job design. However, PCBH work requires in-person teams, so we do not recommend full-time remote PCBH. Remote work can be leveraged when clinics need extra coverage or when a group of remote clinics needs coverage, but resources are not available to staff them individually.

We will discuss the creation of leadership roles in the next section. For now, we recommend that engaging your staff's innate talent and desires is vital to building a successful program. People are designed to flourish, so job designs should consider this. Access strongly focuses on its core model but also allows for and encourages experimentation and creative approaches to solving problems. Staff can use their skills and interests in public speaking, program management, data analysis, writing, multicultural issues, training, etc., as long as they maintain a population-based focus.

Finally, the other characteristic of a job that can make it attractive for staff is room for personal and professional growth. Too often, in our desire to build a program, we forget that people are always in development and going through different phases of their lives. A place of employment that recognizes this and accounts for the impact of this is going to be a place that retains staff effectively.

Access encourages their behavioral health consultant moms to communicate how they feel they will best deal with maternity leave and flexibly manage their re-entry into the workplace. They encourage their behavioral health consultant parents to openly and honestly care for their sick children without apologizing for their personal needs. And they discuss their career desires and goals with leadership, even when some of those desires will not be met within the organization.

The point is people are in development. One of the issues we will likely need to face as a profession is what happens with behavioral health consultants when they grow older. Will older behavioral health consultants sustain the pace of primary care? Will more senior behavioral health consultants be perpetually fulfilled working in primary care? Where is the career growth path for a maturing behavioral health consultant? We need to be attentive to this reality and create a profession that can meet talented people where they are, with the expectation that when we do so, they will produce efficiently over the long term for our organizations. If these strategies are good enough for Fortune 500 companies, they should be good enough for primary care.

Chapter 10: Inclusivity From The Start

By Martha Saucedo, LCSW

As an immigrant from Monterrey, Mexico, I brought with me a degree in counseling psychology and a wealth of experience in providing traditional therapy. My transition to the United States, however, meant starting anew. In Mexico, I was already recognized and established in my field, but in the U.S., I found myself back in the classroom, striving to align my qualifications with the American system. This phase was not just about academic adaptation; it was a profound cultural and professional reset, which included adapting to a work system vastly different from what I was accustomed to, where advocating for oneself was not just beneficial, but essential – a skill I continue to work on. In this new landscape, I was acutely aware of being one of the few students of color, navigating an educational and professional world that was starkly different from what I had known.

What struck me most profoundly in the U.S. was the concept of microaggressions - a term and experience unfamiliar to me in Mexico. Suddenly, I was encountering subtle, often unintentional, expressions of bias that I hadn't faced before. Despite my naturally positive outlook on life and belief in the goodness of people, these microaggressions began to erode my spirit over time. They not only challenged my professional identity but also my integrity as an immigrant. Balancing my aspirations with the exhausting reality of constantly being 'different' was a relentless test of resilience. Advocating for myself, whether it was for recognition, fair pay, promotion, or simply to feel valued and respected in my workplace, became a routine necessity, further highlighting the challenges of navigating a system that at times didn't fully recognize my worth.

These experiences of feeling marginalized and undervalued were what propelled me into action. The journey, fraught with challenges, became my catalyst for change. It drove me to learn more, seek support, and courageously step out of my comfort zone. This path wasn't just about professional development; it was a journey towards reclaiming my self-worth and integrity. I learned that my 'difference' was not a detriment but a distinct advantage. This realization led me to where I stand today - an advocate for the empowerment and sponsorship of women of color in healthcare. My story is one of transformation, resilience, patience, and the relentless pursuit of equality and recognition in a world that often overlooks the unique strengths brought by diversity.

As a team leader, your ability to recognize and support talented individuals, regardless of their background, is a crucial element in building a successful team. Most of you have not likely received any formal training in leading teams or addressing diversity issues on your teams; this is a key deficit in healthcare leadership which we hope to address in this section. Our focus here will be women of color, but many of the lessons of the chapter apply to staff members from different backgrounds. Addressing the needs of women is particularly important because statistically women dominate the mental health workforce and women of color face additional unique challenges in the workplace due to a variety of systemic barriers such as bias, discrimination, and microaggressions. By creating an inclusive work environment that values and supports diversity, you can attract and retain top talent, improve employee morale and engagement, and ultimately boost productivity and profitability.

Taking action on this information is essential, as failing to do so can lead to missed opportunities to cultivate a diverse and inclusive workplace, limit your organization's growth and potential, and even contribute to a negative work environment that can impact your team's morale and productivity. Therefore, as a leader, it is your responsibility to leverage your power and position to create a workplace that values and supports all individuals, including women of color, and contributes to a more equitable and just society.

Notice that we are advocating that leaders of PCBH programs take an active role in developing their staff and in supporting their women/ people of color. It is not enough to claim to have an unbiased work environment. We propose that you aim to create a pro-diversity environment.

Women of color encounter unique obstacles in the workplace due to discrimination and bias. These challenges range from subtle microaggressions to overt prejudice, which can have a significant impact on their personal and professional lives. Women of color may struggle to gain recognition for their accomplishments, receive equal pay, and advance into leadership positions. They may also feel excluded, marginalized, and powerless, which can impede their ability to thrive in the workplace. Despite these challenges, women of color make valuable contributions to their fields and communities, demonstrating resilience and perseverance in the face of adversity. It is important for organizations, especially their leaders, to recognize and tackle these challenges. They should work towards establishing a workplace that is fair and inclusive for all employees. Let us explore these issues and navigate through the most common challenges, as well as examine possible solutions.

Microaggressions In The Workplace

Microaggressions are subtle, often unintentional, forms of discrimination that can make women of color feel marginalized and disrespected in the workplace. It is important to understand that microaggressions are often unintentional and unconscious elements in our communication and that awareness, not perfection, is the goal. Here are some examples of microaggressions that women of color may encounter:

CHALLENGE:
Women of color can be type-cast for their cultural skills and not seen for the totality of their skill set. For example, they

can be told that they are "articulate" or "well-spoken" for their race; this comment suggests that the speaker has low expectations for women of color's communication skills and reinforces harmful stereotypes. Latina and Asian women are often asked where they are "really" from: This question implies that the person does not belong in the United States and can be a way of othering and exoticizing women of color.

Moreover, women of color in the workplace who are bilingual may face additional challenges, such as being asked to interpret or translate materials for their colleagues or clients. While this may seem like a minor request, it can be a burden on these women, as it takes away from their main work responsibilities. Additionally, staff members may not have the same level of language proficiency as trained interpreters, and may feel undue pressure to perform the function. This perpetuates existing disparities in the workplace as these staff have less time and energy to devote to their other job duties, impeding their career growth and limiting their opportunities for advancement.

Being the only bilingual or person of color in a workplace can also lead to feelings of tokenism or being viewed solely through the lens of their linguistic or cultural abilities rather than their full range of skills and expertise. A typical example is the lone African-American woman fielding constant requests to lead diversity initiatives. Being a Black woman does not by default indicate an interest or proclivity to leading diversity initiatives.

SOLUTION:

Overall, healthcare organizations and other institutions must prioritize the use of qualified interpreters and respect the linguistic and cultural needs of patients. Women of color have the right to advocate for themselves and demand that their workplace provides appropriate resources to ensure that patients receive high-quality care. Per CLAS (Culturally and Linguistically Appropriate Services) standards, it is the responsibility of healthcare facilities and other organizations to ensure that they have qualified interpreters available to assist patients who have limited English proficiency. This is critical to ensuring that patients receive high-quality care and can fully understand their health conditions, treatment options, and medical procedures. It is also important to ensure that all staff members are aware of the importance of using qualified interpreters and the potential consequences of using untrained individuals for interpreting roles.

The best way to ensure that microaggressions do not permeate your team communication is to simply ask the women of color on your team how they feel about the communication on the team and the ways their skills are being utilized as team members. The good news is that this line of questioning is helpful for all of your other staff as well. Everyone wants to feel like they are seen for who they are and have their skills respected in the workplace. Conversations in 1-1 settings and team meetings around the issue of microaggressions can set a tone that allows unspoken concerns from festering into resentments.

When working on diversity, equity, and inclusion (DEI) initiatives ensure that the opportunity to work on the project is not solely directed to the women of color on your team nor that there is an unspoken expectation that they will lead the initiatives. Allow staff to self-select for these opportunities.

CHALLENGE:
Appearance-based microaggressions can be particularly damaging to women of color in the workplace. These microaggressions may take the form of comments or judgments about their hair, makeup, or clothing, which can make them feel like they don't belong in the workplace. These microaggressions can impact their job performance, as they may feel anxious or uncomfortable in their work environment.

Moreover, these microaggressions can have long-lasting effects on their mental and emotional well-being. Women of color may feel like they are constantly being judged or evaluated based on their appearance rather than their skills or accomplishments. This can lead to feelings of inadequacy, low self-esteem, and even depression.

Furthermore, the expectation that women of color should represent their entire race or provide insights into issues that affect their racial group can also be a form of microaggression. This expectation places undue pressure on women of color to conform to stereotypes and limits their ability to express their unique ideas and viewpoints. It can be overwhelming and unfair to expect women of color to be spokespersons for their entire racial group, especially when their experiences and perspectives may be vastly different from others in their group.

SOLUTION:

A solution is to implement policies and guidelines that explicitly prohibit appearance-based discrimination and harassment in the workplace. This can be done through the development and enforcement of anti-discrimination policies, including specific language that addresses appearance-based microaggressions. Companies can also create reporting mechanisms that allow employees to report incidents of discrimination or harassment, as well as a system for investigating and addressing those reports.

Encouraging diverse perspectives is essential in creating an inclusive workplace. Women of color should not be expected to be the sole representative of their racial group or to have all the answers to issues that affect their racial group. Instead, colleagues should be encouraged to share their own experiences and perspectives on issues.

This can be achieved through various strategies, such as creating safe spaces for open dialogue and discussion, encouraging participation in diversity and inclusion training programs, and promoting the importance of diversity and inclusion throughout the organization.

In addition, leaders can actively seek out and engage with individuals from diverse backgrounds to ensure that a range of perspectives are represented in decision-making processes. This can include recruiting and promoting diverse candidates for leadership positions, seeking input from diverse employee resource groups, and creating opportunities for cross-functional collaboration and teamwork.

CHALLENGE:

Women of color often face the challenge of being excluded from networking opportunities, which can hinder their professional growth and success. They may feel left out of social events or professional development opportunities, which are critical for building relationships and gaining visibility in the workplace. The exclusion from networking opportunities can have long-term impacts on their ability to advance in their careers, as they may miss out on important information or connections that could help them achieve their goals.

Women of color may experience exclusion from leadership opportunities within their organizations. They may not be given the chance to lead important projects or teams, and their viewpoints may not be taken into account. This lack of representation and recognition can make women of color feel undervalued and marginalized. The lack of opportunities and support for professional development can also make it difficult for women of color to gain the skills and experience necessary for advancement in their careers.

These microaggressions can be subtle and difficult to recognize, which can make it challenging for women of color to address them. Over time, they can erode a woman's self-confidence and trust in the agency, leading to disengagement, decreased job satisfaction, and, ultimately, a higher risk of turnover.

SOLUTION:
To address the lack of representation of women of color in the workplace, it is important to recognize and appreciate their strengths and contributions. Employers can

intentionally seek out opportunities to showcase the talents and achievements of women of color by highlighting their accomplishments in team meetings, company-wide announcements, and internal publications. This can help raise awareness of the valuable role that women of color play in the organization and can help combat any implicit bias or stereotypes that may exist.

Moreover, companies can also take concrete steps to provide more leadership opportunities for women of color. This can include creating mentorship and sponsorship programs that match women of color with more senior colleagues who can provide guidance and support as they navigate their careers. It is also important to ensure that women of color are included in discussions about strategy, planning, and decision-making and that they are allowed to lead projects and initiatives.

Sponsorship is another important way to support women of color in the workplace. Sponsors are typically senior-level colleagues who advocate for and promote the careers of their protégés. Sponsors can help women of color navigate the organization, connect with influential colleagues, and gain exposure to new opportunities. They can also provide guidance and advice on how to overcome obstacles and challenges that may arise. We will explore this role in more depth in a later section of this chapter.

Ultimately, creating a workplace culture that values diversity, equity, and inclusion is essential to supporting women of color in the workplace. Employers can create this culture by ensuring that all employees are held accountable for their actions, that there are clear policies and procedures in place to address bias and discrimination, and that there is ongoing education and training on these issues.

Lack Of Representation In The Workplace

CHALLENGE:
Women of color may experience a lack of representation in their workplace, as they may be the only person of color in their team or department. This can lead to a feeling of isolation and a lack of community within the workplace. Additionally, women of color may feel that their perspectives and experiences are not valued or acknowledged, as their colleagues and managers may not have an understanding of their cultural background and experiences.

Moreover, women of color may also experience a lack of support from management and colleagues. For example, they may not have access to mentors or sponsors who can provide guidance and support in their career development. This can make it difficult for them to navigate the workplace and identify opportunities for growth and advancement. They may also face difficulty in receiving constructive feedback that helps them to improve their performance, as feedback may be influenced by unconscious biases or stereotypes.

Furthermore, women of color may also experience workplace discrimination, such as being passed over for promotions or being subjected to hostile work environments. Discrimination can take many forms, including microaggressions, harassment, and biased hiring and promotion practices. This can create a toxic work environment that can negatively impact a woman's mental health, job satisfaction, and overall well-being.

Overall, the lack of representation and support, coupled with workplace discrimination, can make it difficult for women of color to thrive in their careers and reach their full potential.

Women of color may also face disparities in salary, promotion, and leadership positions that can further hinder their career growth and success. Studies have shown that <u>women of color earn less than their white male and female counterparts</u>, even when controlling for factors such as education, years of experience, and job type. This wage gap can result in long-term financial insecurity and instability, making it harder for women of color to plan for their future and provide for their families.

Furthermore, women of color may have limited access to opportunities for advancement and leadership positions, which can make it difficult for them to reach their full potential and contribute to their organizations in meaningful ways. This can be due to bias in hiring and promotion processes, as well as a lack of role models and mentors who can provide guidance and support.

SOLUTION:
Organizations and leaders need to recognize and address the systemic barriers that may be preventing women of color from advancing in their careers. For instance, organizations may need to address pay equity issues, provide flexible work arrangements, and offer training and

development opportunities that are tailored to the needs and experiences of women of color. These efforts can help to create a more supportive and empowering work environment for women of color, which can, in turn, lead to better job satisfaction, retention, and overall organizational success.

Another important aspect is to create a culture of allyship, where colleagues and managers actively support and advocate for their women of color colleagues. This can involve educating oneself on the unique challenges that women of color face in the workplace and taking steps to address these challenges, such as calling out microaggressions, actively seeking out opportunities for women of color to lead and contribute, and amplifying their voices and ideas. By working together and creating a sense of community and support, organizations can help to ensure that women of color have the opportunity to thrive and reach their full potential in the workplace.

Employers should focus on regular pay equity audits to identify and address any disparities in pay, as well as implement clear and transparent promotion criteria. Providing leadership training and mentorship opportunities specifically for women of color is also encouraged. Employers can work towards creating a culture that values diversity and inclusion by fostering a welcoming and supportive environment for all employees. Actively seeking out diverse candidates for leadership positions and promoting them based on their qualifications and skills can also contribute to a more equitable workplace.

Additionally, employers need to recognize that addressing these issues requires a sustained effort over time rather than a one-time solution. It is important to regularly monitor progress and make adjustments as needed, as well as continue to educate and train all employees on the importance of diversity, equity, and inclusion in the workplace.

Mentoring Versus Sponsoring A Woman Of Color

Mentoring and sponsoring a woman of color is important for several reasons. First, it helps to address the lack of representation and advancement opportunities that women of color often face in the workplace. By providing guidance, support, and advocacy, mentors and sponsors can help women of color to navigate organizational politics, develop critical skills, and build professional networks that can lead to career advancement.

Second, mentoring and sponsoring women of color can also help to create a more inclusive and diverse workplace culture. By actively promoting and supporting women of color, organizations can send a message that they value diversity and are committed to creating a more equitable workplace for all employees.

Finally, mentoring and sponsoring women of color can have positive benefits for the mentor or sponsor as well. It can help to develop their leadership skills and increase their awareness and understanding of diversity and inclusion issues. It can also provide a sense of personal fulfillment by helping to support and empower someone else to reach their full potential. Let's define the difference between these two important concepts:

Mentorship

Mentoring a woman of color means providing guidance, support, and advice to help her navigate her career and achieve her professional goals. A mentor can offer insights into the industry, share their own experiences and lessons learned, and help the woman of color develop her skills and abilities. They can also offer emotional support, build confidence, and provide constructive feedback. The goal of mentoring is to help women of color grow both personally and professionally and to support them in achieving success in their careers.

To successfully encourage open communication, it is essential to create a safe and welcoming space where women of color feel comfortable expressing their opinions and concerns. Employers can achieve this by actively listening to women of color's feedback and taking steps to address any issues they raise. In addition, providing regular opportunities for women of color to share their experiences, such as through focus groups or surveys, can demonstrate a commitment to creating a workplace that values diverse perspectives. Employers should also be prepared to take action based on the feedback they receive, demonstrating that they are committed to making meaningful changes to improve the experiences of women of color in the workplace.

As a mentor, your role is to provide guidance and advice on career development, professional goals, and strategies for overcoming obstacles faced by women of color. You can accomplish this by sharing your own experiences and insights, as well as providing resources and support. It's important to listen actively and offer constructive feedback while also encouraging your mentee to take ownership of their career path. Additionally, you can help your mentee to develop and refine their skills through training and development opportunities and provide introductions to key contacts in your professional network. Ultimately, your goal as a mentor is to support the growth and success of the women of color you are working with.

Mentors play a crucial role in helping women of color develop new skills and take on new challenges to advance in their careers. By recommending relevant training programs and encouraging them to pursue new opportunities, mentors can help women of color gain valuable experience and expand their skill sets. Providing regular feedback and support can also be helpful as they navigate new roles and responsibilities. By empowering women of color to step outside of their comfort zones and take on new challenges, mentors can help them build confidence and grow professionally.

One way to further support women of color in the workplace is by creating affinity groups or employee resource groups (ERGs) that focus on supporting the unique experiences of women of color. These groups can provide a safe and inclusive space for women of color to connect with and support one another, share resources and strategies for success, and advocate for their needs and concerns within the organization. Employers can also allocate resources and funding to support these groups and their initiatives and ensure that they have a voice in decision-making processes within the company. By creating a sense of community and providing opportunities for advocacy and support, employers can help women of color feel valued and empowered in the workplace.

Benefits of Mentoring Women of Color in the Workplace

By investing in the growth and development of a woman of color, you are not only empowering her to achieve her full potential but also actively promoting diversity and inclusivity in your workplace. When underrepresented groups are given opportunities to succeed, the entire organization benefits from the unique perspectives and experiences they bring to the table. This investment can also have ripple effects beyond your immediate workplace, as the mentee may go on to become a role model and mentor to others in their career paths. As a result, you have the potential to create a positive cycle of change that can transform not just your workplace but also your industry and community as a whole. Your investment in a woman of color is an investment in a brighter, more inclusive future for all.

In addition to the benefits that mentoring can provide to the mentee, it can also be a highly rewarding experience for the mentor. By working closely with someone from a different background or culture, you have the opportunity to broaden your understanding of the world and gain new perspectives on important issues. Your mentee's unique experiences and insights can challenge your assumptions and help you see things in a new light, which can ultimately make you a more effective collaborator and leader.

As a mentor, you may also have the chance to learn new skills or gain fresh insights into your industry or field of work. This can be especially valuable if your mentee comes from a different background or has expertise in a different area than you do. By sharing your knowledge and expertise with your mentee, you may also be opening yourself up to new learning opportunities that can help you grow both personally and professionally.

Ultimately, mentoring is a two-way street, with both mentor and mentee benefiting from the relationship. By investing in someone else's growth and development, you can also enrich your own life and contribute to a more diverse and inclusive community.

In addition to the personal rewards of mentoring, being a mentor for a woman of color can also have positive ripple effects on your workplace and industry. By investing in the growth and development of underrepresented groups, you are helping to promote diversity and inclusivity, which can lead to a more innovative and dynamic workplace. This can, in turn, benefit your organization by attracting and retaining a diverse talent pool and enhancing its reputation as an inclusive and socially responsible employer. Nothing will help you attract more talent from under-represented groups than having an energized and diverse staff.

Sponsorship

Sponsoring someone at work means using your influence and credibility to advocate for and support someone's career advancement within an organization. A sponsor is typically someone more senior and experienced than the person being sponsored and who is willing to use their position of power to help their sponsored candidate succeed.

Sponsorship involves more than just mentorship or coaching; it involves actively promoting the sponsored candidate for high-profile projects or assignments, recommending them for leadership roles, and advocating for their promotion. A sponsor also provides guidance and support to their sponsored candidate as they navigate their career path, offering advice on career development, providing feedback on their performance, or connecting them with key stakeholders and influencers within the organization.

Sponsoring a woman of color in the workplace can be a powerful way to promote diversity and inclusivity while also helping your organization attract and retain top talent. Here are some tips on how to effectively sponsor a woman of color in the workplace:

Identify potential sponsorship candidates

When you are looking for talented women of color within your organization to sponsor, it is important to consider a range of factors that can help you identify those with the potential to advance to higher levels of leadership. Some of the key factors to consider include:

1. Skills: Look for women of color who have demonstrated strong skills and abilities in their current roles, as well as in any previous positions they have held. Consider the specific skills that are needed for higher levels of leadership within your organization, and identify women of color who have demonstrated these skills in their work.

2. Experience: Consider the breadth and depth of experience that your potential sponsorship candidates have, both within your organization and in their careers more broadly. Look for women of color who have taken on challenging assignments, demonstrated the ability to learn quickly, and have a track record of success in their work.

3. Potential: Assess your potential sponsorship candidates' potential for growth and development within your organization. Consider their career aspirations, their willingness to learn and take on new challenges, and their ability to adapt to change.

4. Commitment to organization's values and goals: Look for women of color who share your organization's values and goals and who are committed to advancing its mission. Consider their alignment with your organization's culture and vision, and identify those who are likely to thrive in its unique environment.

Build A Relationship

Building a strong relationship based on trust and mutual respect is a critical first step in sponsoring someone. It is important to take the time to get to know your potential sponsorship candidate, learn about their career goals and aspirations, and offer your support and guidance as needed. To do this effectively, here are some points to consider:

1. Get to know them: Take the time to learn about your potential sponsorship candidate's background, experience, and career aspirations. Ask about their interests, hobbies, and personal goals as well. This can help you build a more meaningful connection with them and better understand their motivations and aspirations.

2. Offer support: Be available to offer support and guidance as needed. This can involve providing feedback on their work, sharing their own experiences, and offering advice on how to navigate challenges in the workplace. Show your sponsorship candidate that you are invested in their success and willing to help them achieve their career goals.

3. Be honest and transparent: Build trust with your potential sponsorship candidate by being honest and transparent about your own experiences and career journey. Share your successes and failures, and offer insights into how you overcame challenges along the way. This can help your sponsorship candidate feel more comfortable opening up to you and seeking your guidance.

4. Listen actively: Practice active listening when talking to your potential sponsorship candidate. This involves

focusing on what they are saying, asking clarifying questions, and reflecting on what you heard to ensure that you understand their perspective. This can help you build stronger relationships with your sponsorship candidates and better understand their needs and goals.

Advocate For Them

1. After establishing a strong relationship with your potential sponsorship candidate, it is important to use your influence and credibility to advocate for them. Advocating for your sponsorship candidate can help create new opportunities for them and help them gain visibility within your organization. Here are some ways to advocate for your sponsorship candidate:

2. Nominating for high-profile projects or assignments: Consider nominating your sponsorship candidate for high-profile projects or assignments that will help them gain exposure to senior leaders in your organization. This can help them build relationships and demonstrate their skills and potential to a wider audience.

3. Recommending for leadership roles: If there are leadership roles available, recommend your sponsorship candidate for consideration. This can be a valuable opportunity for them to take on new challenges and responsibilities and develop new skills.

4. Advocating for their promotion: If your sponsorship candidate is eligible for promotion, advocate for them by highlighting their achievements, skills, and potential to decision-makers. This can help ensure that they are

fairly considered for new roles and opportunities within your organization.

5. Introducing to key stakeholders: Introduce your sponsorship candidate to key stakeholders within your organization, including senior leaders and decision-makers. This can help them build relationships and gain exposure to people who can help them advance in their careers.

By advocating for your sponsorship candidate, you are using your influence and credibility to help them succeed in their career. This can be a powerful way to support diversity and inclusion within your organization and create a more equitable and supportive workplace culture. Additionally, it can help you develop your leadership skills and build stronger relationships with colleagues across your organization.

Provide Guidance And Support

As a sponsor, it is important to be available to your sponsorship candidate to provide guidance and support as they navigate their career path. Your support and advice can help them overcome challenges and make informed decisions about their career. Here are some ways to provide guidance and support to your sponsorship candidate:

1. Offering advice on career development: Offer advice on how your sponsorship candidate can develop their skills and advance their career within your organization. Provide guidance on what skills they may need to

develop, what training programs they should consider, and what roles they should aim for.

2. Providing feedback on their performance: Provide your sponsorship candidate with feedback on their performance. Offer constructive criticism on what they are doing well and what they could improve upon. Help them set goals and develop a plan to achieve those goals. Strive to provide specific feedback to your sponsor to ensure that you are both on the same page.

3. Connecting them with key stakeholders and influencers: Introduce your sponsorship candidate to key stakeholders and influencers within your organization. Help them build relationships with people who can help them advance in their careers. Encourage them to seek out mentors and sponsors outside of your organization as well.

4. Advocating for their work and achievements: Publicly recognize and advocate for your sponsorship candidate's work and achievements. Highlight their successes to senior leaders and decision-makers within your organization. This can help them gain visibility and credibility within the organization.

By providing guidance and support to your sponsorship candidate, you are helping them to grow and develop in their career. Your support can help them overcome obstacles and make informed decisions about their future. Additionally, as you support your sponsorship candidate, you can continue to develop your leadership skills and build stronger relationships with colleagues across your organization.

Measure And Track Progress

As a sponsor, it is essential to measure and track the progress of your sponsorship relationship over time. This helps to ensure that your sponsorship candidate is making progress toward their goals and objectives. Here are some ways to measure and track the progress of your sponsorship relationship:

1. Set clear goals and objectives: Set clear goals and objectives with your sponsorship candidate. This can help to provide a clear path forward and establish expectations for both you and your sponsorship candidate.

2. Track their progress: Keep track of your sponsorship candidate's progress toward their goals and objectives. Schedule regular check-ins with them to discuss their progress and any obstacles they may be facing.

3. Celebrate their successes: Celebrate your sponsorship candidate's successes along the way. Recognize their achievements and publicly acknowledge their contributions to the organization.

4. Adjust your approach as needed: Be willing to adjust your approach as needed to help your sponsorship candidate achieve their goals. Be open to feedback from your sponsorship candidate and be willing to adapt your approach to best support them.

Measuring and tracking the progress of your sponsorship relationship helps to ensure that your sponsorship candidate is receiving the support they need to achieve their goals. By celebrating their successes along the way, you can help to build their confidence and motivate them to continue working towards their goals. Additionally, tracking progress can help you to identify areas where you may need to adjust your approach to best support your sponsorship candidate.

The Benefits of Sponsoring Women of Color in the Workplace

Sponsoring a woman of color can be an opportunity for a leader to develop their leadership skills in several ways. Firstly, by providing guidance and support to their sponsorship candidate, a leader can hone their coaching skills. Coaching involves helping someone to identify their strengths and weaknesses, set goals, and develop a plan to achieve those goals. By coaching a woman of color, a leader can develop their ability to ask powerful questions, listen actively, and provide constructive feedback.

Secondly, sponsoring a woman of color can help a leader to improve their mentoring skills. Mentoring involves sharing knowledge, skills, and experience to help someone develop their career. By mentoring a woman of color, a leader can develop their ability to provide guidance, offer advice, and act as a sounding board for their mentee. This can also help to build trust and establish a sense of mutual respect between the leader and the sponsorship candidate.

Lastly, sponsoring a woman of color can help a leader to develop their advocacy skills. Advocacy involves using your influence to support and promote the interests of someone else. By advocating for a woman of color, a leader can develop their ability to speak up on behalf of others, build coalitions, and influence decision-making processes. This can also help a leader to become a more effective ally and support the development of a more diverse and inclusive workplace. Furthermore, sponsoring a woman of color can significantly impact a leader's reputation positively. When a leader invests time, effort, and resources into sponsoring a woman of color, they are demonstrating their commitment to diversity, inclusion, and equity. This can enhance their reputation not only within their organization but also in the larger professional community.

As a leader, sponsoring a woman of color can send a powerful message to others about your values and priorities. It shows that you recognize and value the importance of diversity in the workplace and are willing to take action to support underrepresented groups. This can lead to increased respect and admiration from your colleagues, employees, and even potential job candidates.

From a pragmatic standpoint, by sponsoring women of color, leaders can help to create a pipeline of diverse talent within their organization, which can be a competitive advantage in today's competitive healthcare market.

A Final Message for Women of Color

As a woman of color navigating your workplace, it is important to recognize that your experiences and insights bring a unique perspective that can contribute to the success of your organization. Embrace your unique background and skills, and remember that you are a valuable asset to your team.

To boost your self-assurance and acquire valuable knowledge, it's beneficial to connect with mentors or allies who can offer assistance and direction as you maneuver through your work environment. These individuals can guide ways to tackle obstacles and triumph in your profession. Seek out people who hold similar beliefs and can furnish practical feedback, as they will be your supporters.

Be proactive in seeking out opportunities to develop your skills and knowledge. This can include attending training programs, conferences, or networking events. By actively seeking out opportunities to learn and grow, you can increase your visibility within your organization and demonstrate your commitment to your professional development.

Unfortunately, discrimination or bias may still occur in the workplace. If you encounter such incidents, it is important to speak up and advocate for yourself. Document any incidents that occur and seek out resources within your organization, such as a human resources department or employee assistance program. Remember that you have the right to work in an environment free from discrimination and bias.

It is important to remember that you are not alone in your experiences. Seek out support from friends, family, or professional networks. There are also organizations and resources available to support women of color in the workplace. CFHA, for example, has its Just Medicine Committee which you can reach out to for consultation and support. By staying informed and seeking support, you can navigate the workplace with confidence and achieve success in your career.

Remember that unpleasant past experiences do not define who you are, and they should not hold you back from being true to yourself. When you embrace your uniqueness and show up as your authentic self, you permit others to do the same. By being true to yourself, you inspire others to do the same and create a more inclusive and accepting environment for everyone.

So, never apologize for being you. Embrace your uniqueness and always show up as your authentic self. When you do, you not only empower yourself but also create a positive ripple effect that can inspire and uplift others. Always be YOURSELF!

Resources For Further Reading:

- A Physician's Take On Supporting Women of Color

- Getting Women To Senior Leadership Roles

- Barriers & Bias: The Status of Women in Leadership: Report and Summary

About the Author

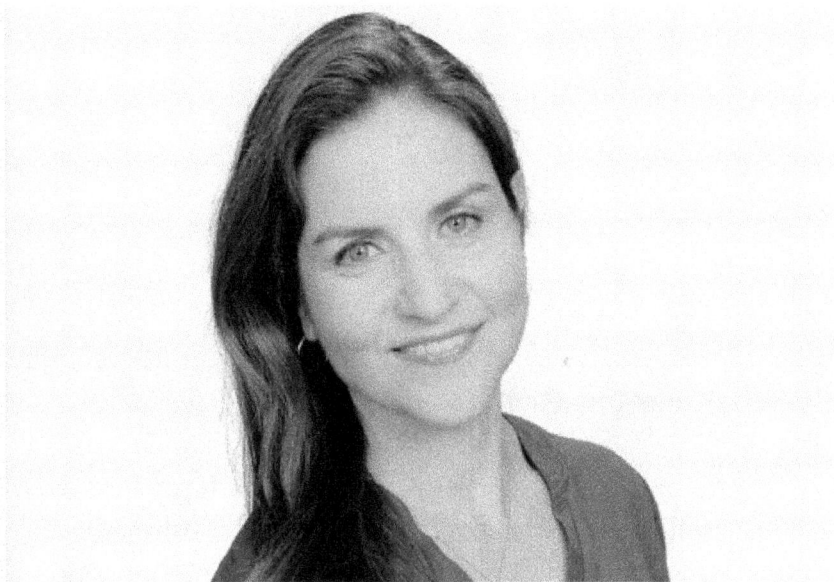

Martha Saucedo, LCSW, is in charge of overseeing the Technical Assistance branch of CFHA, where she loves to share her 13+ years of experience in the integrated care world (mostly in FQHCs). After obtaining a degree in counseling psychology in Monterrey, Mexico, Martha immigrated to the United States rebooting her career in the US healthcare system. As a proud Latina, Martha has always been committed to promoting diversity and empowering minority groups to have a voice. Martha enjoys switching hats from baseball to dance mom (her kid's activities). She finds joy in reading spiritually uplifting material and prioritizes daily meditation.

Chapter 11: Everybody Leads

By Neftali Serrano, PsyD

One of the critical mistakes I made with my first-ever staff person was to see them uni-dimensionally. I saw that staff person, an intern, as someone who would help me see more patients (and thus take some of the pressure off of me); this resulted in a perpetual battle to get her to see more patients and, even worse, to get her to be just like me. It did not go incredibly well, and I take much blame. I learned from that experience that human beings cannot be seen as a means to an end, no matter how noble that end may seem to you. They are unique creatures, each with gifts and talents and ways that will work for them to maximize their innate potential. Tapping into this is the job of any good manager.

Don't get me wrong. I am a stickler when it comes to the core BHC model, and in fact, one of the critical lessons of this text is that you must hire specifically for those core components. But even BHCs with these core skills and characteristics will differ meaningfully. Matching their work to those skills is essential. I have also found that it is important to most human beings that they have a domain or area of ownership. Most call this leadership, but the term leadership can connote having responsibility over others, which is not what I think most people need. Having a domain doesn't mean having a managerial role; it simply means having an area of responsibility and mastery. Most human beings I have met who live functional, well lives have at least one domain - whether it is pie making, house cleaning, or some medical specialty.

To that end, one of the things I set out to do at Access is to hire talented individuals, train them in the core BHC model, and then provide them with domains that match their personal and professional makeup. The best way to tell this part of the Access story is to tell the story of each of my hires during my tenure and how their domains developed over time.

Meghan, Lead & Quality Improvement

Meghan was our first postdoctoral fellow and our first staff member. I got to know her during the postdoctoral year very well since we often worked side-by-side, and thus, I got a sense of her strengths and likes/dislikes related to primary care. One of the apparent things about her was that she was detail-oriented, trustworthy, and timely, and I gathered from her Ph.D. background that she enjoyed numbers. These particular characteristics fit well with one of our early needs in the program around quality improvement and logistics related to our program.

As the director of myself, Meghan, and one practicum student, I handled all managerial responsibilities and seeing patients, so I only did a bare minimum of quality improvement. If I recall correctly, it was a meager attempt to create a spreadsheet to track depression inventory scores. What we needed was to track productivity, begin to track quality outcomes, and, more than anything, have someone familiar with the statistical realities of our program so that we could make essential connections about what we were doing. Eventually, it also made sense to turn over the team's logistical management to Meghan, so she also began to manage scheduling.

Turning over some of these responsibilities to Meghan was not easy for me since I was used to managing them on my own, and there was some loss for me in not being as close to them as I was when I knew each detail of each procedure. However, it gave Meghan a place to flourish and a critical role on our team.

Her success in managing this area also demonstrated her essential skills in coordinating people and responsibilities. So when our team grew large enough, she was given a co-lead role on our team which involved oversight of our interns and procedures at two of our clinics. Essentially, she became responsible for ensuring that our trainees were oriented correctly and had a successful trainee experience. Additionally, she was a point person for clinic managers and other clinic teams to troubleshoot flow issues and facilitate coordination. In all, Meghan's role grew out of what we needed as a clinic, but most importantly, areas where she could excel and enjoy her work. As her domain expanded, my domain changed, and as I said before, each time I handed over responsibility, I sensed some loss. However, I saw her excel and, in many cases, do a much better job than I could by her talent and focus. By this edition's copyright date, Meghan's title was officially changed to Director of Behavioral Health, reflecting her roles in team coordination, quality, and clinical training.

Armando, Lead & Pediatrics

I hired Armando several years into the development of the program mainly because he had a rare combination of good core BHC skill potential and was bilingual and bicultural. The BHC skills were just potential at the outset simply because he had worked for several years at the local community mental health center in a specialty model of care, so I worked hard in the interview process, which also included meeting him in informal group gatherings to see if his skills and temperament would translate well. (I learned of Armando through our first-ever practicum student, Kristina Dell, who was neighbors with him and talked up our model of care to him.)

From the outset, it was clear that Armando had two strengths: a systemic approach that worked well with families and children and a strong interest and affinity for cultural diversity issues. As I got to know Armando better, other strengths emerged, but these were the first areas. It became clear that assigning him pediatrics as a domain would be a great way to utilize this skill set. His task, as I described it to him, was to be our team leader in this area, helping us see how we could improve and monitor our care of children and their families within a population-based approach; this led Armando to visit other primary care clinics to see what they were doing in these areas and adapt his base skills to the primary care behavioral health model. As a result of his leadership in this area, our team developed an aspect of our work where we do the developmental assessment and anticipatory guidance portions of pediatric well-child visits; this is single-handedly responsible for most of our contact with pediatric patients. To make this work, Armando used his clinical skills and ability to work with various personalities on the medical team and co-create flow procedures that the entire team could replicate across clinics. It was a challenging task, but it worked well.

So my decision to have him work in this area was not solely because of his interest but because I knew he had the people skills to work with various team members, including pediatricians, medical assistants, and registrars, to enable the well-child check initiative. I also knew he had the organizational skills to proceed step-wise and create procedures we could all follow and replicate.

Later on, as our team grew, he became co-lead with Meghan sharing intern management responsibilities and being the point person for our clinic on the east side of the city. The intern management also fits one of Armando's other strengths: teaching. I learned from trainees who worked with him that he took time out to do teaching naturally and had good insight into the particular developmental needs of students.

Like with Meghan, handing over these responsibilities to Armando took work. In the first few years, any major initiative like the well child check initiative had my direct imprint. But again, I realized that he did a much better job than I could have from the position of a stretched director, and he brought his potent combination of skills to bear on the development of the program.

It is important to note that Armando was not our most productive BHC, and he tended to be slower with patient care relative to other BHCs and had a more challenging time keeping up with notes. He struggled with the BHC identity, having come from a specialty care background. However, by working with his strengths, providing positive, consistent feedback, and allocating leadership responsibilities, Armando was an engaged, helpful member of the BHC team for several years.

Update: Armando left the Access team to advance his career after several years of service. Given how well he established the pediatric service, the investment in Armando was not lost. He went on to work in various roles, including helping to start an integrated care service at a local HMO, working with the local school district, and advancing cultural competency at a local community mental health center.

Beth, Consulting Psychiatry and Liaison To Specialty Care

No hire I have ever made was as obvious to me as Beth. Beth was born to be a Behavioral Health Consultant. We got to know Beth as our second postdoctoral fellow, so at the end of her year, we knew we had an exceptional clinical talent. She was energetic, easily our most productive BHC, gained the trust of our patients and providers, and loved the model. But right from the outset, I knew the main challenge with Beth would be ensuring that her strength in this area was within the other contributions she could make to our team. She could not just be a workhorse for us since I knew this was a recipe for burnout.

Beth's skill set was clearly in the area of relationships and advocacy. She had a way of making others feel comfortable around her through her friendly, bubbly personality, so I quickly gathered that one area where we could use her leadership was the area of our relationships with external agencies; this also made sense since Beth was always naturally advocating for patients, and few could say no to Beth.

Until handing over this area to Beth, I, as director, was the face of the program. If there was an official meeting with an area mental health clinic, I was the person who would attend the meeting. As Beth became more active in this area, my community activities shifted more to areas related to program growth, such as meetings with local insurance companies or some of the initial discussions with other healthcare entities interested in emulating our work.

Once again, it was not easy to let go of some of these responsibilities, but it was the right thing to do. With all of my duties, I could never obtain comprehensive knowledge of the mental health system and the major players and thus was not very good as an advocate for our patients. Beth amassed a wealth of pragmatic and relational data that she passed on to our team so that we could direct patients appropriately for resources in the community. She also worked tirelessly to ensure that community partners understood the primary care behavioral health model so that their referrals to us were well-informed.

Consulting psychiatry was another area that made sense for Beth because it tied into the stepped care that many patients require. In other words, part of what we do in primary care is determine the level of care a patient needs based on various factors, including patient motivation. Beth's work interfacing with specialty care centers gave us a community-wide perspective of what resources existed. It helped us understand what internal resources we could/should utilize and develop to bridge gaps. Consulting psychiatry is one of those services. So, in many cases where a patient cannot or will not access specialty psychiatry, we utilize our internal consulting psychiatrist to make recommendations to the primary care team. Beth was able to develop a good working relationship with our consulting psychiatrist and then even expanded the program to include psychiatry residents, which expanded patient access and ensured that there is a future pipeline of trained psychiatrists ready to step in should our consulting psychiatrist leave one day.

One key aspect of her job that became an occupational hazard is how stretched someone in this role can become. Working with external agencies and managing an internal consult service requires an essential leadership skill: boundary setting. Some of the boundaries are internal boundaries - that is, learning to understand how many internal resources you have to do the job. Some limits are external - learning to say no to external agencies. One of the areas I worked with Beth on was setting these boundaries to be an effective leader; this, of course, requires good communication and time, but investing in your staff in this way pays off big dividends as these areas of leadership mature and take on a life of their own. I had less and less management to do with my staff simply because we took the time to work on these leadership skills over time.

That work especially paid off when it came time for me to leave Access in the summer of 2015. Beth was promoted to Chief Behavioral Health Officer, fully prepared to lead the BHC team to its following challenges, including building a robust MAT program, advocating successfully at the state level for reimbursement support, and leading the clinic through the pandemic; this is the hallmark of good leadership: that others are prepared to step up as needed.

Chantelle, Specialty Populations

Chantelle came to us through the postdoctoral fellowship (and had a stint with us as a rotating intern), so again, she was well-known to us. Her area of leadership was not difficult to ascertain because she had time to acclimate to the model and also had well-developed interests in the areas of substance abuse and severe mental illness. So when we hired her, we decided that she would assist our team in identifying our needs in this area and developing strategies to improve the care of patients in these categories; this was again fortuitous timing as we were increasingly seeing a higher prevalence of both patients with severe mental illness and substance abuse, issues which can present complexities in any setting, but especially in primary care where time is at a premium. Her mission was to determine how to address population needs while maintaining our population focus and core behavioral health consultant model access. Would groups be helpful? Would protocols help? Do we need some monitoring systems? These were the queries I had for her and her work.

Given room to operate, Chantelle identified one need to connect patients with specialty resources more efficiently. So she collaborated with Beth and various other members of our team to develop an innovative online format that presented the referral information in the community relevant to different patient populations and characteristics. This work allowed our team to discover what resources were available quickly and for whom in a way that a sheet with a list of resources could not.

In addition, Chantelle began to collaborate with a family medicine provider who developed an addictions residency fellowship and internal consultation clinic to help address the substance abuse needs of our patients; this became a forerunner to the MAT services that Access developed years later. She helped design the behavioral health consultant role in the referring process and worked with the clinician on the consult clinic days on patient co-visits.

Once again, this leadership role has incredible potential for growth, so I worked with Chantelle on focusing her efforts on a few tasks or projects to avert diluting her impact. Doing a few things well is one of the critical leadership traits I instill in our program.

Update: Chantelle moved on to direct an inpatient addiction service after many years of service at Access.

Ken, Family Medicine Resident Training

I won't take any credit for assigning or facilitating Ken's leadership role on our team since I had no official supervisory capacity over him and since Ken came to Access as part of a merger with a University of Wisconsin residency clinic for which he was the Behavioral Science faculty. However, Ken's role was crucial for our team.

As our team began rotating through the residency clinic, we needed someone who could be mindful of resident needs and serve as an organizing force for our work there. Ken had already been doing an excellent job with years of experience as an educator. The best thing I did was keep my hands off him. What Ken did so well was to integrate into our team and model of care, even though he had been working in a specialty co-located model before our arrival. He made the transition gracefully and graciously served as our point person for discussing the educational needs of residents, such as working with new residents, having an elective behavioral health rotation experience for residents, and serving as our liaison to the Department of Family Medicine. Ken also provided a valuable specialty service by performing occasional neuropsychological evaluations.

Ken's other vital feature to our team was his connectedness to the University of Wisconsin. Ken's knowledge of and relationship with key people within the university made available resources and possibilities we could not otherwise have obtained. For example, through Ken, our staff were all provided clinical faculty appointments with the Department of Family Medicine, which offers privileges such as library access and generally opens doors when working with other university departments.

Ken was also not one of the most productive BHCs and, like Armando, struggled with his prior identity as a co-located specialty therapist. However, with time Ken became an indispensable member of the team and a key leader in our residency-related efforts.

Update: Ken retired in 2018 after several years on the BHC team.

Ashley, Care Management & Clinic Lead

Ashley came to us through our training program. She excelled as a social work trainee, and when she graduated, we decided to offer her a position as a BHC who also leads us in care management. Ashley had several characteristics that made her an excellent fit for this role, including good attention to detail, a willingness to work with databases (although with little prior experience), a fabulous phone presence, and a strong desire to be helpful to team members.

The care manager role involves a great deal of chart review and phone calls, so picking someone who does well with this is vital. Of note, it is essential not to assume that care management duties are the sole responsibility of one team member. All of our team members had care management responsibilities, though Ashley performed most of the formal care management.

One other aspect of Ashley's hire is that she taught our team of psychologists about social workers; this is important when putting together your team - their particular training backgrounds will bring a different flavor to your team, and just like with multicultural issues, you have to be mindful and aware of biases. It is also important not to exclude team members, purposefully or inadvertently, based on their job titles. For us, this happened more by luck than for any specific reason. Ashley (and Martha) came to us around the same time through our training program. As such, we didn't quite yet know how to transition them to full-fledged staff status, especially since, with social workers, there is a two-year gray period during which they are acquiring hours towards licensure. Should they attend staff meetings? (Yes!) Do we still check in on their patients? (Yes, but providing modified supervision to reflect their developmental needs.) How should they interact with other trainees since they are staff but are not licensed? (Trainees should treat them as staff.) Ultimately, we muddled through these issues, and Ashley and Martha were exceptionally patient with the rest of us. Our team was better off for having three excellent social workers.

Update: Ashley took a role as the East clinic lead when Armando left, earned her LCSW licensure, and in 2023 began to oversee a dedicated care management team as the team expanded into Collaborative Care model work.

Martha, Latino Populations

Martha was our first social worker trainee. However, due to having young children, she decided to extend the time she would acquire her hours toward licensure. As such, after her training year, she worked with us as a PRN provider. Having a part-time staff member posed some challenges for us in integrating her into our team, similar to the issues discussed with Ashley, our other social worker. Again, the key was ensuring good communication around professional developmental needs. For example, after a certain amount of time, it became clear that we were treating Martha as a student but that she had progressed beyond this even though she had yet to obtain her license. So, we made adjustments in the way in which we supervised her and in the responsibilities for supervision that we gave her.

As she was able to make time for more regular work, it also became clear that we should use her best skills for a leadership role on our team. The obvious area for Martha was leading our team in issues related to a significant subset of our population, namely Latinos. Martha's knowledge and passion for this population were self-evident as a Mexican immigrant to the United States. But beyond this, Martha also possessed good teaching skills and was creative about working with our team members. As our leader in this area, Martha helped with raising everyone's competency when working with Latinos and ensured that, over time, our services continued to meet their needs. And, of course, we had a big celebration when she earned her LCSW license in 2014.

Update: Martha continues her part-time work at Access as a BHC and Latinx Community Liaison while adding a full-time role at CFHA as Director of Technical Assistance.

Julie, Consulting Psychiatrist

After a few years of outsourcing our consulting psychiatry needs through a relationship with a local community mental health center, it became clear that we needed to own this aspect of the program internally. The obvious candidate was Julie Nielsen, a psychiatrist we were already working with through our relationship with the University of Wisconsin Department of Family Medicine. She had worked for many years with the Department in a similar capacity but was slightly more co-located in her approach.

Julie has unique skills: she can consult with pediatric and adult patients, is an excellent verbal and written communicator, and is a great teacher for the psychiatry residents we host each quarter. She is also very flexible and can adapt to the needs of our primary care providers and patients. In short, she quickly earned our trust, which is very important for someone whose main job is helping us think critically about how we prescribe medication to our patients.

One other critical factor in a consulting psychiatrist that Julie had was a lack of any professional competitiveness between her discipline and other mental health disciplines. She can exert her leadership as a psychiatrist and be a good team member alongside our psychologists and social workers.

Over time Julie grew her FTE from .25 to .75, adding the supervision of psychiatry residents to her other consulting responsibilities. Julie's impact will be felt across generations of psychiatrists with skills in consulting for primary care.

Growth

Since the original edition of this book was published in 2014, close to a hundred trainees, have passed through Access' training program, and several staff were added. At present, 12 BHCs, ten third-year psychiatry residents, two postdoctoral fellows, one social work fellow, and 2-4 practicum-level interns support the work of over 45 Access providers. The growth of this human capital was made possible through the distribution of leadership responsibilities on the BHC team. The continued growth of Access and the BHC team well past my tenure is a testament to the commitment of the team to continue to nurture and grow its staff.

Making Wise Choices

These staff selections were primarily aided by our experience with them in their training years (except for Ken, Julie, and Armando). As such, it becomes much harder to make poor choices because you have a year to try them out. We have had post-docs we selected who, after their year, realized that primary care was not for them or that our model of care was not for them. That's fine for a post-doc, but costly if you hire staff and either need to replace or live with them. Thus selecting your staff wisely is crucial, and envisioning where they can lead your team is equally vital.

There are times, however, when you will likely err in selecting someone, and so one of the other crucial skills of program development is knowing when to cut ties with staff (later on, we'll also address knowing when/how to cut ties with ideas as well). Usually, organizations err on the side of cutting ties too late. It is not easy to fire people.

However, the cost to an organization and a primary care behavioral health program can be enormous. Consider, for example, a staff member you have hired who does not do well within the model. Perhaps they are slow and prefer lengthy sessions, believing they need hour-long sessions and frequent follow-ups. The problem is that they are not seeing many people and become unavailable to providers. Thus, they begin to train providers to expect unavailability; this impacts other behavioral health consultants who work with those same providers and generally affects the program's reputation. Beyond that, this person can also begin to poison the atmosphere in the clinic if they feel pressure to conform and start to share their displeasure with others on the team and among the provider staff. Such a staff person is not a good fit and will never be a good fit, no matter what rehabilitative efforts you may undertake. The best thing to do is cut ties or reassign them away from primary care if an organization can tolerate it; this can be done abruptly or with some notice, such as informing the individual that they are not a good fit and should start looking for employment elsewhere within a specified timeframe. Either way, it has to happen. Often, I have found that an organization is much better off with a void at the position than with the negative influence of a poor-fit behavioral health consultant.

Sometimes, a behavioral health consultant may generally be a good fit but is less than a superstar. Sometimes staff have lower ceilings concerning their talents, abilities, or motivation. It is important to identify ceilings with your staff to avoid frustrating efforts to make changes in areas where change is impossible or not worth the effort. Often this issue comes up with less productive or efficient staff than an organization may desire. As discussed in other portions of the book, I never see a productivity issue as a function of staff laziness. The strategy with staff like this is to work to remove barriers to productivity; this includes providing support for paperwork, reducing extraneous responsibilities, mentoring in specific areas such as note writing or therapeutic strategies, etc. However, once you have worked at efficiency long enough and encountered enough resistance to conclude that you have hit the ceiling of that individual, it is time to employ acceptance-based strategies as an organization and director. In reality, pushing against that ceiling won't do much good and could harm that individual and the team. Frequently this means focusing on the individuals' other skills and contributions to the team and working on accepting the efficiency level of that individual; this is why, as they often say in sports, there is no replacing or teaching talent. Selecting staff with high ceilings with a predisposition towards the model is the best way to avoid situations where you are trying to fit round pegs into square holes.

In sum, if you combine effective talent selection with an approach that enables their innate leadership skills to shine, you will build a sustainable program like Access. As you can tell from the stories, not everyone stayed with Access forever (I left after nine years and others left after five or fewer years). And in fact, you should always expect staff transition to be a part of your program's life, especially in 20 years like our story covers. However, the foundational health of the program was so strong that it withstood the natural ebb and flow of staffing changes and continued to evolve to benefit the population health vision of PCBH and the benefit of individual staff who found ways to express their unique talents.

Chapter 12: Financing PCBH, The Ideal

By Neftali Serrano, PsyD

W hen creating something, it is essential to consider the ideal at the outset; this allows for creativity, flexibility, and openness to the entire universe of possibilities. It gets you closer to what you want to create or need; this is especially the case when what you create will, by necessity, involve elements of what already has been.

An excellent example of this is the iPhone. When the creators of the iPhone sat down to conceptualize, they certainly had models of existing cell phones, personal data assistants, and music players. But instead of being constrained by these pre-existing devices, at the outset, they allowed themselves to consider what they wanted. Thus something fundamentally different than all of those devices became the one we know as the iPhone. The same is valid for integrated care. We certainly have a history of providing mental health services, and we have a history of providing primary care medical services. But to do our best, we want to conceptualize something new that meets the needs of patients and providers; this is particularly true concerning how these services are funded. This chapter starts with developing a vision for the ideal state of financing integrated care services.

In many settings, this ideal does not exist and may not exist for many years, but program developers must keep the objective in mind and continue to work towards it. In this way, you will create the reality necessary for the ideal integrated care practice. Let's start with some basics.

The Measurement of Service Provision

Historically, customers and insurers have paid for mental health services by the number of encounters or time spent with a mental health professional and the patient. As with much of medicine, this has set up an odd and adversarial relationship between providers and payers of care, with the patient stuck in the middle. It is in the best interest of care providers to have more encounters with patients. And it is in the best interest of payers of care for providers to have fewer encounters and for patients, in general, to utilize these specialty services with rarity. Patients, of course, are not interested in a specific number of encounters with the healthcare provider but rather in the outcome of those encounters, namely their health.

For this reason, integrated care calls for a new way of measuring and paying for a behavioral health consultant's service. One key component of what integrated care calls for is flexible access. For example, it is in the best interest of both the patient and payer for care to occur precisely when it is needed, and in some cases, preventatively, a bit earlier than when intensive care might be required. In other words, insurance companies would be happy to trade a few visits with the behavioral health professional if they knew it would keep patients out of several visits to the emergency department, which are much more expensive. So promoting flexible access is vital. It is also helpful for the mental health provider if a patient has flexible access, and that flexible access does not involve the mental health provider jumping through a bunch of hoops, namely paperwork related to prior authorizations or procedures for re-opening a case.

To achieve this, it becomes essential to decouple the measurement of services from time spent or encounters with patients. In other words, the only way to align the incentives of the patient, the payer, and the mental provider is to stop measuring the work of the behavioral health consultant in encounters. Something is needed that aligns the incentives of the payer, the provider, and the patient; that solution has to have the characteristics of being centered on health outcomes that are important and relevant to the patient, tied to manageable and semi-predictable costs for the payer, and that provide the primary care clinic with enough funding to sustain its service. The bottom line is that we can never achieve the ideal if we measure service provision in the number of times a mental health professional sits down with the patient.

Due to misaligned incentives, there is no way of making integrated care work well in this system. Under this old system, clinics will continually push their behavioral health consultants to see more people more often, and payers will constantly try to manage and restrict the number of sessions and access to behavioral health services. The unfortunate reality is that given the current nature of the system, everyone is behaving logically. The problem is that this is not helpful for anyone - including the patient.

If we eliminate encounters to measure service provision, insurance companies will no longer need to worry about prior authorizations. They will not need to get into the business of limiting the number of visits a patient has with a mental health professional. They can free themselves to make more global judgments around the risk associated with their population and the capital expenditure needed to support that population in a given timeframe. Providers can consider treatment modalities, frequencies, and interventions outside scheduled visits. Suddenly, telephone contact is just as valuable as face-to-face contact. Care management strategies such as using registries become valuable tools instead of being seen as "un-billable activity."

Indeed the success of the collaborative care (CoCM) model is a step in this direction. Payment for that model (though it still needs improvement) is based on work a team performs with a patient over a month. Although time allocation is still counted in this payment scheme, the number of encounters is not, and the payment is irrespective of the specific team members involved (the team is paid even though the official biller is the PCP).

The General Concept Behind Bundling

As you can probably predict, if behavioral health services are not to be paid for by encounters, then there must be a way of quantifying the value of services provided that is more global, or in other words, related to the complete care of the patient for a specific problem area. Something similar to the CoCM approach. To flesh this out, let's walk through an example.

Let's take the example of a 52-year-old depressed female insured by a local insurer and seen at our primary care clinic. The way that a bundled payment might work is that a regional insurer (based on algorithms they create for characteristics of that patient, perhaps including things like age, pre-existing conditions, past healthcare utilization, etc.) develops a dollar figure value for that patient's care including medical, mental health and specialty/hospital care. That dollar value represents the risk they estimate they will take in a given timeframe, say a year. That insurer can then contract with a local provider and negotiate with the provider around the care of that patient (or, more likely, a set of patients) and the reimbursement value associated with that patient(s).

So, let's say, for instance, that the algorithms the insurer uses estimate that the patient will cost the insurer about $7,000 in the coming year. Based on their internal business metrics (insurers know that they will lose money on some patients and make money on others), they can present a global payment to our local primary care clinic to care for that patient. So they might pay our clinic $3,500 annually to provide primary care and behavioral health services to the patient; this means that our job as a clinic then is to keep this person as healthy as possible in whatever way we deem necessary throughout that year, within the constraints of the $3,500 we get for the patient.

It is essential to consider that clinics also make assumptions about their costs, patient utilization, and the staffing required to care for their population. So that patient might incur less than $3,500 of care at our clinic, or more than that, but our job as a business is to work it out so that, on average, we come out ahead - just like the insurer.

It should be obvious how this ideal creates freedom for the primary care clinic and provides some advantages for the insurer. For the primary care clinic, it gives freedom to think creatively about how to care for this individual. This patient could benefit from more frequent contact by phone, which means that provider, BHC, or care manager schedules could be freed up for those patients who need face-to-face contact. And more importantly, it means the clinic can hire behavioral health consultants to provide quality, efficient care that can be integrated into the general business model of the primary care clinic, much like nursing and laboratory staff are. In fact, in most cases, behavioral health consultants provide a cheaper health provider contact for patients than a primary care provider.

In addition, the insurer and our local clinic could negotiate specific incentives. For example, if you consider our example of the 52-year-old female, the insurance company algorithm states that she should cost them $7,000 annually. Their thinking is that $3,500 would be manageable within primary care, but the rest of their risk is likely specialty or hospital-based care. The insurer may then be able to build an incentive for the primary care clinic if the patient does not end up utilizing the remaining $3,500 of care that was projected to be outside of primary care. The idea, of course, would be that if primary care did a great job (and got lucky - let's not forget that much of this is out of our control), then the insurer and the local clinic could share in some of the cost savings. So perhaps an additional $1,500 could be provided as an incentive should the patient be more efficiently managed. Now obviously, these kinds of negotiations are not likely to occur on a patient-by-patient basis but rather across large patient populations - and the judgments made around projected costs of care are rather complex. So, as usual, the devil is in the details. But this is essentially the idea of a global payment.

Ultimately, you are shooting for this nexus in healthcare where everyone's incentives are aligned. In this case, the primary care clinic is incentivized to provide efficient and high-quality care because if they don't, they will spend more than $3,500 worth of staff time and energy on this patient and will not achieve their incentive payment. The insurance company has incentives to fund primary care appropriately to avoid more expensive risk, and they have less incentive to prescribe or interfere with the specific nature of the care (e.g., number of visits, not paying for telephone calls). And all of this aligns much better with what is vital to the patient, which is ostensibly better care, efficiently delivered. One caveat to this Shangri-La scenario is that insurance companies have different risk tolerances and, frankly, different personalities around how flexible they are willing to be.

Additionally, insurance companies may not be incentivized to invest in patients if their panels have a high turnover. For example, why invest in preventative care for a patient whom you may only insure for three years when the expected benefit of the preventive care would only occur after six years? So this is where the single-payer folks (like me) chime in and say that the current system is deeply flawed, and there is not much of a fix for this. But we will avoid that soap box here.

Now you may be wondering where the patient's incentives are in this scenario; this is also crucial and will continue to come to the fore since patients will be asked to shoulder the burden of healthcare costs and decisions to a greater degree than has traditionally been the case. So let's assume that this 52-year-old patient obtains her insurance through her employer, which is how most Americans have health insurance. The most common arrangement is for the employer to pay for a portion of the insurance costs as negotiated with the health insurer, and the employee pays another part of the costs as deducted from their paychecks. In addition to those costs, many patients have co-pays for their specific utilization. And those co-pays vary by the kind of services that patients utilize.

A couple of things are likely to change going forward for patients. First, patients will likely have more information about the actual costs of the services they are incurring. At present, healthcare providers do a horrible job communicating the cost of visits, procedures, or medications to patients. This Wizard of Oz-like veil is what maintains higher prices. One of the reasons why patients are likely to have more knowledge about cost is because they are likely to begin incurring more risk to their finances to cover these costs; this may take the shape of higher co-pays for specific services or simply higher premiums. Concerning integrated care, the ideal would be for patients not to have to worry about separate co-pays but rather that integrated services in primary care are provided in a lump sum (in other words, if you see your doctor and BHC on the same day, no additional co-pay).

One creative way to align incentives is for the 52-year-old woman to have an incentive with the cost savings arrangement between the insurer and primary care provider. For example, suppose the cost savings have been achieved at the end of the year. In that case, a percentage of those savings go back to the patient just as they might go back to the primary care provider, essentially creating a win-win-win situation for all three parties; this would potentially incentivize the patient to work productively and proactively with her primary care team and avoid or use the more expensive services sparingly. Of course, again, as in all these things, the devil is in the details, but this is the general idea.

Participation In Incentives

As if to make what is already a reasonably complex issue more complex (and we should readily acknowledge that our hypothetical scenario is grossly oversimplified), incentives create a further challenge. There is, of course, the actuarial challenge of predicting patient health care needs and utilization (along with projecting stability of patient panels), but beyond this is the challenge of determining appropriate incentives; this is, again, a sticky area concerning how incentives are often aligned.

For example, when we often speak of incentives in healthcare, we speak of clinical quality incentives. These might include diabetes outcomes like hemoglobin A1c scores. My own bias is actually against particular clinical quality indicators such as hemoglobin A1c scores or PHQ9 scores because they are kinds of measurements that are not entirely under the control of healthcare providers and because (if we are being completely truthful) they are not directly relevant to the incentives of an insurance company.

In other words, if an insurance company was making millions of dollars in profit and satisfying their stockholders and their customers' PHQ9 and hemoglobin A1c scores were horrific, it probably would not make a massive difference to them. And I'm not proposing here that insurance companies are draconian enterprises that are heartless. I'm just pointing out that their primary incentive is to be profitable as a business. Those clinical quality indicators are only vital to them in so far as they relate to their profitability. It is possible to argue that poor outcomes on those scores could result in more expensive care provision or that lower scores in those areas could relate to poor customer satisfaction. So there is some rationale for incentivizing insurers in these areas, but it is only a secondary relationship to the primary concern of cost and profit.

For that reason, I've come to believe that the best kind of incentives to create are: A. incentives that are in the direct control of the incentivized party and, B. incentives that are directly meaningful to the parties involved. So, regarding the concept of direct control, it is undoubtedly the case that in the last decade, we have learned some things about managing depression and diabetes in primary care that generally results in improved quality compared to usual care. However, on a patient-by-patient basis, it is also true that what influences outcomes often is beyond the direct control of a healthcare provider.

So, for example, it is possible for a clinic (and this is often the case with federally-qualified health centers that have impoverished patient populations) to have used system redesign principles in diabetes or depression and yet have poorer outcomes than expected due to factors outside of the control of the health center such as poverty, housing, cultural factors, regional issues (e.g., migratory populations), etc. In other words, a healthcare provider can do nothing to decrease a person's scores in these areas directly since formal medical care only accounts for a portion of the variance in outcomes; social determinants of health often account for more of that variance.

What the healthcare provider can do is ensure that their systems are designed to provide high-quality care that will enable their populations to respond. Indeed, on average, it should be the case that these numbers show improvement in general but "should" looks different in different settings and different populations. The point is that it is essential to recognize that the actual outcome (lower A1c) is not directly manipulable by the clinic.

Another good example is depression scores. In clinical practice, it has become clear to me that depression scores are highly influenced by various factors, including the patient's cultural background, the patient's state at the moment, the presence of co-morbid mental health conditions, and many other factors. So it is not uncommon for behavioral health consultants to complain that their patients are getting better but that the scores do not reflect it. And in fact, it is also the case in specific scenarios that patient scores reflect improvement that is not realistic.

For example, I've had many situations where Latino patients who initially scored incredibly high on the PHQ9, with help, very quickly went incredibly low, even down to zero. It is more common for patients to have at least some symptoms even if the depression has resolved (I don't believe any zeros I get on PHQ9s). Even many CoCM programs struggle with metrics that require PHQ9 scores below 5 to count for remission status. So for these reasons, I don't put much stock in these measurements for incentives. The score is not what is under my control as a healthcare provider. So what are things that are under my control?

Generally speaking, the things under healthcare providers' control have to do with their systems of care and what opportunities they provide patients. So I control whether I present a patient with a depression screen. A medical provider controls whether they offer laboratory tests to patients at visits. These procedural elements improve outcomes when consistently applied via evidence-based protocols or guidelines. So internally, I tend to like to measure these elements for clinical quality. However, for our already discussed reasons, they are still not great for incentive arrangements with insurers. For insurers, I believe that things like healthcare utilization make more sense.

For example, although it is not entirely in my control whether a patient goes to the emergency department, we can, as a primary care practice, create systems that make it more attractive to the patient to go through us before they decide to go to the emergency department. And in the case of patients with psychiatric crises, for example, or medical crises related to psychiatric issues such as panic attacks, I believe that our behavioral health model can proactively and preventively address these issues with patients in an efficient manner such that they will be less likely to utilize the emergency department; this then becomes a perfect nexus of incentive with an insurer and our clinic.

For example, we could develop an incentive around the utilization of emergency departments in our community by the patients the insurer entrusts to our care. We could set a threshold either for the total costs incurred by our shared population in emergency department costs or some other threshold related to the percent of the population that accesses emergency care. Again, the devil is in the details. However, the principle here is that an incentive should be under the direct control of the healthcare provider and should be meaningful to both the healthcare provider and the insurer. Access performed a study of emergency department utilization that showed some utilization reduction among patients seen by behavioral health (note, however, how complex the results were).

Despite my overall aversion to metrics outside of direct provider control, I am a big believer in the responsibility PCBH has to develop patient registries that assist in measurement-based care pathways. Increasingly better tools are available to make outcome tools easier to administer (e.g., by text, email). These tools can compensate for one of the areas that primary care (and, by extension, PCBH) struggles with, namely, losing patients to follow-up. We still need some consensus on the best tools, but PCBH adherents must invest in them to demonstrate their value actively. This demonstration of value is critical to moving towards the ideal funding state we envision; we must also make ourselves accountable to continuous quality improvement efforts. CoCM has proven that such efforts yield results. PCBH should follow suit for specific problems PCBH is attempting to solve.

It is also important to note that behavioral health incentives do not need to be specifically related to behavioral health conditions. In other words, the proper measurement of the value of integrated behavioral health services is not just in ameliorating mental health conditions. When choosing incentives, we should not restrict them to traditional mental health outcomes alone, such as depression remission. The goals of PCBH are applicable to outcomes like provider and patient satisfaction, team efficiency, population access measures, equity goals, and others. This is where PCBH is distinct (not better, just different) from CoCM in that the collaborative care model is distinctly oriented toward specific mental health outcome improvement (thus why the two models run side-by-side effectively).

As an organizational consultant, I have noticed that mental health professionals often make the mistake of setting unrealistic grant goals. When these goals don't align with the core objectives of the consultant model they can be challenging to achieve. For example, PCBH is not the best way to reduce PHQ9 scores, CoCM is. So I would not write PHQ9 score reduction into a PCBH grant. I would be more likely to write a goal related to increased access for targeted patient populations with evidence of functional improvement on a relevant survey tool. In the same way, one should avoid setting oneself up for failure when negotiating incentives with an insurer. Choose metrics that match the strength of the model.

Where There Is Money, There Is Regulation

As the subtitle suggests, healthcare financing goes hand-in-hand with regulating healthcare. In many states, this regulation is largely the reason why integrated care has yet to progress further. For example, payers will not reimburse medical and mental health visits in some states on the same day. In several states, funding for mental health services (through programs like Medicaid) is separate from funding for medical services. This can lead to integration issues due to varying payment systems and regulatory requirements. The same problem can arise when insurance companies assign separate management for mental health services (carve-outs).

So our ideal concerning integrated care is for it to exist in the same payment and regulatory structure as our medical counterparts; this seems to be a relatively obvious solution to many of the integrated care problems that exist in many states, but as with most of these apparent solutions, humans get in the way. There are decades worth of regulatory structures and jobs associated with those regulatory structures that are at stake should integration occur. In other words, those state agencies and carve-out agencies that manage the funding stream for mental health services can often see integrated care as a threat to their existence.

They may be correct in some cases, but in most instances, logical accommodations that do not necessarily threaten the wholesale elimination of departments are possible. For example, in many cases, these departments make allowances or arrangements for places like federally qualified health centers to be reimbursed through medical funding streams. Alternatively, they may align or use their regulatory practices with what medical centers already do. In some cases, it should be possible for a simple distinction between integrated care and specialty mental health care, with integrated care coming under the regulatory practice of the medical funding side and specialty mental health continuing to exist on the mental health side.

It is increasingly agreed upon that individuals cannot be easily segmented based on their care needs. Therefore, combining funding and regulation is as logical as the concept of integration itself. The existence of these distinct entities on state, federal, and private levels is a result of our professional boundaries and the power structures implemented to safeguard them. They have very little to do with protecting patients.

The advantages of being included in the medical regulatory and financing structure are numerous. First, clinics do not need to learn a new set of billing or practice management rules. Second, practices that are odd to primary care, such as the practice of prior authorization of visits, intakes, treatment plans, discharge plans, etc., are not imposed upon the behavioral health consultants working in the primary care practice. Third, billing is more straightforward. And last but certainly not least, the sad reality is that the regulatory structures associated with medical payment and oversight tend to be much more up-to-date, well-developed, and responsive than the structures in place for mental health systems; this is due to years of neglect, underfunding, and a general lack of innovation. Much of the same applies to private insurers who carve out mental health services. So, it seems true that it doesn't look very pretty whenever you isolate mental health, whether in practice or regulation.

Conclusion

Therefore our ideal environment for integrated care includes one where we are free to work with patients creatively, unencumbered by arbitrary visit limits or pressures to have face-to-face contacts, and yet intimately involved in a clinic's efforts to provide cost-effective and efficient care with incentives aligned with patient goals and with the business models and practices of both the insurer and the primary care clinic. And ideally, the environment includes no separate structures for the oversight of the behavioral health practice other than the structures in place for supervising the primary care practice since our goal is to do primary care excellently.

In practice, there are a great many barriers standing in the way of this straightforward vision. But I can imagine back in the early 2000s when the engineers and software developers and executives at Apple Computers sat down to consider what they wanted to create when they considered the functions of a cell phone, a personal data assistant, and a music player, that they too faced a great many hurdles. How do we create a device that makes all of these things work equally well without sacrificing one function over another? How do we do so in a cost-effective manner? How do we make it so anyone can learn to use it, from a grandparent to a teenager? How do we make it fit easily in someone's pocket?

Well, history has already determined the efficacy of their efforts. They envisioned a product that was better than the sum of its parts and created something special. Each practice's steps to reach this ideal will ultimately change the financing and regulatory structures needed to develop this extraordinary thing called integrated care. Our job is not just to survive in the current systems but also to teach the existing structures about what could be better and to begin to set the community standard now. It is undoubtedly true that regulation in financing will follow the successful implementation of behavioral health consultant practices, not vice versa. So if you're waiting for the ideal to exist before you begin an integrated care practice, you're not in the right game.

The good news is that there has been significant progress towards value-based purchasing in the primary care space and reduced regulatory barriers impeding integrated care in the last decade. The momentum is definitely towards integration, not away from it. But some realities still need to be confronted. We turn to those realities in our next section.

Chapter 13: Financing PCBH, The Current State

By Neftali Serrano, PsyD

Healthcare economics is anything but simple. As such, beginning with a basic explanation of how healthcare is funded is helpful. The fee-for-service approach is the most common way mental health services are paid for; this means that behavioral health providers are reimbursed by the insurance company based on a face-to-face encounter. So, suppose a behavioral health provider sees a patient today for 20 minutes. In that case, they will provide the insurance company information on the diagnosis and associate that diagnosis with a level of service code otherwise known as a billing code (or CPT code). When a behavioral health provider spends 20 minutes with a patient, they use a 90832 code. This code is used for visits that last between 16 and 37 minutes. See Table 1 for all the psychotherapy codes reimbursable in this fee-for-service system.

Each insurance company or payer of medical services sets its fees for reimbursement. In other words, the insurance company decides how much they will pay for each code; this probably seems odd since, in most cases, the purchaser of services doesn't dictate the cost, such as when you go to a store to buy a shirt. In the case of healthcare, although there are the invisible (and it often feels like, theoretical) market forces which help to set prices, the insurer holds much of the power. If Medicare will pay a certain amount for a service, there is not much an individual provider can do about it.

The way that health insurance coverage is usually structured is that the insurance company pays a percentage (usually the majority) of the healthcare provider's service charge, and the patient pays the other portion of the costs. The patient's payment comes in co-pays for each visit or service and regular premiums paid to the insurer, often directly from a paycheck. Some plans also have deductibles or a cap amount the patient is responsible for before their insurer pays for services. So, if a patient is responsible for 20% of their costs for a visit that costs $100, they would pay a co-pay of $20, and the insurer would pay the remaining $80. In the case of a deductible, the patient may have to pay up to a certain amount before the insurance company begins paying for services. For example, if a patient has a $1,000 co-pay, they must accrue that much before the insurance company begins paying for their health care.

In other words, the main difference between what we consider a more normal marketplace and the healthcare marketplace is that instead of individuals purchasing services independently, insurance companies buy the services and share the burden of paying for those services with the patient. Of course, the idea is that the money that the patients pay monthly to the insurance companies collectively (meaning the aggregate of all the patients that pay into a specific insurance company) is enough for the insurance company to pay the different healthcare costs of individuals while still making a profit. The advantage for the individual is that they can afford healthcare, especially healthcare outside of their financial means (this would occur when the cost of services they receive is more than what they pay in). It is the power of group purchasing.

Another common way mental health services are paid is when a patient belongs to an insurance company that provides the actual medical care or at least portions of it. These kinds of insurance companies are often called health maintenance organizations or cooperatives. In this case, the idea is that the insurer can not only manage how much they pay for services but also how those services are provided, often aiming to provide services in the most cost-efficient fashion, as this would directly impact their profitability. So these companies hire their mental health providers and pay them a salary; this allows the insurer to know exactly how much it will cost them to provide care (assuming they have staffed themselves adequately) and enable them to manage how patients access that care more readily.

Insurers who do not offer medical services manage care in through rules they place on providers they contract with. This insurance system may still use psychiatric payment codes like in Table 1. Still, they will not pay providers directly since they are paid based on salary (the code may just be used for record-keeping). Again, there are many variations, and the various plans may still include a copayment that the patient is responsible for on a visit-by-visit basis.

A third important variant of how mental health services may be paid is when a provider group contracts with an insurer in a capitated model. In such an arrangement, an insurer will arrange for a mental health provider to provide services for a subset of patients. They will pay that provider a certain pre-negotiated amount to care for that subset of patients, usually a year. Again, in this case, the application of billing codes would not result in a payment for that visit since the provider has already been paid but rather may be used for record-keeping or monitoring of services under the contract. In other words, a specific clinic may negotiate a contract with a particular insurance provider who then assigns that clinic 1,000 patients. To provide services for that 1,000 patients (note that neither the insurance company nor the clinic can predict which patients will need services), the insurer will pay $100,000 to the clinic; this is why this is called a capitated model because payment is "capped" at a certain amount. In other words, the clinic can't make more money, and the insurer will not pay more than the predetermined amount. There are many variants of this model, including models where the clinic can make less money than the capitated amount and others where the insurance company can arrange to provide incentive payments to the provider of services if costs are kept below the capitated amount.

For example, if the capitated payment is $100,000 and the clinic "bills" for $80,000, the insurer can pay the clinic

$10,000 of that remaining $20,000 as an incentive to keep costs low. In sum, there are about as many different payment arrangements as insurance companies and, worse yet, about as many rules and forms.

The critical thing to remember here is that the design of your primary care behavioral health service will largely depend on how services are paid for. As such, some of the beginning homework for a new program is to catalog the insurers that pay for services for the primary care clinic, determine the payment arrangements that the clinic has with those insurers, and identify the relevant rules for that payment; this may sound daunting, and it certainly can be, but once you become well-versed in your particular patient population and its mix of payers, it will all make some sense. The beginning program director will often have to partner with a key member of the billing department or the organization's chief financial officer to put this information together and make sense of it.

However, it is essential to understand that medical clinics have existed in a very different business environment than mental health clinics. As such, their billing personnel often do not have ready answers or understanding about billing for mental health services. So, don't be surprised that you and the billing people will begin a learning process. And don't be surprised when billing people speak pessimistically or present obstacles to learning about these new processes. It may be a gross generalization, but it has been my experience that billing people are good rule followers but are not necessarily very good at investigating these things or being creative about developing or adapting systems. Doing this kind of work requires figuring out particular rules and identifying or creating loopholes (legal, of course) while building actual human relationships to bring it all together. (Check out this tool for more specific information on state-by-state billing practices and additional decision support.)

It may also surprise you to know that billing personnel may not have a handle on actual income received from payers. There are a variety of reasons for this that don't necessarily have to do with their incompetence. First, insurance companies make it challenging to submit claims for payment (which is why some specialties including many mental health professionals make patients do it). Each insurer also has their own systems. And many insurers deny claims for technical reasons (eg. wrong modifier codes). Add to that labyrinth the reality that payment can take weeks or months to get back to the practice and you have an inexact understanding at any given time as to how the business of the practice is actually doing. It is not uncommon, for example, for some payers to aggressively deny claims submitted to the tune of 50% or more of mental health claims denied. So, be nice to your billing people.

Final Pieces to the Payment Puzzle

Once you have figured out who the payers are and what some of their rules are, you have to figure out how each payer recognizes the providers of services it pays for. In other words, you have to begin the process of what is called credentialing your providers. Credentialing is simply the process by which a payer of services recognizes that a valid professional is providing services to their patients. So a behavioral health consultant may have a licensed clinical social worker license, but that does not mean that Blue Cross Blue Shield has credentialed that individual to work with their patients. This credentialing process often includes an application, background check, and approval process, which can take a significant amount of time.

Many organizations have administrative individuals who are in charge of helping their staff complete these credentialing applications. Some regions have consortiums or organizations that will organize credentialing information for such organizations and thus make it easier to apply to multiple payers. In either case, services will only be reimbursed if the insurance company recognizes the provider.

Another term similar to credentialing is called panel enrollment; this refers to this process where a provider of services becomes part of the set of authorized providers or panels within an insurance company's offerings to their customers; this can present somewhat of a quandary since theoretically, if you are on an insurance panel, any patient with that insurance could access your services. But of course, in the integrated model, the only people that should have access to services are patients of your particular clinic. Thus it is essential to have conversations with specific insurers during or before the application process so that they understand that you will not be accepting new patients from outside of your particular clinic.

In most cases, this is not an issue. You could even set up a screening process at your front door (your registration process) so that any patients who might see your name on the insurance website, for example, might be turned away when they attempt to make an appointment specifically with your behavioral health consultant. However, it is a good idea to discuss this with the insurer as they might get feedback from customers who are unhappy that they are being turned away. You don't want to get kicked off their insurance panel inadvertently.

Another word you may hear in this process is called privileging. Privileging is a process by which a provider of services' scope of practice is determined; this is perhaps easiest to identify in medicine. For example, there are medical providers who, by their training, perform specific procedures. So a medical provider in a primary care clinic may be privileged or allowed to perform particular procedures by the clinic under a pre-set of standards. Such procedures can be things like colposcopies. In the mental health world, privileging can include being authorized to do things such as perform psychological testing or engage in certain specific forms of treatment such as hypnosis or EMDR. For behavioral health consultants, privileging is usually not a vital issue, but it is helpful to understand the terminology if an insurance company or a clinic brings it up.

The other key issue to investigate with payers is whether they allow for and pose any barriers to warm handoffs. Since behavioral health consultation is centered on warm handoffs, with 50% or more of the patients seen coming via the warm handoff, it becomes essential to ensure that these same-day visits are reimbursable. Some insurance companies require 'prior authorizations' for service, which usually come with procedures and paperwork that must be followed before the behavioral health provider can see a patient. If this is the case, working with the payer to eliminate or modify their procedures will be essential. For example, we worked with a local insurer to allow us to see the patient first and then submit a shortened form for prior authorization after the fact; this made the prior authorization process doable within the constraints of our work day.

The key when talking with insurers is to explain the benefits of the model, many of which go very well with some of the goals of insurers, including preventing poor utilization of healthcare resources such as emergency departments and retaining as many patients in primary care as possible. It also helps to explain that patients in this model typically average one to three visits per patient, which makes one of the reasons for a prior authorization less relevant (many insurers use the process to determine an initial set of authorized visits, often less than six visits). In the end, as with any business deal, you want to create a win-win situation where the insurer gets what they need, but you also get what you need to ensure the model's integrity. It is also important to advocate with insurers based on the 2008 Mental Health Parity Act, which should outlaw most prior authorization procedures for outpatient mental health services.

Another potential barrier that sometimes applies to specific insurers, but most often applies to certain states and how they regulate Medicaid, is the prohibition of billing a medical and behavioral health visit on the same day (this can sometimes apply to a dental visit). This arbitrary and puzzling restriction means that if a patient has seen their primary care doctor and then sees a behavioral health professional, only one of those will be paid, irrespective of where those appointments occurred. I have yet to discern the precise reason or advantage of this rule. Fortunately, it only exists in a minority of states – but it is puzzling and severely damaging to integrated care efforts. In these cases, there is not much more one can do than attempt to lobby one's state representatives and decide to take a hit financially on unreimbursed same-day visits. It is essential to understand and distinguish that these are state rules, not federal rules.

While I have suggested that you investigate these issues in each instance, that does not mean one must have all these questions answered before beginning work. It would be ideal to do so, but in many cases, it is difficult to answer any of these questions, partly because often, the people working within these systems, whether private or public, don't know the answers. As a result, it is often the case that the best way of figuring out what the rules are is to play the game first and see what happens. In other words, seeing some patients and billing for those patients is a good way of figuring out what will and will not work. Working through those cases when they are not reimbursed can be the easiest way to diagnose the issues.

What All This Means For the Design of Your Model

 With all of this said, I don't want you to forget our central premise, which is that the integrity of the model and its singular focus on supporting primary care providers and creating access for patients through the flexibility of the behavioral health consultant should remain your central focus. So, by describing the reality of the current financial situation, I don't mean to imply strict conformity. In this respect, your mantra should be to skate where the metaphorical puck will be, not focus solely on where it is.

To this end, programs need to balance promoting encounter-based productivity and concentrate on the true metric of behavioral health consultation, namely population penetration. Let's take a few moments to flesh this out, considering how payment occurs today. A fee-for-service model, in particular, encourages encounter-based productivity; this is not antithetical to the behavioral health consultant model since a consultant, on average, should outperform a therapist in a well-functioning clinic. However, encounters are not an accurate measure of the core of the behavioral health consultant model, so a focus on encounters can derail program goals and confuse staff. But let's consider how you might assess income based on a fee-for-service approach.

If you work in an environment that is 100% insured (no uninsured patients), you have successfully credentialed all of your behavioral health consultants with insurers, and those insurers do not pose any obstacles for same-day warm handoffs, you can create a model with an estimate of productivity that should give you a reasonable estimate of your income potential. It would be helpful to do so with an understanding of the usual ramp-up time that is part of program development. In other words, given the above factors, you would potentially plan for the productivity of an average of 6 to 8 patients per day per behavioral health consultant for the first year and then plan for up to 10 patients per day per behavioral health consultant for subsequent years. Then all you need to know is how much the insurers pay for the relevant codes. The most commonly used code in most environments is 90832 - the 30-minute code - so this should be used in planning the business model. A key piece to consider when making such projections are hidden factors that can bring averages down, such as employee time off, administrative time, scheduled holidays, and variations in clinic productivity (for example, if there are certain days with few medical providers). While these factors may not seem like a lot, they can add up and significantly affect your bottom line.

Of course, many environments present challenges. You may work in an environment that has a percentage of uninsured patients. You may also work in environments with many payer sources, in which case it becomes a challenge to estimate which patients and in what proportion are likely to access behavioral health services. For example, let's imagine that 10% of your population has insurance through Medicare, 50% has insurance through one form of state Medicaid, 20% has insurance through another form of state Medicaid which does not cover behavioral health services, 5% of your population has private insurance primarily through four different insurance carriers, and the remaining are uninsured. You can imagine then the complexity of developing a model based on the various factors related to each payer and anticipating the utilization of the patient population.

In general, without any other form of data, you should be able to assume that behavioral health services will see a proportionate number of patients from each group. There's not much use in assuming that patients with one type of insurance will access services more than others, especially since you hope you are working with all kinds of patients in this generalist model.

One of the keys to developing the business model in this instance is identifying the impact of uninsured patients on your bottom line. With uninsured patients, assuming your clinic has a general policy for their billing, behavioral health services billing should be concurrent. In other words, if the policy at a clinic is that uninsured patients pay according to a sliding fee scale, then behavioral health services should fit along the same sliding fee scale. So you will have to determine the existing policy, project utilization, and income based on that information. Another critical issue to address is the issue of co-pays. At our clinics, we have dealt with the issue of co-pays by developing the philosophy that behavioral health consultation services comprise one aspect of all the possible services a patient may interface on a given medical visit. For example, the patient may see their primary care provider and visit our laboratory on the same day, but they will not be charged a separate co-pay for their visit to the lab.

In the same way, if the patient pays one co-pay for the medical visit, then we do not charge them a separate co-pay for a visit with the behavioral health consultant; this is particularly helpful in removing a barrier to a patient who may find themselves put off by having it announced to them in the room that if they want to see a behavioral health consultant, they will have to pay an additional $20; this, however, does not remove the co-pay obstacle for many insured patients. What will happen is that their insurance company will bill them after the fact for the co-pay amount; this makes it essential to have informed consent procedures at the time of registration (when a patient registers to become a patient of the medical clinic, not at the time of the medical visit) so that the patient understands their responsibilities. It is not an ideal situation by any stretch, but it is also not unusual in the crazy healthcare world we live in.

For example, I'm sure many readers have received bills after their appointments with charges on those bills that they knew nothing of at the time of the appointment. Since Access is a federally qualified health center, most patients don't encounter this co-pay issue, but a subset do, and occasionally Access has to work with the upset patient. And more often than not, the patients who are upset are not those who have co-pays to pay (patients are used to this by and large) but rather patients who do not know about their particular mental health coverage and have to pay the entirety of their visit (such as patients with high deductibles for mental health coverage).

As a reminder, while you will be building business models based on the reality of your payer mix and on encounter projections, in practice, the metric that should guide whether your program is developing well is the metric of population penetration. This metric is not a metric that will necessarily help your bottom line in a fee-for-service system, but it is a metric that can have a significant impact in a capitated model. As a reminder, population penetration is simply the number of unique patients who have seen behavioral health consultation services in a given time frame, divided by the total number of individual clinic patients, often expressed as a percentage.

In a capitated model, it is best to distribute resources across the entire population of patients who need those resources. In other words, you wouldn't want a few patients using up all of the resources, which is what can happen in a specialty model of care. The reasoning is that since you are entrusted with the care of the entire population, you want to ensure that everyone has access to timely and effective care. If you do an excellent job of this with a correct and efficient amount of resources (staffing efficiently, for example), then you will fulfill the terms of your capitated contract and turn a profit. For example, if you have $200,000 in staff costs (salary plus benefits) and capitated contracts that can net you $300,000, then you are doing well. Of course, the norm is that, more often than not, you're working in mixed environments where you have a mix of capitated and fee-for-service contracts, and each of these contracts may have different incentive-based payment structures; this is why no one has been able to figure out the perfect approach to funding integrated care models and why your job is to be as creative and innovative as possible in bending the current reality to the will of the core simplicity of this model. In short, never take no for an answer, never assume the present reality is immutable, and never forget that what you are attempting to accomplish is more important than rules created to preserve the current system.

As our explication of the ideal displayed, ultimately, population penetration will be the metric of the future, not encounters, but for now, you have to be well-versed in both. In addition, one of the errors that program directors make is to allow their teams to feel the pressure of the encounter-based present-day reality; this pulls the team in two directions. One force pulls them towards seeing more patients by filling slots, while the other pulls them towards simply being the best consultants they can be for their primary care providers. These are not necessarily antithetical, but they can be, and the pressure to see patients can be a corrosive influence on the team. As stated in this book, I never try to motivate my team based on encounters. My job as program director is to look at encounters and address the business component, not theirs. I want them to focus on being the best behavioral health consultants they can be and continue making themselves as accessible as possible in every way possible; this means that I highlight for them the pieces of their work that are not billable, such as the number of care management calls they make and the population penetration they have achieved at their respective clinics; this is what should drive your behavioral health consultants, not the mess of the current healthcare setup.

No matter your current setup, a key feature of your work as a program director will be to work with your local insurers. Within your organization, you'll have to develop a good relationship with your chief financial officer and often your chief executive officer. Additionally, getting to know the people who do billing for the organization and have expertise in this area will be critical. Some subset of those individuals in organizations usually create contracts with insurers, so they may already have relationships you can leverage.

In those cases, it will be helpful for you to sit down with them and formulate a plan of action, including collecting information on that insurer's current processes and procedures, what the prospects might be for contracting with them to provide mental health services and developing a best-guess business plan. I always focus on whether there are barriers to same-day warm handoffs, prior authorization requirements, and excessive paperwork (for example, paperwork for treatment initiation, treatment plan, and treatment discharge). Those are the real backbreakers. If those are in place, you want to collect that information, clarify it perhaps with phone calls or simply a patient test case, and then work with a contact at the insurer to discuss your concerns and see if you can generate possible solutions. In the case of Access in Madison, Wisconsin, in a reasonably small community, we only had to deal with one insurer who posed such barriers to warm handoffs. However, our chief financial officer had worked hard over the years to develop a good relationship with this insurer and was able to invite them to talk with us about these barriers. We learned why prior authorizations were a helpful feature for them, and they learned about our model, how it could potentially keep some of their costs down in the long run, and how we needed to provide patients with same-day access to do so. We worked out a compromise that included having us fill out the prior authorizations after seeing the patient. We included a reasonably efficient setup that used our electronic health record to send the reauthorization (so no dreaded faxing!).

In addition, they were willing to accept a key component of our model, our group management of patients. (Since our behavioral health consultants do not have individual panels, it would make no sense for the insurer to authorize visits for a patient with a specific behavioral health consultant). We were able to educate them about how we manage patients as a team. Thus with each authorization, all providers in our group were authorized to see that patient. We still had visit limits imposed, but even those were negotiated and generous enough that we rarely had to re-authorize care. After a few years, that insurer finally removed all prior authorization requirements. The moral of the story is that forming good relationships is essential. A sub-moral is that intelligent, practical, win-win processes for the payer and clinic often win out (assuming you continuously present the data and story as part of the relationship).

The primary strategy for a good program developer is to build something great, not wait for an invitation for it to be made. In other words, these details will not be worked out before the first patient is seen. Convincing others, including insurers, of the importance of this model to them and the patients is very difficult without having any lived experience to speak from. So while some planning is essential and helpful in developing a business model and setting up these arrangements with local insurers, the reality is that you must build and start working, which means taking on some risk and trying things before you know that they will work. The truth is this is how most businesses are built anyway. Therefore, although there might be a day when primary care behavioral health programs are so well-established as a standard of care nationally that one could develop a comprehensive business plan and have all of the variables predefined, that day will not arrive if clinics and programs do not take certain risks today. In today's environment, if your strategy is to wait until the climate changes, you will be waiting a long time.

Final Thought: Starting With "Free" Money

The section title should tip you off to the reality that there is no such thing as free money; this is true generally speaking of grants as well. Many primary care behavioral health programs developed today have started with private and public grant funds. Again, The key is to focus on the consultation service's mission rather than allowing funding sources to derail your core intentions. Therefore, choosing grants wisely and communicating bluntly with funders about your intentions is vital.

I've witnessed many clinics use grant funding that placed so many requirements on their staff that their access to providers and work satisfaction suffered significantly; this can take the form of reporting requirements, paperwork, cumbersome research protocols, etc. In addition, although grant funding can be an excellent way to get things started, the cushion provided by such funds sometimes keeps organizations from working as diligently on developing a sustainable strategy such as those discussed in this chapter. So, be wary of free money - because it is rarely free.

Table 1: Typical Billing Codes, PCBH & CoCM

Code	Description	Billing Parameters
Psychotherapy Codes		
90832	Individual psychotherapy, 30 minutes	Time-based code (16-37 minutes)
90834	Individual psychotherapy, 45 minutes	Time-based code (38-52 minutes)
90837	Individual psychotherapy, 60 minutes	Time-based code (53+ minutes)
90846	Family psychotherapy without the patient present	Time-based code (50 minutes)
90847	Family psychotherapy with the patient present	Time-based code (50 minutes)
90853	Group psychotherapy	Time-based code (90 minutes)
Health and Behavior Codes		
96150	Health and behavior assessment (e.g., HRA, screening)	Typically billed as a one-time service
96152	Health and behavior intervention, individual	Time-based code (16-37 minutes)

Code	Description	Billing Parameters
96153	Health and behavior intervention, group	Time-based code (90 minutes)
CoCM Codes		
99492	Initial psychiatric collaborative care management	First 70 minutes of service at initiation of care within first month
99493	Subsequent psychiatric collaborative care management	First 60 minutes of service in subsequent months
99494	Initial or subsequent psychiatric CoCM, add-on	Additional 30 minutes of service per month
99484	General behavioral health integration	Billed once per patient per month for 20 minutes of care management work

Chapter 14: Financial Skills

By Neftali Serrano, PsyD

There are some basic skills that you may not have been taught overtly in graduate training which nonetheless are crucial for managing programs. Here we will review a few of them and present some of the tools you need to navigate your team's budget.

Budgeting

Every organization has a budgeting process which you need to become familiar with. Some organizations have a structured way of determining the upcoming budget, but not all do. An interesting question to ask administrators is how exactly a budget gets put together. Often, few people know the mechanics, and fewer still likely know why. Regardless, it is often true that the Chief Financial Officer and the accounting department provide the parameters for the budget, most often based on the organization's performance in the previous year. Some organizations have a more democratic process of developing their budgets with input from department heads. Others include only a few key players in deciding their budgets.

Behavioral health consultants should be more leaned upon to help put a budget together. So, as quickly and politically expedient as possible, a new behavioral health consultant should become familiar with how the organization runs; this does not mean that the behavioral health consultant needs to have a seat at the table right away. Often, this takes some time as the organization develops trust, knowledge, and experience related to the model of care. However, learning allows the behavioral health consultant to speak the organization's language and understand key stakeholders' thinking. The error many mental health professionals make is sticking their heads in the sand and complaining when productivity demands are made of them. A knowledgeable behavioral health consultant can shape the destiny of the primary care behavioral health program. A whiny behavioral health consultant has no power.

A critical factor in understanding the budget is that these documents have multiple purposes, audiences, and data sources. Budgets are one of many accounting tools for an organization that helps to allocate funds, provide transparency to external groups (such as a board or auditors), and provide direction to staff regarding organizational priorities. In their raw form, budgets are often difficult to understand except to their creators. A significant amount of translation is necessary to understand the document, which means asking many questions, even if they sound dumb.

Budgets have basic elements, including the inputs and outputs of the organization. The inputs represent the organization's sources of income; the outputs represent the organization's costs. Each category will have subcategories, including recurring or one-time line items and specific line items for administrative and clinical expenditures.

The budget associated with primary care behavioral health services will often mimic the budget for medical providers, and many organizations treat them as the same. You will have staffing costs (salary plus benefits), expected income per provider (by FTE), administrative overhead, and a bottom-line expectation of net result (profit or loss). Administrative overhead can include various line items that may not make much sense or even specifically apply to the program because budgets often have an equal arbitrary division of overhead costs (space, supplies, administrative support) for each department or staff. Nonetheless, the PCBH model intends to be slim and trim financially, so it may be worth reviewing how these charges are allocated to ensure that they do not unfairly affect the costs associated with the team. For example, PCBH does not require additional registration staff support in most instances.

Another language to learn when reading budgets is the language of charges, encounters, and net revenue. Charges refer to the billable work that a behavioral health consultant engages in; this differs from the amount of money the organization brought in or expected to bring in. An organization may bill for a service but not get paid, and a charge is what the organization bills for. Reasons for not getting paid include individuals not willing to pay, insurers not willing to reimburse, billing errors, or a differential between what an organization sets as its price for a service and what an insurer will pay. In community health centers, this is especially important, as the number of individuals who are self-pay or uninsured is exceptionally high, so there will be a significant difference between charges and actual income. The net revenue is the actual income minus the costs associated with the service. Ideally, you want this to be positive. Most often, in the current financial environment, you are doing great if you break even.

Finally, encounters are the face-to-face billable visits that a behavioral health consultant has with patients. It is important to remember that the budget represents only the work the organization does, which is directly billable; this means that telephone encounters, unbillable visits such as well-child visits, care management work, etc., are not represented in the budget; your job will be to find other ways of helping the organization remain aware of this other valuable work that is going on. At Access, we did that by tracking metrics, reporting on them at least annually, and celebrating milestones (e.g., "We've made our 1,000th care management call!").

Figure 1 provides an example of an Access budget. Contextually, it is crucial to understand that while the organization cares about financial solvency, it does not think of the behavioral health service as an independent service but rather an extension of its primary care services. As such, financially, they do not place an undue amount of pressure on the service to sustain itself; this is a very progressive stance that has paid off on multiple levels for the organization. Financially, the robust nature of the service has resulted in community attention (positive) for the organization, external funding (United Way grants), and interest in collaboration from community insurers and providers. And, perhaps most importantly, the service has been responsible for keeping many of its providers sane while working with a very complex, often seriously mentally ill population.

The PCBH service began as a budget-negative entity and worked toward positive net revenue, including grants and fee-for-service activity. The organization is focused on its margin, the bottom line differential between revenue and costs, which usually runs between 2-4%. It is not a large margin, but the behavioral health service alone does not jeopardize that margin. This attitudinal stance is vital for organizations in this in-between time of payment reform. Until the costs of integrated behavioral health services are funded on a global payment system bundled with medical care, most programs will have numbers like those in the figure. Each program will progress at different rates, but a well-functioning program can often reach budget neutrality in 2-5 years. Of note the budget presented in the figure shows deficits in large part due to investments Access made in expanding FTE and staffing. The payoff (in terms of increased billing revenue) is expected to more than make up for the losses shown.

When looking at budget actuals, especially when you have a net deficit, it is vital to identify the specific causes of that deficit. These can include situational variables that inflate costs in a given year, staff outages, or other variables. One clear nuts and bolts skill to accomplish the above analyses is working with spreadsheets. The most commonly used is Excel, but Apple has a program called Numbers for more basic needs, which I prefer for light-duty analysis. Excel is much better for really complex or large files. I never went to school to work with spreadsheets, so don't let a lack of formal training deter you. Play with the programs and figure out how to get the information you want out of it. Another good strategy is to ask someone in your organization with good experience with these programs to tutor you. One universal truth is that all organizations have at least one expert in Excel and that these experts typically love to share their knowledge about how Excel works. Almost all financial data eventually ends up in an Excel spreadsheet, so ignore it at your peril.

A couple of tools will help you in your journey toward building the financial infrastructure of your program. A financial planning tool like this one created by the National Council can be a helpful generic start. When you are ready to get down and dirty for a more granular analysis, this tool designed by psychologist and financial guru Lesley Manson can help you create a pro forma (expected financial performance). Additionally, this CFHA session led by Mary Jean Mork, LCSW is a good place to start learning about the basics of billing.

It's Still About People, Stupid

Ex-President Bill Clinton had a saying in the Oval Office that it was the "Economy Stupid!" Well, the most basic nuts and bolts skill for managing finances is still about "People, Stupid." Building relationships with stakeholders to understand and interpret their concerns and agendas and educate yourself about the functioning of the entire organization is the most basic and essential skill; this requires spending time with key players, formally and informally. One of the things I started doing with some of my administrative time was spending it camped out in a central conference room at Access' administrative offices (which are apart from our clinics). I did this to be available to have unscheduled face-to-face time with individuals. Note that I am not talking about manipulating individuals for your purposes but rather taking a learning posture and building genuine relationships of trust. The more you learn about others and create that trust, the more common understanding and common goals you will share with them. One of my most important relationships at Access was with the CFO, Joanne Holland, and she became a champion of PCBH and worked with me and the subsequent Chief Behavioral Health Officer to grow the program.

Together Joanne and I took risks. Risk is an essential concept in business; this is both a financial factor in business development and an emotional factor. Successful companies take risks because of a sense of internal trust and confidence, usually a combination of trust and confidence in their product and talent. Unsuccessful companies either take foolhardy risks or no risk at all. When it comes time for your organization to take risks, relationships of trust will need to be in place, and shared values and understandings about the nature of the business will need to be present to make those difficult decisions.

So, spend time formally and informally with people within your organization. Also, do so with key financial stakeholders outside of your organization. Access to insurance personnel, other healthcare partners in the community, etc., may not reap benefits immediately, but these connections are worth their weight in gold over time. And it's okay to feel intimidated by them and not to understand everything they talk about; they might feel the same way about you. Just hang around long enough, and you'll get it.

Figure 1. Exemplar Budget

	December			Prior Year Monthly Actual	Year to Date			Prior Year YTD
	Actual	Budget	Variance		Actual	Budget	Variance	
Operating Revenue								
Net patient revenue	63,648	84,988	(21,340)	117,452	448,656	542,008	(93,352)	572,868
Total Operating Revenue	63,648	84,988	(21,340)	117,452	448,656	542,008	(93,352)	572,868
Expenses								
Personnel	117,624	117,731	107	106,299	707,298	741,419	34,121	653,558
Fringe benefits	31,858	40,347	8,489	33,125	169,078	184,118	15,040	172,853
Facilities and space	2,724	2,586	(138)	2,467	13,408	15,168	1,760	13,993
Other	848	2,696	1,848	1,166	23,776	16,176	(7,600)	13,847
Supplies	21	6	(15)	56	185	75	(110)	694
Contractual	775	958	183	835	5,275	5,868	593	6,100
Equipment	81	153	72	163	681	822	141	1,031
Travel	-	168	168	-	7	555	548	-
Uncollectible patient accounts	439	-	(439)	3,544	3,618	174	(3,441)	34,777
Admin Support Allocation	26,642	23,830	(2,812)	21,695	162,589	158,837	(3,752)	131,287
Clinic Support Allocation	17,290	15,504	(1,786)	20,222	89,394	95,578	6,184	121,674
Total Expenses	198,301	203,979	5,678	189,573	1,175,305	1,218,790	43,485	1,149,814
Operating Income (Loss)	(134,652)	(118,991)	(15,661)	(72,121)	(726,649)	(676,782)	(49,867)	(576,947)
Nonoperating Income								
Federal grant	44,112	47,793	(3,681)	32,947	206,683	223,895	(17,212)	206,718
Community benefit grant	30,531	30,531	-	29,007	183,188	180,354	2,834	174,044
Fundraising revenue	-	-	-	100	-	-	-	200
Other revenue	-	-	-	-	14	-	14	84
Total Nonoperating Income	74,643	78,324	(3,681)	62,054	389,885	404,249	(14,364)	381,046
Net Profit (Loss)	(60,009)	(40,667)	(19,342)	(10,067)	(336,764)	(272,533)	(64,231)	(195,901)
Encounters	396	444	48	553	2,697	2,799	102	2,905
NPR per Encounter	$161	$191	$30	$212	$166	$194	$28	$197
Cost per Encounter	$500	$459	(541)	$336	$434	$435	$1	$384

Note that budget format may be quite different across organizations, but the categories will be typical. Familiarizing yourself with the budget and it's parts and definitions is work you need to do in order to advocate for the PCBH service.

Chapter 15: Introduction To Special Populations

By Chantelle Thomas, PhD

I came to work in the BHC model due to my interest in primary care settings, particularly the intersection of medical and psychological factors. I came from a family of physicians and observed the high percentage of mental health needs that my father, as a family physician, addressed with his patients. Additionally, I have always been interested in doctor-patient communication styles and how information is conveyed in medical settings. As a result, I chose health psychology as my specialty track and area of interest during my graduate school training.

Previous to my work in primary care, my clinical experiences stemmed from residential substance abuse treatment, traditional outpatient therapy, and medical/surgical inpatient consultations. I have always been interested in adopting a collaborative multidisciplinary approach. Still, I have often felt frustrated with the need for proper integration in treatment planning and patient management in other settings. Working with varied medical disciplines in a primary care setting provides a unique opportunity to observe individuals in different environments, in real-time, when dealing with varying issues of life. When working closely with a physician, nurse, or midwife, I can see an individual through another provider's eyes and gather a new perspective on their coping and what matters to each patient.

While working as a consultant in the hospital setting, I was rarely able to speak to providers face to face. Most importantly, I rarely had the experience that what I said mattered or would significantly impact their treatment planning. Several unique aspects of our model aim to facilitate improved integration between medical providers and the BHC team. The immediate "warm handoff" (involving direct discussion between BHC and provider) and the abbreviated length of our patient sessions allow me to consult, meet, and develop an individualized treatment plan in less than 30 minutes. This time-sensitive consult also enables the provider to personally "wrap up" with the patient to incorporate our impressions, inform treatment, and reinforce recommendations.

It is no secret that mental health work, in general, can be challenging, demanding, and draining. So why would I choose to work in a setting that treats individuals with the least resources and harrowing psychosocial barriers? The group of providers surrounding me. Having worked in various "team" settings, I have come to appreciate and distinguish the difference between a true team approach and merely working with other clinicians in the same facility. What initially brought me to Access was a curiosity about the PCBH model. What largely kept me at Access was the experience of working in a supportive, integrated care environment where I felt valued and respected. As a result, I discovered how many professional and personal growth opportunities come from working with this population when an extraordinary team genuinely supports you. The authentic compassion of our medical providers and their desire to be of service to the underserved is infectious. Day after day, I could witness the brilliant and dedicated people who cared deeply about their patients and were devoted to improving their quality of life. The fast pace of our setting requires a level of energy that is only sustained by efficiency. We don't work in isolation; our very job title implies collaboration. To remain relevant, your accessibility must keep pace with that of your primary care providers; this requires constant "on the fly" skill development to hone and tailor your craft. You don't have three to six sessions to gather your first impression of a patient. The provider referring you to the patient awaits your impressions and recommendations today.

Don't Short-Change Your Ability To Make A Difference As A Team

While initially daunting, this dynamic, symbiotic relationship between the provider and myself can be exhilarating. In doing this work, you also realize the powerful impact that one present-focused, 20-minute visit can have on those without anyone else listening in their life. This work has led me to appreciate the resiliency and the tremendous need of marginalized people. It has dramatically shaped my sense of duty and drive to advocate for those in greatest need. Not to mention, it offered invaluable cultural exposure to the range of diverse challenges unique to the underserved. This work continually reminds me that we all desire the same things at the end of the day: to be heard, respected, and valued.

Working in our setting has significantly shaped my clinical practice by choice and necessity. When you don't have the luxury of a 60-minute visit or the default of weekly sessions (though this appears to be a fading reality in traditional outpatient mental health as well), you are forced to zero in on critical and relevant information with a different form of intensity. Sometimes, this has resulted in taking risks in my sessions that I would have otherwise second-guessed; this means rapport is immediately essential, and our contacts must quickly arrive at patient-relevant conclusions or insights. Many patients we met did not attend the clinic intending to talk to a therapist or counselor. Additionally, they may hold concerns about the meaning of "going to therapy" or fear the stigma of being labeled "crazy." Many patients may lack the funds, and the time, have more pressing life issues and believe things are "not bad enough" to warrant therapy. Consequently, many patients are ambivalent about whether treatment is needed or helpful.

In my sessions, I have learned (and continue to learn) how to constantly recalibrate what is needed within the context of what the patient is ready for. Allowing myself to be genuinely authentic and using humor at times can provide excellent opportunities to defuse a patient's natural defenses to being "in therapy." Additionally, working with individuals who live in survival mode has taught me how to address my patient's highest values and needs. This realization led me to expand the scope of my knowledge and interventions into "social work" territory. Understanding and recognizing relevant community resources allows me to ensure that our patient's basic needs are not ignored. I have learned that sometimes less overtly sophisticated interactions can provide a platform for important therapeutic change. When I help patients understand their resistance to "calling the food bank," I can increase their insight while addressing their avoidance (by calling in the room). Ultimately, I need to know what food bank exists in their area and how to reach them best; this need led to developing flexible software solutions for housing referral information.

In doing this work, I have realized that the most critical intervention you make is the intervention that happens. I cannot spend my time and energy developing an elaborate treatment plan because a treatment plan only works if the patient returns. I often ask myself, who is this intervention for? Is it crafted for what I think is needed, or is it tailored to the patient's expressed needs? I have often had to scale back the extensive list of things that I believe should or must change and identify one thing, at this moment, that could change. Interventions must be practical and functionally driven because many of our patients are not invested in the "theory of change" but rather in the reality of what will feel different or change in real time.

Expand Your Knowledge Of Psychopharmacology

I have always been interested in psychopharmacology as a fascinating facilitator of change and treatment. I love the science and mechanisms of medication, but most importantly, I have learned that medication is only part of the equation. Increasing my familiarity with the mechanisms of action, categories, side effects, and monitoring precautions has provided me with a valuable currency in the primary care world. It allows me to provide helpful consultation and informed discussions about how we understand the role of medication for patients. When an anxious patient asks solely for a benzodiazepine, my working knowledge of various anxiolytics allows me to offer relevant alternatives that do not reinforce anxiety avoidance. It has aided me in raising awareness and questions about the intent and goal of polypharmacy that are often overlooked due to more pressing medical issues.

Additionally, it has facilitated more targeted functional discussions with patients about how they view the role of their medication. Once again, a discussion about "Are you taking your medication" can be unfolded to reveal so much about a patient. A patient's approach to medication can inform the patient's view of themselves, their ability to consistently implement behavior change, their environment, their cognitive capacity, and their understanding of their condition.

You Don't Have To Be An Expert In Special Populations To Work With Them

Soon after I began working at Access, Neftali officially tasked me with identifying strategies for treating "specialty populations" at Access. I soon discovered that almost every patient at Access could be classified as falling within a special population! Everything we do at Access hinges on understanding the most pressing concerns of our providers. Observing our providers in action, I see them often most challenged by our patients with:

1. Severe and persistent mental illness
2. Co-morbid drug and alcohol issues
3. Chronic pain

Fortunately, I had a fair amount of experience working with two of these populations in particular (chronic pain and drug and alcohol treatment) based on my previous training experiences. The SPMI population was relatively new to me, and developing an understanding of the best strategies for working with this group of patients was primarily informed by my knowledge of community treatment programs and resources; once again, developing community resource maps was essential. Additionally, unique aspects of the mental health treatment culture in Dane County presented us with unexpected challenges (I will elaborate on this later).

I developed my first clinical exposure to alcohol and drug treatment while obtaining my master's in psychology at Pepperdine University, amongst Malibu's numerous residential treatment centers that line the Pacific Coast. Through a fellow student at Pepperdine, I started volunteering at a dual-diagnosis residential treatment center. This experience was invaluable in leading me to understand better the various modalities utilized for substance use treatment, including group, milieu therapy, individual therapy, and community-based sobriety groups. Additionally, my father (a general practitioner) was one of the first physicians in the United States licensed as an addictive medicine specialist. My father decided to pursue licensure in addiction medicine because he observed how many patients sought help for problematic alcohol or drug use in primary care. I can recall having or overhearing so many conversations growing up about the nature of drug and alcohol addiction and treatment. My father's knowledge provided an invaluable and seminal training ground for my learning.

While working at the dual diagnosis center, I began developing a strong base of compassion and a deeper understanding of how to support the healing process of drug addicts and alcoholics. I was often inspired by the resilience, compelled by the "larger than life" personalities, and amazed by the resourcefulness of these individuals who were often mislabeled as selfish. I came to appreciate the high co-morbidities of untreated depression, bipolar disorder, and trauma found in this population. So many of these individuals believed the only way to survive painful feelings was through the numbing of alcohol and drug use.

This training experience helped me to realize the tremendous societal need for better-informed and educated clinicians. After watching the devastation from countless years of self-destructive substance use, I recognized the necessity of identifying those suffering so much earlier. Patient's primary care homes could allow them to speak openly to trusted professionals who would not judge or minimize their struggles. In working with those in recovery, I was also acquiring an invaluable skill that would serve me well in behavioral health consulting: the ability to authentically and compassionately voice what is painful while supporting empowering opportunities for change. My experiences helped me learn how to empathically identify (sometimes with humor) entrenched patterns of avoidance and reveal that so many excuses perpetuate unnecessary suffering.

Demystifying Chronic Pain & Substance Abuse

My first exposure to chronic pain populations came through my graduate training program. I opted for the Health Psychology track, which provided the opportunity for the necessary curriculum, training, and clinical experience to become a biofeedback practitioner. In these classes, I learned about the high percentage of individuals seeking treatment for chronic pain conditions through primary care. In this training program, I began to appreciate the limitations of Western medicine for managing chronic conditions.

My graduate program offered an internship rotation through the Sharp Multidisciplinary Pain Clinic in San Diego, California. During my internship year at Sharp, I was exposed to a multidisciplinary program that local referring physicians heavily utilized as a tool to improve patients' functioning and decrease their reliance on narcotics; our treatment team at Sharp involved health psychologists, a physical medicine and rehabilitation physician, and a physical and occupational therapist. This program relied heavily on education, medication management, and behavioral interventions (such as water therapy, biofeedback, massage, and relaxation techniques) to shift patients' reliance on narcotics as the sole treatment modality. This training also taught me how to understand better patients who developed narcotic dependence without addiction or aberrant drug behaviors. My sessions with patients titrating down their narcotic regimens also highlighted the extent to which patients (often unintentionally) medicate their emotions.

As I mentioned, my exposure to the SPMI population came through the relatively high percentage of patients seen at Access meeting criteria for these diagnoses. I came to appreciate how the complexity of these patients' mental health needs often removes the need for referral to more traditional outpatient mental health settings. Additionally, I observed how many individuals in greatest need of community, federal, and state assistance were least capable of obtaining it. Many of these patients struggle with few resources, homelessness, active mental health symptoms, and no transportation, making it impossible to follow through with scheduled referrals/appointments to other agencies.

Despite their interpersonal struggles (often marked by paranoia), I also observed the deep bonds and trust that many of these patients experienced with their primary care providers; for some individuals, their doctor/patient relationships were the most meaningful and sustained in their life. I also observed our providers' great need for consultation when making important decisions about which patients were appropriate for management in primary care. We at Access continue to work on models for determining the needed level of care, what services the patient's insurance (or lack thereof) entitles them to, and, most importantly, the patient's motivation for additional services. We developed a patient severity grid to serve as a visual and informational guide for making treatment decisions based on each patient's varying levels of complexity.

ADHD As A Special Population

Also falling under the umbrella of specialty populations are patients presenting with reports of attention deficit with or without hyperactivity. By its very nature, a primary care setting is the first line of referral for intervention, assessment, and diagnosis of problematic behavior and attention concerns. When schools and parents are concerned about a child struggling to succeed in school, they are sent to their physician for further evaluation; this provides a valuable opportunity for intervention on multiple levels extending well beyond medication. These clinical complaints of inattention and problem behavior are often unpacked to reveal relevant information about mood, anxiety, trauma, and the individual's home environment.

I have observed provider challenges in deciding psychostimulant prescribing in children and adolescents but have found decisions about adults to be even more perplexing due to several other complicating factors. In a subsequent section, I will elaborate on some of the strategies and approaches we have developed for dealing with the complexities inherent to this diagnostic category.

Career And Personal Growth Related To Working With Challenging Populations

Before joining Access, I recently completed a postdoctoral fellowship at the University of Wisconsin Hospital Clinics. My work there was primarily focused on providing medical-surgical consultation to patients in the inpatient medical hospital setting. One day per week of my fellowship was devoted to primary care behavioral health consultation at

Access. As I began looking for employment opportunities, I became aware of available hospital positions and Access positions. One factor that made my decision relatively easy was Access' offering of a very reasonable and competitive wage for early career psychologists.

Additionally, as a federally-qualified health center, employment at Access offered student loan repayment, a strong incentive due to my accrued graduate school loans. During my fellowship Access rotation, I found the pace demanding and the patient population often in various forms of crisis. I knew this work could take a significant emotional toll on me, but I could also feel my skill level and competence deepening. Most importantly, at Access, I knew I would never bear the sole burden of responsibility for caring for my patients. I had an excellent, compassionate, intelligent group of medical providers and behavioral health consultants who were "in it" with me daily. I deeply respected the clinicians I worked with and connected deeply with the sense of meaning the work for the underserved provided. Access was an environment where my impressions would be valued and used to inform treatment decisions.

Knowing the challenges of the pace and intensity inherent to BHC work, I learned my self-care was not only invaluable but essential to the sustainability of my work. I also realized previously effective "stress relievers" no longer functioned as decompression outlets. I became fiercely protective of my private time and did not overcommit to social outings. Once a highly social person, I discovered that I craved silence during my downtimes (much to my and my husband's surprise). I found regular exercise, yoga in particular, was an absolute necessity.

When Neftali introduced the option for using Skype between our clinics for consultation with each other, I questioned the utility. I could not have been more wrong. I have learned an essential antidote to burnout is not sharing the patient burden alone. Consult, consult, consult. With my most challenging cases, I had the luxury of consulting with talented, professional, non-judgmental, and supportive clinicians (face to face, regardless of location, thanks to Skype).

Additionally, I learned that attending to my emotional health was essential to my resiliency. That meant having regular involvement in therapy. Knowing I have dedicated time to process my internal struggles helps insulate personal issues from unintentionally seeping into my work. Regular sleep also became paramount; when my sleep levels are depleted, so are my internal reserves, and my therapeutic "center" is challenged. Having an excellent social support network and time away from work (without checking my inbox or email) for travel and decompression often restores my stamina while refueling my reserves immeasurably.

In the day-to-day moments, I found different strategies for keeping myself grounded amid the pace and stress of a workday. I came into work feeling fueled (fed, rested, exercised, etc.) and ready to see patients. I tried to arrive early. I found that on days when I arrived on time or late, I felt set back for the entire day; consequently, my frustration and tolerance levels were directly impacted. I tried not to let my notes accumulate. Unfinished notes from the day before are sometimes unavoidable but will impose stress and pressure that ultimately permeates your current work day. I learned to become comfortable with strategies such as documenting in the room with patients to reduce my note-writing times. With certain consults, I kept with the pace of the day by having my note virtually finished before I left the exam room.

I did not hesitate to consult with my colleagues about challenging cases to provide me with alternative perspectives or immediate feedback about my impressions. I remembered how invaluable humor can be during times of exasperation. I tried to be mindful of how I labeled my experience. A hectic day can be viewed as miserable or, if you choose, as exciting and stimulating. I tried to remind myself that I could set limits when I felt over my head (sometimes, this means saying no to a provider for a face-to-face consult, making it a curbside instead, or clarifying your timeline). I recognized that my ultimate goal was to do no harm. It helps to realize sometimes, it's okay to be a "good enough" behavioral health consultant.

Learn To Communicate With Medical Providers By Learning Their Experience Of Caring For Challenging Patients

Coming from a family of physicians, I realized my family background directly shaped my communication strategies with medical providers. I learned to temper my ability to wax eloquent and get to the point. There is an art to relaying information in a concise, relevant manner, highlighting only what is essential to your provider. No provider will consult if consulting with you consistently delays their work cycle. Shape your communication style by carefully studying your providers and what matters to them. Some providers want to hear details about an individual's psychosocial history; others, not so much. With certain providers, I know my medication knowledge has been central to their confidence in my ability and competence. At the same time, other providers appreciate my emphasis on behavioral strategies.

Medical providers care deeply about their patients, and they want to help. They are eager to provide a patient with something to alleviate their suffering. As a result providers often lack the skill of delivering a compassionate "no." This is an area that needs improvement. How do we empathically offer care when we believe the patient's request (or demand) is inappropriate? In my experience, these struggles are almost surrounding medication. This conflict can become even more significant when we (or the provider) know medication could temporarily relieve the patient's ailing issue. I believe an invaluable role for behavioral health consultants is to share the burden of difficult decisions and uncomfortable conversations with providers. As a team, behavioral health consultants and providers can more fully fulfill the mission of primary care even with the most complex patients.

With those generalities in mind, we now focus on the specific categories of patients in complex populations most likely to present in primary care.

A Personal Update From The Author

Chantelle left Access to pursue her passion for working with patients with trauma and substance abuse as Executive Clinical Director at Windrose Recovery, a comprehensive treatment facility in the midwest.

About the Author

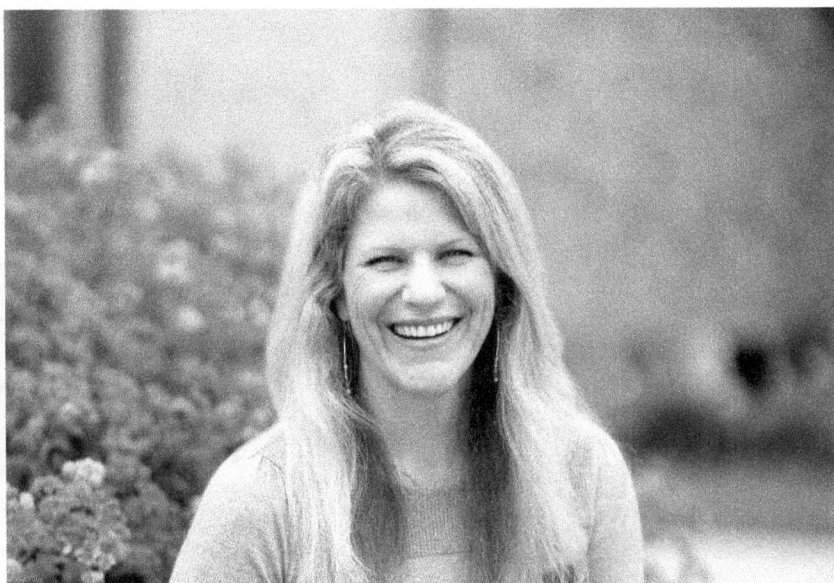

Chantelle Thomas, PhD, is a licensed Health Psychologist and has worked for the past 15 years in a range of different environments that include outpatient, residential, and hospital based settings. Her current endeavors include clinical research, consulting, and direct patient care primarily in the domains of trauma work and substance use disorders. Additionally, Dr. Thomas has been engaged in clinical research exploring the therapeutic use of psychedelics over the last 10 years through the University of Wisconsin-Madison, working as a therapist, educator, and consultant in this space. She is deeply passionate about treatments that address and dismantle problematic health care and diagnostic biases that unwittingly contribute to shame and isolation for those who seek healing and recovery. She loves skiing with her two girls, performing with her local band, and traveling with her family.

Chapter 16: Substance Abuse In Primary Care

By Chantelle Thomas, PhD with edits from Meghan Fondow, PhD

B arriers exist to accessing substance use treatment, similar to mental health treatment, leading patients to present to primary care for assistance in treating substance use concerns, including opioid use disorder (OUD) and alcohol use disorder (AUD). These factors led Dr. Randy Brown, family medicine physician and addiction medicine specialist, to begin an outpatient addiction medicine service (Health Promotions Clinic or HPC) within one of our Access clinics around 2010. The HPC provides ongoing, specialized treatment to patients interested in changing their alcohol and drug use but who may not 1) be ready for more intensive treatment and 2) have access to treatment. The HPC was a forerunner to the office-based Medication Assisted Treatment (MAT) care available within our Access clinics as more providers have sought out training for MAT and data waivers to prescribe suboxone (no longer required).

The HPC has undergone many changes. Initially, it was the only resource for MAT within our clinics. The Behavioral Health Consultants (BHC) would assist in providing referrals to HPC in collaboration with medical providers when patients motivated for MAT were identified during clinic visits. We gathered information regarding patients' history, current use, motivation for change, and treatment history and screened for any comorbid mental health concerns. The HPC team (consisting of the Addiction Medicine Specialist, a BHC Lead, and resident trainees) reviewed the referrals and determined suitability for the clinic. If the severity of the concerns were determined to be beyond the scope of primary care, the recommendation would be for patients to seek care in specialty outpatient substance use treatment, often with visits with BHC as interim support. If patients were not beyond the severity criteria, they would be scheduled directly with the HPC team, which met weekly or bi-weekly with patients, depending on the need. Patients would meet directly with the addiction medicine physician and often the BHC team to provide MAT and behavioral interventions.

In recent years, more and more primary care physicians have been interested in providing MAT and have completed the required training to get their data waivers to prescribe suboxone for OUD. Now, many more patients can receive MAT directly within primary care. The HPC team has served as a resource for consultation, assisting primary care providers with specific questions for patients they are seeing in the clinic. Referrals to HPC are now focused on the more complex cases.

There are several essential components to improve the treatment and management of substance use populations in a primary care setting, beginning with patient identification. Generally speaking, the more severe the drug and alcohol addiction, the easier it is to identify, but not consistently. Even patients who are not suspected of having problems with drug or alcohol use can be profoundly suffering. It is essential to ask all patients about their substance use at some point in their care journey.

At Access, we have a universal screening protocol for adults that consists of administering the AUDIT-C and the NIDA screening questions to screen for alcohol and substance use and misuse. Patients complete the full AUDIT and DAST measures if either or both are positive. These can further provide information about a patient's use, combined with BHC and primary care visits, to assess the patient's use status and severity.

Currently, when a primary care provider meets with a patient and substance use concerns are identified either through our annual universal screening or during the visit, the BHC team is likely to receive a handoff to collaborate in the patient's care. The BHC will implement brief interventions for patients to educate and provide a better understanding of their patterns of use, typical triggers, relapse reduction strategies, and environmental factors contributing to their use cycle. Part of this process may often involve accurately identifying and treating comorbid mental health conditions previously untreated.

For patients ready and interested in pursuing outpatient specialized drug and alcohol treatment, our team members can provide options for treatment in the community based on their needed level of care and insurance status. Our Behavioral Health Care Coordinators can assist with connecting patients with resources, making calls with patients, and checking in on the status of connections. We often provide patients with resources outlining options for sober living, outpatient treatment, and community recovery support groups (AA, smart recovery, etc.).

Initially, our most high-risk substance-abusing patients were referred to the HPC, regardless of their readiness for treatment, to evaluate their candidacy for MAT and harm reduction strategies and to provide medical providers with a clearer picture of the severity of their diagnosis. Currently, this is done on a case-by-case basis, depending on the comfort of the primary care provider. Therefore, if a patient is seen with high-risk substance use, the medical provider can request a referral to HPC (see Table 2 for note template BHCs use for referral), where the patient may be seen once or multiple times before transitioning back to primary care. Examples of complexities might include pregnant individuals, adults with severe use and small children, IV drug users, and individuals who are physiologically dependent with complicated detoxification histories. The HPC team is currently the only option if patients are interested in Sublocade, the injected buprenorphine that lasts 3-4 weeks.

With many of these complex patients, the HPC team will provide continued contact for treatment readiness until they are ready for more intensive treatment. These patients continue their general medical care through their primary care clinic and retain their primary care provider while having ongoing access to BHCs at their primary care clinic home. In the interim, we often also facilitate the involvement of other treatment resources (family support agencies, housing assistance, community support agencies) to mitigate risk or harm while eliminating some factors contributing to the cycle of use.

Hopefully, it is clear to the reader why we gave the clinic its name. Our approach to substance abuse issues in our patient population is centered on a harm reduction philosophy and, even more, an essential primary care approach. In short, we treat substance abuse as a chronic health condition. In doing so, we respect our patients and equip all our staff to work with patients suffering from addiction.

In our case, our journey began with the interests of a family medicine provider turned addiction medicine specialist. Your journey may start with an effort to start or expand MAT services or screen patients with the above screeners. In either case, adopting the cultural harm reduction framework will be the key to your success. Once you adopt a chronic disease mindset as a team, establishing clinical workflows, policies, and procedures will be seamless and often uncomplicated; this does not mean you will not encounter challenging patient situations or thorny ethical issues. However, these are surmountable if you all share a solid philosophical framework centered on harm reduction and chronic disease management as the primary goal of care.

Table 2. HPC Referral Note (Embedded In Full BHC Note)

Note Element	Choices
Statement of purpose	Patient here for referral to Health Promotions Clinic for consideration of medication for {Opioid Use/Alcohol Use:51165} disorder and verbally consented to meet with BHC. Pt reported the following symptoms/concerns:
Current Use	Substance drop-down Method of intake drop-down Duration of use drop-down
Severity of Illness	Drop-down for severity indicator
Impaired Control	Yes, No, Needs More Assessment (for each of the below) Larger amounts or longer than intended Persistent desire or attempts to cut down or stop Excessive time using, getting, recovering Craving
Social Impairment	Yes, No, Needs More Assessment (for each of the below) Failure to fulfill a major role Continued use despite social/interpersonal conflicts Withdrawal from activities

Note Element	Choices
Risky Use	Yes, No, Needs More Assessment (for each of the below) Use in physically hazardous situations Use despite knowing it's doing harm
Pharmacological (for abuse of prescription medications)	Yes, No, Needs More Assessment (for each of the below) Tolerance Withdrawal
Severity indicator (score above items marked Yes)	Mild: 2-3; Moderate: 4-5; Severe: 6+
Duration/ Trajectory or History of Use	Free text
Trigger for Use	Free text
What happens when you don't use/ withdrawal symptoms?	Symptom drop down
History of OD/ hospitalization	Yes/No
If yes, when:	Free text
Goal regarding use:	Goal drop down
Motivators toward goal	Free text
Previous treatment history	Yes/No
If yes, when and effectiveness:	Free text
What would be different this time?	Free text
Actively engaged in MH treatment?	Yes/No

Note Element	Choices
Social Factors	Known Medical and/or Psychiatric Co-morbidities: ***
	Other Health: {Other Health Areas:51170}
	Social Supports/Connections: ***
	Personal Interests/Fun: ***
	Employment/Work: ***
	Housing: ***
	Transportation: ***
	Financial issues: ***
	Awareness of use disorder/lack of awareness: ***
	Other: ***
	Functional Impairment: {Functional Impairment Areas:51169}
	Progress towards prior plan: {BHCprogress:24228}
	Duration of problem: {Duration of Problem:39176}
	Severity: {BHCSeverity:24227}

This note is used by BHCs when seeing a patient in need of referral to the HPC clinic. This EPIC smartphrase is pulled into a standard BHC note. We have left the EPIC smartlist elements to lend greater authenticity to the ways in which you may wish to craft the options. You will need to create your own smartlists in your EPIC instance.

Chapter 17: MAT From The Provider's Viewpoint

By Walker Shapiro, MD

From 2013 to 2016, I was a resident physician in Family Medicine residency at the University of Wisconsin. During this time, the pain management pendulum was swinging rapidly away from the liberal prescribing of opioids toward a sobering recognition of the harms caused by this approach. We accepted that long-term opioid therapy (especially at high doses) was neither effective nor safe for many patients with chronic pain.

During my first two years of residency, nearly every day in the clinic, I engaged patients in difficult conversations regarding risky high-dose opioid prescriptions. At times, the doctor-patient relationship would take on an adversarial quality. Patients were hesitant to disclose risky drug and alcohol use, fearing we would discontinue their pain medications.

As doctors collectively backpedaled on prescribing opioids, the epidemic of overdose deaths from opioids was in full swing, driven first by prescription opioids, then heroin, and later by fentanyl. During residency, I was fortunate to be mentored by physicians prescribing buprenorphine for opioid use disorder as part of their primary care practices (which is uncommon now and was even less common at that time). Following specialized training required by the DEA (fortunately no longer needed as of 2023), I could start prescribing buprenorphine for a small number of patients. I found the work immensely satisfying.

The improvement in health and quality of life some patients could attain through recovery was astounding. For many chronic conditions we manage in primary care, the best we can hope for is "control" (slowing the disease's relentless progression firmly established in a patient's body). By contrast, with opioid addiction, a person who can achieve and maintain recovery will dramatically improve their quality of life and reduce their chance of premature death by overdose.

It was also refreshing to have patients discuss their substance use openly and honestly. The adversarial relationship I had frequently encountered in treating chronic pain was nonexistent. It felt much more like we were "on the same team." (There were still challenges in the doctor-patient relationship, such as suspected medication diversion or lack of consistent engagement in treatment).

While I know that many primary care physicians are hesitant to become involved in managing substance use disorders (and mental illness in general), my residency training had the opposite effect on me. I attribute this to my residency clinic's highly skilled integrated behavioral health providers, who could meet with patients as needed. I came out of residency confident of two things: (1) I would make substance use disorder treatment a central part of my practice, and (2) I needed to work in a setting with integrated behavioral health.

When I started working at Access Community Health Centers in 2016, I was the only provider prescribing buprenorphine. As demand for medications to treat opioid use disorder soared, we worked to expand our capacity. Three years later, in 2019, at least seven of my colleagues also actively prescribed buprenorphine. Since then, most providers have learned to incorporate medical management of substance use disorders into primary care. This success is attributable, in large part, to our integrated behavioral health team. Our PCBH colleagues support recovery and harm reduction for our patients through the following:

- Motivational interviewing
- Emotional support and problem-solving
- Addressing co-morbid mental health conditions
- Coordinating referrals to a higher level of care (e.g., residential treatment) when warranted

All of this allows the medical team to focus on medication management and maintaining relationship with the patient.

The PCBH team of highly experienced psychologists and social workers are available daily to meet with our patients struggling with substance use disorders and other mental health issues. This "on-demand," highly flexible model is critical for working with people dealing with the psychosocial complexity and chaos that often accompanies SUD. Physical co-location and shared medical records ensure accessible and open communication between medical providers and our PCBH colleagues. In contrast, our patients often find that specialty SUD services have limited availability and poor communication with the primary medical team.

Our experience at Access Community Health Centers has demonstrated that medical management of SUD can (and should) be provided in the primary care setting for many patients. A fully integrated PCBH team is essential to making this approach successful and sustainable for primary care providers.

About the Author

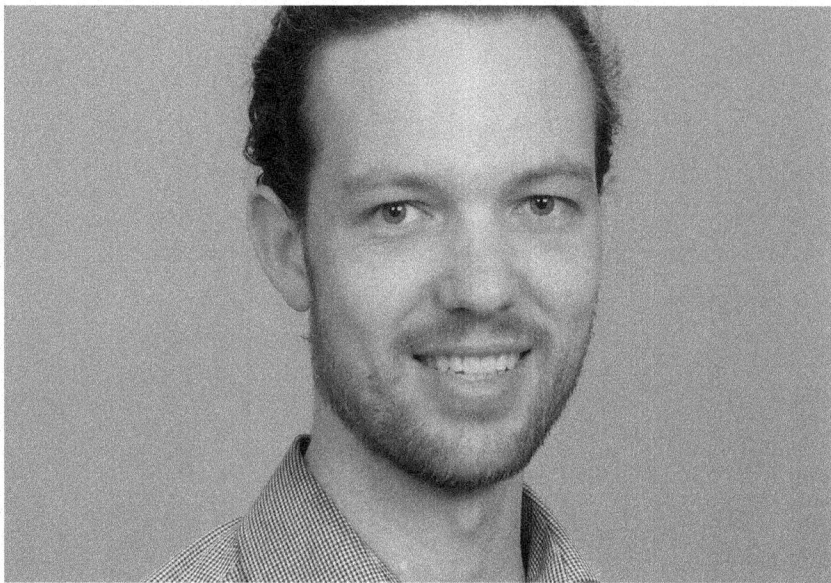

Walker Shapiro, MD, is a Family Doctor at Access
Community Health Centers, an FQHC in Madison,
Wisconsin. In his role as Substance Use Disorders Provider
Lead, he endeavors to make treatment of SUD a routine
part of primary care. Originally from California, he
obtained his medical degree and residency training at the
University of Wisconsin, and has been living in Madison
ever since. He enjoys spending time with his wife and three
children, meditation, cycling, skiing, and pretty much
anything outdoors.

Chapter 18: Chronic Pain

By Chantelle Thomas, PhD with edits from Meghan
Fondow, PhD

When working with chronic pain patients, most of your behavioral health intervention relies on explicit collaboration with the medical provider. In my training at a pain clinic, I came to appreciate one fundamental principle that has shaped my interventions moving forward: patients and providers must speak the same language. The patient's beliefs about their pain, what it is, where it comes from, and the appropriate treatment options can not be contrary to the opinion of their medical provider. Agreement between the patient and medical provider through diagnostic clarification is essential and directly informs the recommended treatment approach.

Additionally, treatment implications for an acute injury should differ from treatment decisions to manage a chronic condition, and nerve pain should be treated differently than myofascial pain. Most importantly, having these conversations is crucial to shifting the unhealthy dynamic in many medical provider/patient dialogues surrounding pain: the patient believes that the doctor holds the only key to alleviating their suffering through pain medications.

How We Started Our Work In Chronic Pain

Discussions with medical providers about chronic pain management have never been dull. Most primary care providers are exasperated and conflicted about their role in treating chronic pain. Medical providers will quickly tell you there is a subset of their patient population for whom they are uncomfortable prescribing narcotics; this is typically due to several "red flags" that have surfaced during their treatment.

To keep an open dialogue about these issues, I set up meetings with the medical directors of two of the Access clinics to review their concerns. As a result of those meetings, we dedicated several all-provider sessions to chronic pain treatment to begin a dialogue among providers about their primary concerns. These provider meetings resulted in 1) an opportunity to share knowledge/perspective from my experience working with chronic pain conditions and 2) the ability to identify the providers' primary concerns.

A recurring theme emerged: providers were uncomfortable saying 'no' to patients. This struggle was most pronounced for providers who felt they were saying 'no' to patients and offering them nothing to manage pain in return. Our medical providers consistently voiced concern about how to compassionately deliver news that will likely make patients uncomfortable (or angry!) and, consequently, make providers uncomfortable (worried, sad, guilty). While we all know most medical providers have experience delivering difficult news that could be painful, chronic pain discussions often take a different tone. The distinguishing difference between delivering news of a terminal diagnosis versus denial of narcotics for chronic pain is that, in the latter conversation, a patient may believe you are withholding treatment.

Systemic Interventions To Improve Consistency Of Chronic Pain Management

After several provider forums on chronic pain, I met again with medical providers to provide information on the risks and questionable efficacy of long-term opiate prescribing, particularly regarding chronic, non-cancer pain conditions. Several critical points developed for discussion:

1. The need for a different barometer beyond a patient's report of pain levels to evaluate the efficacy of a narcotic regimen
2. The need for increased patient accountability in managing their pain
3. Increased provider awareness regarding the role narcotics serve for a patient

Our discussions focused on encouraging providers to ask whether narcotics increase a patient's day-to-day functionality by asking questions such as, "What are you hoping to do in your life that you cannot do now?" We also reviewed the importance of physical therapy, stretching, and exercise for improving function and decreasing pain from inactivity. Most importantly, we discussed how narcotics might inadvertently treat patients' anxiety, sleep, and mood and even help them to "tune out" from life stressors and chaos; this is a critical reminder, as it can become unclear over time, for both patient and provider, what type of pain (emotional vs. physical) you are treating. In this regard, having a BHC involved in teasing out various aspects of mental health or coping challenges subsumed under chronic pain is essential. As a team, we also discussed the importance of identifying the following risk factors:

- Co-morbid substance use
- Patient's expectations of having no pain
- No awareness of or resistance to the connection between stress and pain
- Sole reliance on medications for pain relief
- Failure to treat co-morbid mental health issues

It has been essential to involve medical providers in every step of the process. At the outset, our approach included providing a series of chronic pain forums where providers could bring their most challenging cases to collaborate about new treatment directions. We also started discussions on our internal social networking site, particularly with our triage nurses, around new strategies for triaging pain management patients. The BHC team also processed their experience working with providers to ensure that our consultation service kept pace with current team needs in this area. Having a person dedicated to the issue on the team helped us organize ourselves as we interfaced with the medical providers on a consistent approach to chronic pain.

What Has Happened Since Our Initial Efforts

These initial efforts took place in the 2010s. At the time of this writing, 2023, we no longer have regular meetings with medical providers as we received feedback that they were no longer needed. We offer chronic pain group medical visits to give a treatment alternative to patients. These visits included a medical provider, behavioral health provider, and dietician. The content includes psychoeducation on pain and chronic pain, behavioral interventions, including training in mindfulness strategies, gentle movement activities, and nutrition education.

We also have a chronic pain care management program that includes regular outreach calls by a BHC for patients with chronic pain receiving narcotic pain medication to check in on patient status and satisfaction with their care, offer BHC visits, or connect patients to a medical provider to see if they could benefit from other non-medication options for care such as OMT.

While we no longer have regular meetings, we certainly have curbside consults regularly between BHC and medical providers to support providers when they want to debrief after a difficult conversation or are planning a difficult conversation. Offering this support from BHC to the medical providers has been well-received, as medical providers don't have to feel they are navigating complicated patient dynamics and competing demands independently.

These curbside consults take time but are worth it to decrease medical provider stress and reduce burnout. The whole tone of medical providers' approach to chronic pain has shifted significantly, related to the earlier work in the 2010s. Several factors, in particular, have contributed:

- Increased focus on discussing patients' functioning concerning chronic pain.
- Increased confidence/comfort of our medical providers in declining to start or continue patients on narcotics while offering treatment alternatives.
- The environment changed: both our providers and providers nationwide are more conservative in starting patients on long-term narcotics.

Chapter 19: ADHD

By Meghan Fondow, PhD, Elizabeth Zeidler Schreiter, PsyD, and Chantelle Thomas, PhD

Our team has taken several steps to improve our work with patients with ADHD and attention concerns in our child and adult populations. This work has been ongoing for years, and was accelerated during the COVID-19 pandemic as we saw a large increase in patients with concerns around focus and concentration, particularly in adults. We continue to think about efficient and timely methods of ADHD assessment in the primary care setting. The influx of information on social media in recent years around ADHD has provided both helpful and unhelpful information for patients. We found ourselves in need for a more routine screening process for adults, similar to what we have in place for children, which included a fair amount of time dedicated to psychoeducation for patients and providers.

Pediatric ADHD Management

When children present with attention concerns, we assess functioning at school and at home with both clinical interviews and assessment tools. At the current time, all children considered for a diagnosis of ADHD must first: 1) have their parent (or primary caretaker) complete a Vanderbilt regarding the behavior observed in the home setting, 2) have at least one but preferably two to three teachers complete Vanderbilts based on behavior observed in a school setting, in addition to 3) obtaining a release of information to exchange information between Access and the school.

To better streamline communication with the schools, we identify the school nurse or social worker as the primary person of contact or a school representative. If the child is working with a counselor or psychologist, we may include their name on the release forms if the family provides that information. In many instances, we will call those individuals directly to inform them an evaluation is ongoing and request feedback about their impressions or observations. While we initially started with paper and pencil Vanderbilts provided to families during medical visits to bring to school and then return or mail to Access once completed, we have transitioned to an all-electronic format; this has allowed us to alert teachers immediately through secure email (which we can easily find on the school's website) and provide them with a link to complete the survey online via a HIPPA compliant platform. All we need from the patient is the first and last name of their teacher, school, and current grade.

Beyond obtaining collaborative information from the schools/teachers, our consults aim to consider all other differential diagnoses contributing to the observed attention and behavior problems. We explore possible co-morbid diagnoses patients including depressive disorders (we most commonly use C-ESD as a screening tool or PHQA), anxiety disorders, trauma/PTSD, sleep disturbances, autism spectrum disorder, and other developmental disorders, learning disorders and substance use.

The patient's home environment and other contextual factors are the second area we explore as we know adverse childhood experiences, changes in home environment and changes in caregivers can have a significant impact on behaviors in children. We gather relevant diagnostic information via clinical interview related to behaviors seen in the home. In addition, we explore the responses of the caregivers, providing psychoeducation and support positive, developmentally appropriate interventions to assist in improving target behaviors. Sometimes caregivers have unrealistic expectations for their children. It is also not uncommon that we find that the caregivers of children with reported behavioral concerns also have caregivers who may struggle with organization skills and planning.

Encouraging parents to structure their expectations and reward good behavior can be facilitated through behavioral charts. Finding free access to behavioral charts online is relatively easy, or some BHC providers will make their own. Other strategies we may use include: assisting parents in identifying additional community resources (parenting clubs, homework clubs, available after-school programs, in-school tutoring, Boys and Girls Club, and family resource centers) and advocacy with schools for IEP (Individualized

Education Planning or 504 plan) consideration. In-home strategies such as increased consistency and predictability of the child's schedule can be very effective. We often start with attempts to establish a bedtime routine and consistent bed and wake times, and have seen many children show large improvements in behavior once sleep is regulated. If other contextual factors such as housing instability are a factor, we partner with our Patient Services team to assist in finding safe and stable housing for the patient and their family, which also has a significant impact on patient behavior.

We collaborate with the patient's PCP when families express interest in medication options. Our internal consulting psychiatrist is also an excellent resource when PCPs are not sure how to proceed. When a psychostimulant is prescribed, PCPs will talk with caregivers about administration and whether any administration will happen at school, as coordination is needed for this. Several non-stimulant options may be helpful when deciding what medication to trial for the patient. Some providers may need to become more familiar with non-stimulant options, so increasing your familiarity with this class may be beneficial. Some medications with primary indications for anxiety, tics, and sleep may also improve attention as an "off-label" indication. As such, leveraging the expertise of the consulting psychiatrist for additional guidance related to pharmacological options is highly beneficial.

It is vital to overtly clarify target behaviors that can be reliably monitored before initiating a medication trial. Be careful to note whether hyperactivity, impulsivity, or inattention may be the primary targets (or all three). Visits with children who have started on medication focus on areas of improvement and possible worsening in symptoms or any adverse side effects. It is always important to monitor for increased irritability, moodiness, decreased ability to sleep, and weight loss. Lastly, it is crucial to have an informed discussion with caregivers about realistic expectations for medication and the role of other behavioral supports.

Adult ADHD Management

With the COVID-19 pandemic and changes in people's routines, habits and coping strategies, combined with social media, we saw a dramatic increase in the number of adults seeking screening and treatment for ADHD. As such, as a team, we decided to create a more robust functional assessment and screening process to support both patients and our PCPs. We begin by asking why patients are presenting now, what is their motivation: are they seeking medication, a diagnosis for a sense of validation, or accommodations for school or work? Understanding the reason the patient is seeking this care can shape the tone and approach for the visits dedicated to this presenting concern.

Diagnostic identification and treatment of adult ADHD is another presenting concern that can be particularly challenging to our providers, likely due to multiple factors including comorbidities, life context factors, substance use and more. Often these individuals do not have a documented history of ADHD in childhood. In some instances, there can be co-morbid substance use, particularly marijuana. It is essential to consider all other psychiatric conditions that could manifest with inattention, task completion challenges, restlessness, inability to relax, and difficulties with concentration. Some of the most common co-morbidities include untreated PTSD, depression, bipolar disorder, and anxiety disorder. We developed a more standardized protocol for patients presenting with ADHD concerns and for stimulant prescribing in adults, particularly those presenting with some of the above mentioned concerns.

Similar to the process for pediatrics, we try to combine a clinical interview with standardized tools to understand the patient's concern. We developed a smartphrase embedded in our template in EPIC to assist with the clinical interview that includes prompts for the various areas to assess. Our team uses the ASRS, WURS, and another form that gathers collateral information from a caregiver or other adult who knew the patient as a child. Gathering all of this information generally takes several visits, which we explain to the patient before we start. Once we have gathered all of the information, we share the results with both the patient and the PCP, who will decide next steps for any prescribing.

As a standard of practice, we generally try to follow the following steps:
1. Obtain a childhood history of ADHD if available.
2. Ensure there is no consistent and significant substance use occurring (active substance use disorder impacts ability to make a definitive diagnosis as well as influences pharmacological options).
3. Rule out and treat any other co-occurring mental health conditions.

4. Determine the level of impairment secondary to attention/concentration concerns on the patient's emotional, interpersonal, and occupational state.
5. Ask for specific examples where deficits have resulted in a loss of or damage to a job or relationship.
6. Identify a clear set of target behaviors for intended modification and monitoring during the stimulant trial rather than just a subjective sense of improvement.

The protocol for stimulant prescribing is straight-forward: no patient will receive a stimulant medication at a first visit with a PCP and several visits with the BHC are needed to obtain a stimulant prescription via the PCP if clinically indicated; this allows for adequate information gathering (as indicated above) and observation of the patient's functioning deficits over a period of time. Non-stimulant options and certain antidepressants are available to target cognitive/concentration concerns and have the secondary benefit of targeting co-morbid mood symptoms. As with pediatric populations, we leverage the expertise of our consulting psychiatrist as needed.

There are no magic bullets for perfectly identifying and treating adult ADHD. Your goal should be consistency across all care providers, so your first step will be to work with all BHCs and medical providers to achieve consensus on a process that everyone can agree to.

Chapter 20: Severe & Persistent Mental Illness

By Chantelle Thomas, PhD, Elizabeth Zeidler Schreiter, PsyD & Meghan Fondow, PhD with edits from Neftali Serrano, PsyD

What does managing patients in primary care with severe and persistent mental illness (SPMI) mean? It depends on the provider, the care team, the patient, the patient's needs, and the available resources in the community. There are no easy answers, but there are some ways to think about complexity that can help you in developing boundaries for your clinic in this area.

What Is Too Severe For Primary Care?

In our clinics, one area of great debate involves the question: when is a patient too "psychiatrically severe" to be safely managed solely in primary care? Psychiatric complexity extends beyond individuals with psychotic spectrum disorders or bipolar spectrum disorder and often includes those with pervasive instability in the context of personality disorders, extensive polypharmacy, multiple psychiatric hospitalizations and/or mandated orders for treatment. The questions these patients pose are numerous. What will be the care team's role? Does the care team have the resources and expertise to safely manage? Is the provider willing to take on medication prescribing for this individual? What will be the BHC's role? What will determine whether a specialty care referral is needed? Psychiatric complexity poses a lot of difficult questions for the care team.

External factors also make this question complex, namely the limited availability of psychiatric care. In Dane County WI, finding a psychiatric provider can be complicated due to increased demand in the context of lack of supply of psychiatric prescribers. Further, those that are uninsured or underinsured face even greater barriers. Typically connection with a psychiatric specialist may take up to 6-12 months regardless of insurance type or lack thereof.

An additional challenge includes policies of closing patients to care for perceived lack of motivation or engagement. As you can imagine, patients with complexity in their lives often cannot follow through with appointment attendance due to unpredictable life circumstances (transportation, housing, lack of child care), which change daily. This raises the question: how can we best help these individuals in primary care while also maintaining our focus on the overall health of those medically homed at our clinics (i.e., population health). We want to maintain our identity as a primary care clinic, not a speciality mental health facility.

So, the question of what is too severe for primary care is: nothing. There is nearly always a role for primary care in caring for any patient that walks through its doors. A care team should be equipped to work with a patient with SPMI, even if the treatment of the SPMI is not the main domain of the team in the same way that a cancer patient will still see their primary care provider while receiving chemotherapy from their oncologist. The best question to ask is not what is too severe, but rather what is our role in this patient's life. Rarely is the answer a zero-sum answer.

Strategies That Help The Care Team Be Ready

A BHC may determine that the best role they can play is to support a patient with schizophrenia with simple interventions like helping them communicate their needs effectively to their medical providers, and providing in-the-moment skill training (eg. grounding exercises, daily self-management). A PCP may determine that their best role is to ensure that an extra set of eyes are monitoring the patient's weight and blood glucose levels to protect the patient's health. Together they can be part of the community of helpers surrounding the patient even if they are not "officially" treating schizophrenia.

There are all kinds of variations of the above strategy that a care team can take to engage patients with all kinds of complexity in their lives. In some cases the medical provider could choose to prescribe psychiatric medications based on the patient's relative stability and the provider's comfort level. Based on the clinical information and other contextual factors there may be times in which providers set boundaries that primary care is not able to safely prescribe psychotropics for a patient. With the education and support of consulting psychiatry, the need for these hard boundaries are minimized.

Due to increased difficulties in accessing long-acting injectable (LAI) anti-psychotic medications in the community and the growing body of evidence related to their efficacy in improving the quality of life of individuals living with chronic mental illness, we have started providing access to these medications within the primary care setting. As a medical home we strive to support the on-going stability of the patients that seek care in our facilities. Thus, when access to care changed in our community we quickly engaged in reviewing our internal resources and expertise via consulting psychiatry to ensure we would be able to support this need for our patients. Further, our care teams have grown to include behavioral health care coordinators (BHCC) that are able to track patients receiving LAIs to support optimal engagement and outcomes. Our past lack of care management capacity, before the BHCCs, had been a barrier to taking on LAIs in our clinic. Further, we were able to leverage the expertise of our consulting psychiatrist to provide education and training for our medical providers and nursing triage team to ensure we have consistent processes and workflows related to monitoring and providing the injection via our triage team.

We determined that our efforts were most effective in helping patients with complex psychiatric needs when we prioritize meeting their basic needs, advocating for their healthcare and disability rights, providing training in social skills, building trust, and connecting them with relevant community resources, while caring for their physical health needs.

It is important to remember all that the care team and BHCs can do to support a patient even if medication is not part of their treatment, or being prescribed by a psychiatrist in the community. It can be a common pitfall for mental health professionals to think medications are all we have to offer for patients with complex psychiatric concerns. Even for those individuals with more severe psychotic issues, our aim should be to increase our application of behaviorally-based interventions. In other words, we can aim to increase function in patients with these conditions even in situations where medication is not part of the solution. This is a common need due to:

1. Many patients with complex psychiatric issues struggle with consistency in taking their medications
2. Many do not want to take medications
3. Non-medication-based interventions can effectively improve their quality of life

So, don't short-sell what your behavioral health toolkit can accomplish even with psychiatrically complex patients. The PCBH model is predicated on a functionally-oriented approach that actually lends itself well to working with complexity in patient lives. Using Functional Acceptance and Commitment (FACT) based principles a BHC can have a values-driven conversation with a patient with schizoaffective disorder and determine areas where behaviorally-oriented functional improvement might be helpful. So one of the steps you could consider with your BHC staff is to offer training in FACT as it applies to patients with psychiatric complexity.

Specialty Mental Health Resources

Working with this complex populations also requires familiarization with community resources. The expansion of the behavioral health team to include behavioral health care coordinators was key into ensuring knowledge about available community resources and speciality psychiatric care providers. The BHCCs have created a list of smartphrases in EPIC for various resources including specialty mental health and substance care in the community by insurance type, clubhouses, social/peer -base community programs, and more. Our patients also benefit from our Patient Services team, who can provide information on housing resources, shelters, disability advocacy, financial counseling, low-cost legal assistance, domestic abuse, rape crisis, and crisis home options.

Supporting Our PCP Colleagues

The role of the BHC provider is to help providers say "Yes, and..." In other words, we want to empower providers and their care teams to be engaged with complex patients and we want them to set appropriate boundaries in situations that exceed the limits of their ability to provide safe and effective care.

We encourage providers to consider their decision and not feel pressured to provide a definitive answer during a patient's first visit. Once again, this decision is primarily dictated by the provider's comfort level depending on the diagnoses, complexities and medications involved. Many of our providers have grown in comfort and competence with the support of our consulting psychiatrist. The ability to easily access psychiatric expertise for curbside consultations, e-consults, or face-to-face evaluations increases the willingness of our providers in managing more complex cases. Our consulting psychiatry services will be discussed in greater detail in the next chapter.

Specialty Mental Health Referral Practices

While this discussion addresses some of the complexities inherent to providers' medication management decisions, another related issue involves a BHC's decision on when to refer a patient to a more traditional therapy setting. This issue resurfaces for our team repeatedly as we notice patterns or trends emerging with our trainees. We noted the tendency of trainees and occasionally staff to refer patients too quickly when they are feeling overwhelmed. We teach them to consider several important factors when making a referral: 1) Is the patient motivated for more intensive therapy? 2) What is the goal of the referral (what can traditional mental health/specialty care do that you cannot do) 3) What options are available (dependent on insurance or lack thereof)? Here too we emphasize a nuanced approach to a complex set of questions.

Another critical factor prompting an outpatient referral may be the patient's lack of perceived progress in the primary care setting. When making this decision, it is essential to question what the expectations are for progress. We need to keep in mind the idea of meeting patients where the are, and avoiding placing our own biases, expectations on the patient's care.

278

Some patients do exceptionally well if referred out at the right time. Referring someone too soon can set up a patient for failure or turn into a referral to nowhere. In many situations, patients may benefit from more intensive therapy but remain inappropriate for a referral because they do not demonstrate the consistency in follow-through required to establish a therapeutic outpatient relationship. Patients can be barred from returning to an agency if they miss too many appointments, further contributing to feelings of hopelessness. Often our therapeutic agenda may involve "testing out" various interventions to see what may be a good fit for a patient and what they may be ready for. In this regard, one part of our work is to facilitate treatment readiness or readiness for more intensive therapy when clinically indicated, something often referred to as bridging care. However, many patients remain in the primary setting and thrive with behavioral interventions by the BHC. We want to provide a positive experience for the patient, to build their trust and confidence in working with behavioral health providers broadly.

Even if a patient would benefit from more intensive services in the community, if they do not want this or have other barriers, it is important for the the BHC to focus on interventions and support that meets the patient where they are related to readiness while honoring their preferences. Regardless, it is imperative to emphasize your willingness to continue working with your patients, in a PCBH style, even if they decide they are not ready for more intensive therapy. The most important question for a BHC before a referral occurs may be: Who is the referral truly for, you or the patient?

Primary care has an important role to play in working with patients with complex psychiatric needs. It is tempting to want to assume that primary care only works with mild to moderate patient complexity. The reality is far more nuanced. So, as you start your program, you want to embrace this complexity with flexibility. Determine the resources of your care teams, assess for gaps in knowledge or training for working with this population. Over time, examine any boundaries to care in place, and consider changes and expansions that makes sense for your setting.

Chapter 21: Consulting Psychiatry

By Elizabeth Zeidler Schreiter, PsyD

I first encountered primary care behavioral health in graduate school. I was lucky enough to have mentors such as Drs. Tina Runyan and Stephanie Wood during my training. The training program provided me with a specialized track that exposed me to various opportunities for integrated healthcare; this included practicum opportunities in primary care and coursework focused on working in a medical setting. Some of the topics covered included psychopharmacology and medical literacy. They assisted with fueling my passion for working with the underserved and reducing barriers to care. When I started reading about integrating behavioral health services, I felt a sense of kinship with this model and thus began my journey toward becoming a behavioral health consultant.

I fully grasped behavioral health consultation and appreciated the impact of providing services within the medical home when I had my first practicum experience at a Federally Qualified Health Center (FQHC) in Springfield,

MO. Working in an FQHC dramatically opened my eyes to the volume of patients seeking mental health services within primary care. It increased my awareness of potential barriers to accessing needed care in other settings.

Given my exposure to primary care behavioral health during graduate school, working as a behavioral health consultant on an integrated care team was the career path I wanted to pursue. Still, I needed help finding an internship that allowed further exposure and training in this model of care, so I secured an internship at the University of Kansas Medical Center. While the main focus was not on primary care, numerous learning opportunities helped to increase my comfort in medical settings and my ability to communicate with medical providers. I also had the opportunity to function in a medical setting as part of a healthcare team and work collaboratively with various disciplines. Given my challenge of finding an internship that provided exposure to the primary care behavioral health model, I feel strongly about working in a healthcare home that has a robust training component.

I am comfortable and thrive in primary care's culture, pace, and collegial atmosphere. I function at a higher, more effective level when I have multiple demands. I enjoy social interaction with others as part of a team and find these interactions energizing. I am always open and eager to learn new information from my colleagues in primary care and truly value my interactions with others with a different knowledge and skill set than my own. I am very fortunate to have had exposure and training within this model of care early in my career, as I have found great satisfaction in working as part of a multidisciplinary team. I have always been interested in health and wellness and learning ways to empower others to take an active role in their healthcare. My interpersonal style and ability to build rapport quickly with patients and providers alike have served me well, as relationship building is a core component of the PCBH model. While primary care can be a fast-paced and intense work environment, I have found the extraordinary dedication and compassion of the providers I work with to be contagious as they tirelessly support their patients in improving overall health and wellness. Being part of a well-functioning team with mutual respect for each other's disciplines and talents has made this work sustainable and highly fulfilling.

Joining Team Access

I met Dr. Neftali Serrano by chance at the Collaborative Family Healthcare Association's annual conference. I was seeking a post-doctoral fellowship and heard him present on integrated care, where he referenced Access Community Health Centers. At the time, the post-doctoral fellowship was offered in collaboration with the University of Wisconsin Hospital and Clinics. The community-based track allowed for training opportunities in hospital-based health psychology and primary care behavioral health consultation. This opportunity was a natural fit for me, as it offered additional training within primary care and further exposure to health psychology interventions in the hospital setting.

I was not initially interested in moving to Wisconsin and was unsure I could handle the ferocious winters; this was tested further when I arrived for my interview on a cold and dreary winter day with more than 20 inches of snow on the ground. There was something unique and inspiring about observing these tenacious Madisonians riding bicycles between the snowdrifts. At this moment, I considered the benefit of living amongst people who could persevere and produce the best-case scenario from what some might view as an inclement nightmare.

Additionally, the training program matched my professional goals seamlessly. So, I packed my snow boots and headed to Madison, excited to join their growing team and program. Fifteen years later, after purchasing a snow blower, I continue to work happily with my primary care colleagues in providing comprehensive, integrated treatment focusing on all aspects of health. My role within the team at Access has changed significantly since the first edition of this book. Many changes have occurred on the team involving growth, staffing changes, re-defining of roles, and professional development.

We now have a team of 12 Behavioral Health Consultants, 2 Behavioral Health Care Coordinators, and one consulting psychiatrist. The team has a wealth of experience, ranging from early career professionals to veteran BHCs. I assumed the role of the Chief Behavioral Health Officer 8 years ago when Dr. Neftali Serrano, founder of the PCBH program at Access, transitioned to other opportunities. Shifting to supervising my previous peers and stepping into the shoes left by the founder of our program had a steep learning curve. However, I embraced my leadership style and harnessed my voice to continue to grow and evolve as a provider, leader, and human.

Leadership in healthcare settings is challenging, difficult, painful, and immensely rewarding. The patient populations, my fellow behavioral health consultants, my primary care colleagues, and the organization's overall health, with a deep commitment to behavioral health integration, have sustained me over the past 15 years and counting. I am passionate about our mission at Access Community Health Centers to increase access to care and advocate for the underserved to improve health and lives. I am humbled by the resiliency of the people we serve and take great pride in providing quality care to those in greatest need. Daily, I am grateful for the opportunity to share this work with behavioral health consultant team members who are all clinically competent and diverse in their knowledge base. A great sense of support is readily available via my fellow behavioral health consultants to consult about challenging clinical situations or decompress after a hectic day. The passion and drive of my colleagues are infectious, and we can learn from one another and develop additional skills continually.

The primary care clinicians I work alongside daily strongly influenced my decision to continue and sustain my career at Access. They are a talented, compassionate, and hardworking group of individuals devoted to improving the lives of each patient they treat. Access, as an organization, has provided tremendous support for the behavioral health program by providing genuine buy-in from the top down. It is truly remarkable to be part of an organization where your co-workers and administration value your contribution to the team; this has been made evident through the constant financial support of the behavioral health team during its inception and ongoing growth periods.

Since starting as the Chief Behavioral Health Officer on the Senior Leadership team in 2015, I have been part of critical decision-making related to strategic planning, organizational investment, and how and where we allocate resources. I appreciate the ability to share my voice and advocate for behavioral health expansion and be met with overwhelming support to grow to meet the ever-increasing need for comprehensive behavioral health services within primary care. I was intentional when I took on more leadership responsibilities at Access to continue my clinical duties as a BHC. While my clinical versus administrative time allocations have changed over the years, I remain steadfast in my commitment to staying connected to the clinical aspect of our work; this fuels my values related to service to others and affords me a greater understanding and connection to the challenges and joys of clinical work with underserved populations, which also assists with my leadership style and relational currency with my team. There is an implicit trust that each behavioral health consultant will work hard and do the work that needs to be done each day to meet the needs of our population. We each have a sense of duty to ensure we contribute to the best of our ability and are ready, willing, and able to see the number of patients needed during each clinic.

Leadership Opportunities

Access invests deeply in career pathways and professional development/growth opportunities; this was evident in the early years of our program under Neftali's leadership, in which team members were given additional responsibilities and areas of leadership related to community-based pathways, consulting psychiatry, clinic-based leadership, etc. In the early years of my career at Access, I was tasked with being the "Liaison to Specialty Care." In this role, I was responsible for building our resources and information to assist with navigating the behavioral health resources in our community. Working in primary care with patients with limited resources has revealed how crucial patient advocacy can be. Additionally, we needed to understand what options exist in the community so we could connect patients with the appropriate resources. To effectively connect patients to these resources, we also need to understand what structural barriers may impede successful referrals. This information also assists us in determining what we need to do internally to meet the needs of our population.

What I quickly realized was the amount of time, energy, and effort that goes into developing and sustaining healthy relationships with the community. I also appreciated how complex it was to understand our county's more extensive mental health system. Change is inevitable; thus, it is necessary to have an accurate and up-to-date understanding of what the community's mental health system offers. This information vitally informs care planning and allows us to set realistic expectations for both patients and providers. Over time, we added additional team members to serve in this role. We hired 2 Behavioral Health Care Coordinators (BHCC) who are Bachelor's level trained in psychology, sociology, or human services to serve as the critical navigators of community resources and assist patients directly in making needed community-based connections; this has enhanced the care we provide as well as free up clinician time for more direct patient care/ clinical service delivery to best allocate resources and have the most significant impact on our patients.

I have always had an interest in psychopharmacology, and the role medication serves as a tool in the treatment of mental health issues. I am keenly aware of the high volume of patients seeking psychiatric treatment and receiving prescriptions via primary care clinicians. I also appreciate the difficulty many patients have accessing psychiatry services via our community's specialty mental health sector. Primary care clinicians need increased support in managing an increasingly complex patient population. Thus, an additional area of leadership I took on early in my career was as the lead of the consulting psychiatry service to assist with stepped care and triaging of patients to our amazing consulting psychiatry team.

As the consulting psychiatry service has matured, we expanded to involve psychiatry residents from the University of Wisconsin Department of Psychiatry. Involving medical residents has increased our capacity and expanded our reach for our existing patient population. The residents are exposed to a functional psychiatric consult model in primary care. As this aspect of our program has grown and my leadership role has shifted, we have elevated other BHC team members to take on additional leadership in collaboration with our consulting psychiatrist (more on the development and growth of a consulting psychiatry service later).

Access' Consulting Psychiatry Model

Numerous models exist utilizing psychiatrists within primary care; thus, consulting psychiatry is not unique to our setting. However, how we have structured the service is designed to maximize the consulting psychiatrist's time and provide the most significant benefit to the population in our setting. The consulting psychiatrist is utilized for face-to-face consultations, chart reviews/written consultations, and verbal curbside consults. The expertise of psychiatry is often sought for various intents and purposes. These include:

- Behavioral health consultant or primary care clinician needs additional support related to diagnostic clarification
- A desire to explore medication options
- Guidance for monitoring parameters for specific psychotropics and
- Further consultation regarding treatment options in complex co-morbid psychiatric and medical issues

Our goals for the consulting psychiatry service include:

- Increasing support to primary care clinicians in managing patients with complex mental health issues
- Increasing access to care
- Guiding the use of evidence-based treatment and medication algorithms
- Improving primary care clinicians' comfort and competency in managing psychiatric illness

A key to consulting psychiatry at Access involves our *primary care clinicians always retaining prescriptive authority and ultimate responsibility for the ongoing care and management of the patient.* The behavioral health consultant is the conduit for all referrals to consulting psychiatry. Ultimately, face-to-face consultations compose a smaller percentage when compared with verbal and written consults. Typically, the written and verbal consultations per quarter are two times greater than the face-to-face consults - meaning the psychiatrist's reach into the patient population is much greater than the number of direct patient contacts. This reach is further amplified by the growing knowledge of psychotropic medications shared with the primary care clinician through consultation. As primary care clinician's psychotropic competence increases, so does their comfort related to prescribing. We have written an article on our consulting psychiatry service entitled <u>Consulting Psychiatry within an Integrated Primary Care Model</u>.

When embedding a psychiatrist within your clinic, you should assess the clinic's needs and examine the patient population to gauge the amount of psychiatry time needed. You can develop a hiring strategy once you determine the required or desired time. Previously, at Access, we had 0.25 FTE psychiatry time, which equates to an average of 10 hours per week. However, increased demand during the pandemic led us to raise this FTE to 0.75, which provides population-based care to an annual patient population of approximately 33,000+.

I highly recommended creating a job description that clearly outlines the needs and expectations of a consulting psychiatrist. Consider including not only the allotted hours the psychiatrist is in the clinic but also their potential availability via telephone or secure chat in the EHR for more immediate concerns when off-site. Include specifics related to their responsibility to write recommendations based on chart review or conversation with the PCP alone. This helps weed out candidates who are not willing to adopt a consultative approach or are too risk averse.

Payment for the psychiatrist's time should be commensurate with psychiatric services provided within your community. Competitive compensation is warranted to attract a high-quality and talented psychiatrist.

When looking to hire a psychiatrist, there are two main options: 1) contracting with an outside agency for psychiatry in which the psychiatrist then remains employed by the outside agency and is a contracted worker within your setting, or 2) hiring a psychiatrist directly as an employee of your clinic. This is a crucial decision that hinges on various factors, internal and external to your organization.

The benefit of contracting with an external agency is that hiring is simplified, and all costs are rolled into the contract. Sometimes, an individual's connections to the external agency may be valuable, such as a relationship to specialty services you may want to leverage for your patient population. The main con of this arrangement is that a contracted worker can be more challenging to manage organizationally (where do they fit in the chain of command?) and may have less investment than an employee. Sometimes, hiring externally is essential due to a limited pool of psychiatrists.

The benefit of hiring an employee consulting psychiatrist is that you have more say over who to bring into your team and more management potential and oversight; this allows you to monitor performance more readily and make adjustments within the supervisory structure. The downside is the risk of hiring any staff member, namely the difficulty of hiring and retention. This decision is an important decision and should be considered carefully. Regardless of the strategy chosen, clear communication around expectations and parameters with the specific psychiatrist and the external organization is vital to success.

A variant of these two options is hiring a tele-psychiatrist. In this instance, the same issues apply but are complicated by the arrangements needed to sustain the technology and billing requirements around the work itself. For example, clinics may find it easier to hire a company with telehealth expertise.

We encountered several challenges and experienced many learning opportunities while growing our consulting psychiatry service. We initially contracted for a psychiatrist's time via a local mental health center and thus were assigned a psychiatrist rather than individually selecting a candidate. Fortunately, the designated psychiatrist was passionate about working with the underserved. At the time, our organization did not have a formal management structure to assist our psychiatrist in acclimating to our organization. Consequently, our lack of clarity surrounding the position's expectations complicated our ability to provide the appropriate level of oversight. Psychiatrists contracted with outside organizations could quickly feel "caught in the middle" of two organizations with competing priorities. Despite these challenges, we had a successful and productive six-year relationship with our psychiatrist, who provided vital consultation regarding hundreds of psychiatrically complex patients. This experience taught us several important lessons:

1. To be intentional about our approach.
2. To communicate expectations clearly at the outset of the relationship.
3. To take the necessary steps to integrate our psychiatrist into our organization's lifeblood fully.

Choosing the Right Psychiatrist: A Goodness of Fit in Primary Care

To successfully implement a consulting psychiatry service, there should be careful consideration of the ideal characteristics of a consulting psychiatrist. Clinically, the psychiatrist should be able to function as a generalist, given the diversity in presenting problems and referral questions. Having an appreciation and awareness of the impact of co-morbid medical issues on psychiatric presentation is also vital. They should be comfortable with assessment and diagnosis in the context of one-time consults and also be able to think stepwise when providing recommendations to primary care clinicians. Awareness of patient resources is also essential when making medication recommendations. Suppose the psychiatrist is unaware of what is feasible for the patient given their insurance (or lack thereof). In that case, the recommendations are not helpful to the primary care clinician or the patient.

The ability to build rapport quickly with patients is also crucial to the environment in which they will be working. In our setting, the consulting psychiatrist must have awareness and sensitivity to the patient's cultural background, socioeconomic status, medical status, and other contextual factors. Having a solid psychopharmacology knowledge base is valuable but insufficient alone, as the psychiatrist must also be able to convey this information to primary care clinicians effectively. Therefore, it is essential to have clear and concise verbal and written communication skills and a collaborative interpersonal style.

The psychiatrist should be comfortable working collaboratively with a team and in their role as a consultant. When functioning as part of a team, having mutual respect for all team members and understanding each other's roles is warranted. An ideal candidate would also have program development skills and leadership potential to develop quality improvement initiatives; this may be particularly crucial if the psychiatrist also functions in a supervisory role.

Description of Consulting Psychiatry Service at Access

The consulting psychiatry service at Access has been in existence since 2007. The service has evolved to accommodate the growing needs of our population better and to ensure we continue to provide high-quality care. We have also become more efficient by developing a streamlined process for triaging patient needs, scheduling, and communicating information back to the primary care clinician. Patients are seen first by the behavioral health consultant and, if clinically warranted, may make a consultation request for consulting psychiatry. This request may be for an initial face-to-face consultation, a re-consultation in situations where the patient has been seen previously, or for written recommendations (now called psychiatry e-consult) via a chart review with comprehensive written recommendations. Suppose the primary care clinician or the behavioral health consultant desires a psychiatric consultation. In that case, the behavioral health consultant submits a formal written request for consultation via an "in-basket" message, the equivalent of email within our EHR. The consult request will include the following:

- Information about who requests the consultation (e.g., name of primary care clinician)
- The specific consultation question
- Information about target symptoms
- Patient history of medical and mental health issues
- Current medications

These requests are then managed by a lead behavioral health consultant who maintains an ongoing list of patients needing psychiatric consultation, and these patients are triaged based on severity for scheduling. The behavioral health consultant then contacts the patient via telephone to make an appointment with the consulting psychiatrist. While a phone call is the typical means of making an appointment with psychiatry, if a patient does not have a working telephone, we can schedule a future consult while the patient is in the clinic to streamline care coordination. BHC staff can also leverage their clinical judgment if clinical presentation warrants real-time scheduling versus future outreach calls.

The consulting psychiatry schedule includes three patient appointments per half day (when the psychiatrist is working alone) or four patient appointments (when psychiatry residents are in the clinic). Each face-to-face consultation is approximately 45-60 minutes in duration. In the event of "no shows" or if the schedule is not full for the day, the psychiatrist will complete written and verbal consultation requests received. Following face-to-face consultations, the psychiatrist creates a consultation note that is documented directly into the EHR and viewable by the care team. A request for written or verbal recommendations (in which the patient is not seen directly) also includes formal documentation in the EHR with specific recommendations and the rationale for such recommendations.

Options for reimbursement for these valuable services have evolved over the years. Recently, payment for non-face-to-face services, including the Interprofessional Telephone/Internet/Electronic Health Record Consultations CPT Codes: 99446, 99447, 99448, 99449, and 99451 were added by Medicare as well as Medicaid in the state of Wisconsin for reimbursement. As such, we developed a psychiatry e-consult workflow to support payment for the value added of non-face-to-face consultation to move care forward and provide enhanced quality and support of evidence-based treatment. At Access, we have been providing unbillable written consultation to support PCPs for over a decade, before the addition of these codes. Now the codes further support the fiscal sustainability of the psychiatry service and enhanced reach into the population.

At the outset of each clinic involving psychiatric consultation appointments, the first 30 minutes are reserved for a multidisciplinary team meeting involving the psychiatrist, psychiatry residents, behavioral health consultants, and primary care clinicians as appropriate. The goal of this meeting is to provide additional information to the psychiatrist regarding the referral and what information is being sought. A brief overview of the patient, relevant history, reason for referral, and insurance status is provided to psychiatry by the behavioral health consultant. This face-to-face interaction between the primary care clinicians, behavioral health consultants, and psychiatry has led to increased satisfaction and understanding of the referral reasons and potential nuances associated with the referral, including provider comfort with possible options for care (e.g., benzodiazepine not being an option due to provider preference or patient risk factors). Previously, all messages were sent to the behavioral health consultants and the consulting psychiatrist via the "in-basket." Still, it was found more efficient to have the consults triaged by the behavioral health consultant and presented to the psychiatrist during the weekly meeting. The lead behavioral health consultant can also gauge the psychiatrist's workload better and better inform the behavioral health consultant team about potential response times for consultation requests and scheduling availability.

Typically, most consultations with psychiatry are one-time consults and re-consultations (if needed) that occur six months to years later. However, we also have the option for closer follow-up with the consulting psychiatry service to monitor highly complex or acutely unstable patients better.

The parameters of this brief follow-up psychiatric consultation include:

1) Primary care clinicians will always retain prescriptive authority.
2) Possible monthly visits for up to three consecutive months to continue assessment of psychiatric symptoms and response to medication.
3) Open communication with primary care clinicians related to the rationale for additional follow-up with consulting psychiatry, with clear communication that consulting psychiatry is not taking over care of the patient but instead providing more robust assessment and monitoring related to response to treatment.
4) Open communication with the patient regarding the rationale for additional follow-up with consulting psychiatry and that the primary care clinician will maintain prescribing and ongoing management.

We monitor the type of consults with psychiatry (initial, re-consultation, brief follow-up) to ensure the addition of a brief follow-up consultation does not impact the accessibility of consulting psychiatry service for new consults or re-consultation requests.

While consulting psychiatry services allows us to provide care to more psychiatrically severe patients, we must be mindful that the primary care clinician is still responsible for ongoing care.

Important points:

1. The behavioral health consultants are the only people with scheduling access for consulting psychiatry to avoid patients being inappropriately scheduled via the call center or front desk staff,
2. To minimize the no-show rate and ensure timely access to high-acuity consultations, patients are not scheduled to see consulting psychiatry more than two weeks in advance,
3. If a patient has been on the list to be seen by consulting psychiatry and is unable to be scheduled or has missed a scheduled appointment, there is the option to complete an e-consultation with initial pharmacological recommendations by the psychiatrist to move care forward,
4. Patients are given a reminder call the day before their scheduled appointment and encouraged to bring in all medications to get a more accurate picture of medication adherence.

The psychiatrist at Access is a vital team member with an on-site, in-person presence to build relationships with providers and the larger medical care team. The consulting psychiatrist is given workspace alongside the primary care clinicians and behavioral health consultants; this allows for informal discussion and knowledge sharing. A support staff (MA or LPN) is assigned to the consulting psychiatrist and rooms all patients on the schedule, checks their vitals, and reviews the current medication list with the patient. The consulting psychiatrist will then see the patient in one of the clinic exam rooms.

Psychiatry Resident Training

In 2010, we collaborated with the University of Wisconsin Department of Psychiatry to become a residency-training site for psychiatric consultation within primary care. This collaboration has provided residents greater exposure to a diverse patient population concerning patient demographics and diagnostic complexity. Access hosts 10 PGY-3 psychiatry residents annually.

During their rotation, residents become part of the multidisciplinary team and learn valuable primary care consultation skills. These skills include clear and concise communication and documentation, algorithmic thinking related to pharmacological recommendations, increased appreciation for the impact of socioeconomic and psychosocial stressors on diagnoses, and the experience of functioning collaboratively within the primary care team.

By having residents in the clinic, we are also contributing to the primary care psychiatry job force of the future and hopefully inspiring others to consider a career of service to the underserved. The residents' presence has expanded our capacity to see additional patients for consultation and complete more written and verbal consultation requests. To prepare the residents to function within the primary care setting, we offer a seminar at the outset of their PGY3 training year that serves as an introduction to primary care behavioral health and the role of consulting psychiatry while also providing education on the culture of primary care.

Each resident also has the opportunity to participate in a lecture series for the primary care clinicians, nursing staff, and support staff on a topic of their choice to provide ongoing psychoeducation to the team. Previous topics have included:

- Treatment Options for Adult ADHD
- First Generation Anti-Psychotics: A Review of Their Uses, Side Effects, and Monitoring
- Evidenced Based Interventions for Insomnia
- Diagnosis and Treatment of PTSD
- Diagnosis and Treatment of Eating Disorders
- Meditation and Yoga as Adjunctive Treatment for Depression
- Medical Workup for New-Onset Psychosis and Early Medication Interventions
- Managing Psychiatric Medications During Pregnancy
- Patient Risk and Safety Assessment

Residents are also taught how to think and document in a stepwise manner. Working in primary care requires a cognitive shift from functioning within the specialty mental health sector, where a psychiatrist often has the option of ongoing follow-up. With the consultation model, we train residents to anticipate the next steps if there is a lack of treatment response, thus providing first and second-line interventions/treatment recommendations.

In this regard, we require "in the moment" recommendations that anticipate the possibility of future aversive side effects or sub-optimal responses to a medication trial. A consulting psychiatrist in primary care is most helpful when recommendations include multiple medication options and behavioral recommendations with a biopsychosocial lens. When provided with several treatment options, primary care clinicians can exhaust the recommendations before re-consulting and actively engage in shared decision-making with the patient.

When documenting, the psychiatrist will provide several medication recommendations with the typical starting dose, titration plan with target dose, potential side effects, possible drug interactions, and needed monitoring parameters; this is of great benefit to the primary care clinician, who can reference this note in the future, as well as review the risks and benefits with patients before providing a prescription. Upon completion, the note is routed electronically to the primary care clinician for consideration of recommendations. Suppose a more immediate response is needed (e.g., in cases of acute psychosis). In that case, the psychiatrist may approach the primary care clinician the same day and provide recommendations to be implemented while the patient is still in the clinic.

Residents are taught how to introduce themselves to patients within primary care to ensure an appropriate understanding of their role as a consultant on the team. An example of the introductory script used in our clinic by residents:

Hello, I am Dr. _____. I am a psychiatry resident working with Dr. (supervisor). I will complete your evaluation today, and then Dr. (supervisor) will review the plan. Both Dr. (supervisor) and I are consultants in the clinic and, therefore, will not be prescribing any of your medications. We will communicate with your primary care provider with recommendations to assist with your overall healthcare. You will need to see your primary care provider for ongoing care and prescriptions. All information you provide me today will be documented in your shared electronic health record and visible to others participating in your care, including your primary care provider. Do you have any questions before we start today?

Implementing the Collaborative Care Model (CoCM) at Access

As noted in earlier chapters, Access was an early adopter of the PCBH model in 2006. Access' team has long had consulting psychiatry as part of the integrated behavioral health team (since 2007), borrowing components of the CoCM model but not fully engaged in model fidelity in leveraging CoCM or billing using the codes. I previously referred to the robust service offerings at Access as PCBH+, including consulting psychiatry as a key team member and collaborator.

Why Pursue CoCM at Access?

- There are numerous benefits of incorporating CoCM into our already robust integrated care offerings at Access, including:
- Supporting team-based care
- Increasing UDS measures associated with depression screening and follow-up
- Improving patient outcomes related to treat to target for depression and anxiety
- Already well-established PCBH+ program with all necessary team members for the CoCM model, including care coordinators and psychiatrist on the team

- Opportunity for revenue generation for care coordination efforts for BH conditions
- Supporting the use of evidence-based treatment
- Access was a key advocate for CoCM reimbursement for Medicaid members and securing reimbursement at the PPS rate within FQHC settings.

In June of 2022, the Wisconsin Department of Health Services (WI DHS) provided a Forward Health Update related to reimbursement for CoCM codes for Wisconsin Medicaid. As a Community Health Center (CHC), most of our patients have Medicaid as their insurance; thus, the benefits of formally implementing the CoCM model alongside our robust PCBH model were clinically and fiscally relevant.

Community Health Centers in Wisconsin are reimbursed using the Prospective Payment System (PPS), meaning that each eligible encounter with a provider (Medical, Dental, or Behavioral Health) is reimbursed at the same rate. To flag that the CoCM services are rendered within a Rural Health Clinic or Federally Qualified Health Center, the code G0512 must be used. It is important to note that for Wisconsin Medicaid, this was defined as a minimum of 60 minutes or more and that the majority rule related to time does not apply (meaning it must be 60 minutes, no less). It is also important to note that the initial iteration of approval of the CoCM codes by WI DHS only included CoCM CPT codes 99492, 99493, and 99494 (G0512 for Community Health Centers). We were able to successfully advocate with Wisconsin DHS regarding the benefits of the General BHI code 99484 (G0511 for Community Health Centers).

For Those In Wisconsin: Links to Forward Health Updates
2022-25: Collaborative Care Model Policy
2022-40: Collaborative Care Model and New Billing
Procedure for Community Health Centers

Assembling a Workgroup

Implementing CoCM into an already established integrated care program took planning and collaboration across multiple areas on an organizational level. While I am a seasoned BHC, I needed to become more familiar with CoCM and the core competencies of building a CoCM program. Therefore, we sought out opportunities for expert consultation via the Collaborative Family Healthcare Association (CFHA) and collaboration with the Wisconsin Primary Health Care Association (WPHCA) to use Access Community Health Centers as a springboard for learning and sharing with our sister health centers across Wisconsin. We also included other Access staff and leaders, including those from the BHC team (Consulting Psychiatry Services Manager, Primary Care Behavioral Health Manager, Consulting Psychiatrist, etc), Revenue Cycle, Coding/Compliance, IT, and UW Health as a community partner and being on their shared Electronic Health Record (EHR).

We collaborated on developing the project scope and work plan. We obtained additional project management support/ resources to ensure the ability to move this project forward as part of our organizational strategic plan. This workgroup began formal meetings in January 2023, and our Go-Live date of providing actual provision of CoCM and billing for said services was August 2023; this is important to note as having clear workflows and role definitions, as well as automated billing and core documentation tools established were essential to have in place before starting the pilot project. I want to extend my thanks and gratitude to Dr. Shanda Wells at the University of Wisconsin, who leads a robust CoCM program and was generous in sharing her knowledge and workflows with Access to adjust and tweak to meet the needs of our clinics.

WI DHS has now formally approved the General BHI code (CPT code 99484; G0511). Access, in collaboration with other agencies (WPHCA, Wisconsin Psychiatric Association, Wisconsin Collaborative for Healthcare Quality), was a crucial advocate for the inclusion of this code in addition to the other CoCM codes to support the ability to leverage reimbursement for other essential behavioral health care management services outside of CoCM and when the dose of treatment (e.g., care management/care coordination time) is 20 minutes or more. The General BHI code is used for billing monthly services delivered using Behavioral Health Integration (BHI) models of care other than CoCM that also include the following:

- Systematic assessment and monitoring
- Care plan revision for patients whose behavioral health condition isn't improving adequately.
- Continuous relationship with designated care team member

Overview of the Collaborative Care Model

The University of Washington AIMS Center is the national authority on the Collaborative Care Model.

Collaborative Care emphasizes being patient-centered with effective collaboration between the behavioral health care manager and the primary care clinician to incorporate patient goals into the treatment plan. In addition, CoCM is also measurement-based, with clear and measurable treatment goals and outcomes defined and tracked for individual patients (PHQ-9/GAD-7). Treatment and interventions are adjusted until the clinical goals are achieved. Since this is registry-based, it also ensures patients know about follow-up and supports evidence-based interventions.

Core Team Members in CoCM

Treating (Billing) Practitioner - A physician or advanced practice practitioner (PA, APNP, CNS, CNM), typically in primary care (maybe other medical specialties). The medical provider's role includes the ability to introduce CoCM to the patient, obtain verbal consent, initiate a warm handoff to the behavioral health care manager, collaborate with the care manager and psychiatric consultant to develop a treatment plan, implement and make treatment adjustments including medications as appropriate, and continues to oversee all aspects of the patient's care.

At Access, given we already have a robust PCBH program, the PCP refers to the BHC team, and we assess for appropriateness of engagement with the CoCM program, introduce CoCM services, obtain verbal consent, and then connect with the care manager.

Behavioral Health Care Manager- designated care team member with formal education or training in behavioral health, working under the oversight and direction of the billing practitioner. This position is titled Behavioral Health Care Coordinator (BHCC) at Access. The BHCC is responsible for coordinating the overall effort of the treatment team and ensuring effective communication among team members. The BHCC will engage with the psychiatric consultant to obtain recommendations for the patient's provider and support moving care forward. BHCC will also be a point of contact between provider visits to support medication monitoring, adherence, and psychoeducation. This vital team member offers brief behavioral health interventions (using evidence-based techniques such as motivational interviewing, behavioral activation, and problem-solving treatment). They may also collaborate with patients to create relapse prevention plans, participate in systematic case reviews, and support the treating practitioner in providing proactive follow-up of treatment response, alerting the treating practitioner when the patient is not improving, and supporting the engagement of the psychiatric consultant when there is a sub-optimal treatment response.

Psychiatric consultant- a medical professional trained in psychiatry with strong collaboration skills and psychiatric knowledge (qualified to prescribe a full range of psychotropic medications). However, in this model, there is a consultant only; thus, all prescribing authority is retained by the treating provider (PCP). The psychiatric consultant supports the treating practitioner and BHCC in treating patients. They meet weekly with BHCC to review and focus on treatment planning for patients not adequately responding to the current treatment plan. In our setting, since our psychiatric consultant is on-site and in the clinical care team workspaces, they are available for ad-hoc/verbal consultations as needed; this has been highly beneficial in building trust and relational currency between the medical practitioners and the psychiatric consultant (this is relatively unique as in many settings, the psychiatric consultant may not be on-site and provides remote consultation/support via the EHR.

The Patient/Beneficiary- The individual with a behavioral health condition receives support from the care team. The patient/beneficiary is a core care team member, and all care/support should keep the patient at the center.

Benefits of CoCM & PCBH Models

As mentioned above, I trained in the PCBH model as a behavioral health consultant. However, as a psychologist, organizational leader, and administrator, I was intrigued about ways to harness the positive impacts of both CoCM and PCBH to promote population health and provide a comprehensive, whole-person health approach to care. The PCBH approach as a generalist and being open to seeing all behavioral health conditions across a lifespan ensures access to needed services for our populations. Adding CoCM to our current BH service offerings allows us to better support our patients with specific, defined behavioral health conditions of depression and anxiety with a registry-driven systematic process to provide increased support and outreach for engagement in treatment and stepped care. By blending these models, we have the most significant potential for impact on the populations we serve to promote health and wellness.

CoCM in Action: Building the Workforce

To accommodate the additional clinical care demands of a CoCM program, we increased the clinical FTE of our consulting psychiatrist from 0.25 to 0.75. We also hired 2 Behavioral Health Care Coordinators (BHCC). While initially, the BHCC positions were Masters in Social Work (MSW) level of education, we adjusted the minimum requirement to have a Bachelor's degree in Social Work, Psychology, or Human Services with additional training provided in Motivational Interviewing to increase the pool of applicants; this supported increased applicants as well as the diversity of care team members. Having an intentional focus on workforce development and training has been critical to the growth of the behavioral health program at Access.

Educating Providers About Our Services

Our medical providers are accustomed to working collaboratively alongside behavioral health providers as team members and fully embrace the psychiatric consultant role. However, we had to ensure training and education for the providers related to adding CoCM program offerings. Messaging was simplified to decrease confusion about the roles of BHC and BHCC: Continue referring to BHC as usual. The BHC staff member would then meet with the patient, assess, and determine if CoCM may benefit and, if patients are interested and motivated to connect, would make the warm handoff to the BHCC for enrollment in the CoCM program; this has been highly successful as a means of recruitment and role clarity for both patients and providers. Since the BHC and BHCC staff each have defined roles, it is also possible that a patient may access support from both the BHC and BHCC based on their unique needs; this allows flexibility in treatment offerings based on the needs of each patient, taking into account their treatment goals and preferences.

We also leveraged the support of our CFHA Technical Assistance, Daniela Vela Hernandez, LMFT, to create a brief 1-page summary of the CoCM program at Access.

Scaling the Work and Shared Learning

Our workgroup continues to meet to review the current workflow, make adjustments as needed, and monitor the revenue cycle to ensure no errors or need for adjustments. We are following a Plan-Do-Study-Act (PDSA) process to ensure the success of the initial pilot program and then broader scaling on an organizational level, in addition to sharing key learnings with other Community Health Centers (CHCs) in Wisconsin. Key learnings we will be sharing include:
• Inclusion criteria recommendations
• Workflow examples
• Documentation recommendations
• Training materials
• Recommendations and considerations for implementation

Collective Impact and Gratitude

We want to extend our gratitude to Access Community Health Centers for investment and support of integrated behavioral health services and opportunities to continue to grow and enhance the services we offer to support our community. Thank you to all members of the Access BHC team for sharing their skills and talents to improve the health and lives of those we serve. In addition, thank you to the Collaborative Family Healthcare Association (CFHA) for their Technical Assistance related to CoCM implementation, specifically Daniela Vela Hernandez, LMFT, Technical Assistance Associate. Thanks to Kay Brewer of the Wisconsin Primary Health Care Association (WPHCA) for managing this project effectively.

I want to express my gratitude to Molly Jones and Sashi Gregory from WPHCA for their invaluable assistance in advocating for the fiscal sustainability of integrated care practices in Wisconsin. Their efforts have contributed to supporting whole-person health and creating a healthier community. Ultimately, we aim to scale this work at Access and across Wisconsin to support integrated behavioral health care as a routine part of primary care for all Wisconsinites.

In closing, as I always say to team Access, we truly have the "best BHC team in the land."

About the Author

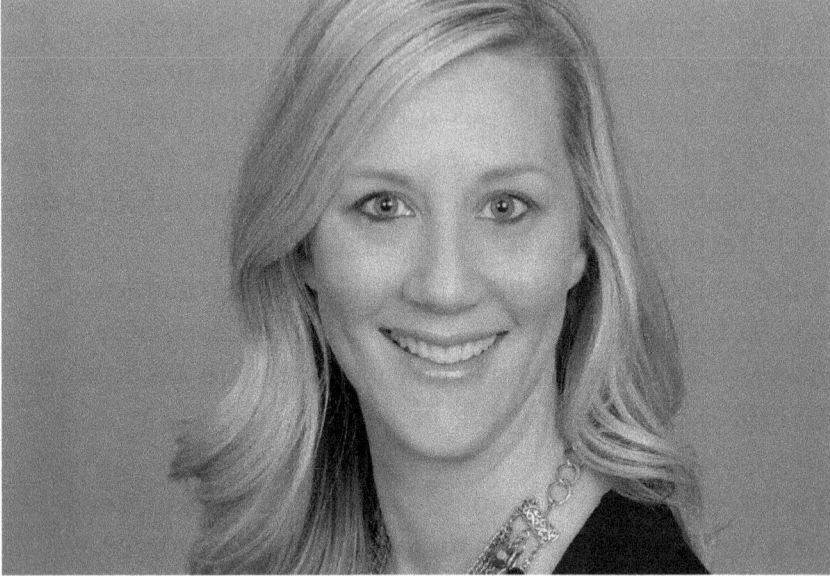

Dr. Zeidler Schreiter is the Chief Behavioral Health Officer at Access Community Health Centers. She is a seasoned clinical health psychologist and Behavioral Health Consultant (BHC) with over 15 years of experience on integrated healthcare teams. She is passionate about teaching future BHCs as well as spreading the benefits of integrated behavioral health care to support whole person health. She has published numerous scholarly articles and book chapters related to primary care behavioral health integration as well as served as a consultant to organizations nationwide to support integration efforts. She is a key collaborator with the Wisconsin Primary Healthcare Association (WPHCA) to assist moving forward state-wide initiatives to promote integrated behavioral health services in the state of Wisconsin via advocacy, education, and collaboration.

Chapter 22: CoCM & PCBH At Cayuga Health System

By Laura Sidari, MD & Trisha Patrician, PhD

The human experience hovers at the blurry emotional, behavioral, and physical health intersection. A strained primary care system is tasked with providing whole-person care, resulting in a heavy focus on physical health care, with relatively scant resources available to care for emotional and behavioral health needs. As all these needs are inextricably linked, an effective health system must include support that can meet a broad range of changing and often ambiguous care needs across the general population.

In 2021, Cayuga Health System acknowledged the critical role of integrated behavioral health services as part of its mission to meet the needs of the primary care population across more than ten practices. The Cayuga Integrated Behavioral Health (CIBH) program was very much a passion project, a somewhat wild idea born from the chaos of the COVID-19 pandemic for one local psychiatrist, Laura Sidari,

MD, as well as her colleagues Kaitlin Lilienthal, PhD and Trisha Patrician, PhD. In a serendipitous moment of "right place at the right time," Drs. Sidari, Lilienthal, and Patrician united to bring integrated behavioral health "home" to their local communities in the central New York region. Using knowledge and experience cultivated from various integrated care practice backgrounds, these three professionals partnered with health system leadership to create a program prepared to serve diverse care needs in a largely underserved local community. In under three years, this team of professionals has harnessed the spirit of localism to engage evidence-based national models of integrated care and build from the ground up a sustainable care framework with the potential for a broad population reach.

Characteristics Of The Cayuga Health System

Cayuga Health System (CHS) is a not-for-profit community healthcare network comprising outpatient and inpatient medical partnerships across the Finger Lakes and Central New York regions. The service region is broadly rural, with three small cities, including a college town, separated by many miles. The health system comprises two small hospitals and a blend of specialty and primary care outpatient clinics. Most of the health system's 10+ outpatient primary care offices consist of 5-10 primary care providers. However, health system priorities include clinic consolidation towards fewer, more extensive group practices of 10+ practitioners in the next five years.

CHS cares for approximately 65,000 primary care patients across Cortland, Tompkins, and Schuyler Counties in New

York State. Within Tompkins County, the community population is 76.8% White (non-Hispanic), compared to >90% of the population in neighboring Schuyler and Cortland counties. The vast majority of patients cared for within the health system are insured (~98%, evenly split between Medicaid/Medicare and commercially insured), and community non-insured rates are around 5% across the region. Patient cost-sharing for medical and behavioral healthcare ranges from no out-of-pocket costs to several thousand dollars in deductible with an additional coinsurance percentage.

Specialty mental health services are minimal within the care network, including no in-network outpatient mental health clinics and one in-network 20-bed inpatient psychiatric unit. At the time of integrated care service development, typical wait times for patients to establish with the county mental health clinic were approximately six months. Most of the alternative care options for therapy or psychotropic prescribing in the region contract with a minimal number of insurance plans, and many are cash pay only.

Features Of Cayuga Integrated Behavioral Health

Cayuga Integrated Behavioral Health (CIBH) provides training, care infrastructure, and behaviorist staffing for affiliate primary care clinics to deliver an effective and replicable combined model of integrated behavioral health. Processes build off best practices for the Patient-Centered Medical Home (PCMH) and are customized to the local health system. CIBH combines nationally recognized Primary Care Behavioral Health (PCBH) and Collaborative

Care Model (CoCM) services to create a unified care delivery system that aims to meet the needs and care objectives of the health network.

Within this blended framework, primary care providers (PCPs) identify when areas of the patient's treatment plan may benefit from behaviorist support and elicit the patient's consent to participate with the integrated team. PCPs "prescribe" the service that best meets the patient's needs as a part of their patient-centered primary care treatment plan, with support from the team's integrated behaviorists.

Providers on the integrated team include Behavioral Health Consultants (BHC), Behavioral Health Care Managers (BHCM), and Consulting Psychiatrists (CP), who partner with PCPs to match the level of care provided to the patient's needs. Using principles of the PCBH model, the BHC is rapidly accessible for warm handoffs from the PCP and typically meets with patients over one to several sessions to provide a brief (typically 20-30 minutes) focused assessment or treatment for acute and routine primary care behavioral health concerns. Patients treated by their PCP for a Depressive or Anxiety Spectrum Disorder are recommended to CoCM to receive robust wrap-around supports, focused interventions, and measurement-based care to help them improve more effectively. Service options are defined by care need, and therefore, a single patient may require and receive support from one, both, or neither care model at a given time in their primary care journey.

Evolution Of CIBH

In February 2021, CIBH development began with contract development for Dr. Sidari, Dr. Lilienthal, and Dr. Patrician as core members of the clinical directorship team. From February – July 2021, this core leadership team partnered with health system stakeholders to gather information about health system characteristics, complete needs assessments in collaboration with benchmarking recommended in the integrated care evidence base, foster buy-in for integrated care delivery, and develop preliminary workflows for clinical services.

In June and July 2021, the CIBH team began implementation meetings with two pilot sites, then launched clinical services at one site in August and one in September 2021. The initial few weeks of services were provided by the two assistant directors, one in the BHC role and one in the BHCM role, and the director as the consulting psychiatrist. By September and into October 2021, an additional BHC and three BHCMs were hired and onboarded to support PCP teams of approximately eight full-time equivalents for each site. Also, in October 2021, the program gained a program manager, Sherry Huddle, with two decades of experience in general dentistry and primary care practice management.

In the first year of program piloting, the team worked together to train and develop effective care delivery in alignment with integrated care model best practices, improve primary care infrastructure in alignment with PCMH best practices, and create local processes and procedures to help effectively deliver both care models within a single care system. The team closely tracked benchmarking data to monitor team progress and identify areas for improvement.

The formation of implementation teams was crucial, with stakeholder champions from critical primary care and behaviorist roles such as practice management, front desk staff, clinical support staff, nursing, PCP, and CIBH team involvement. Implementation meetings were held weekly at first and later every other week to help track team progress, build cohesion, and identify areas that would benefit from improvement. Even after the service establishment, these high-impact teams continue to meet monthly, focusing on sustainability. Benchmarking data gathered from the first year of services reflected a sustainable model of care delivery, with staffing costs able to be fully covered through fee-for-service reimbursement for BHCs and BHCMs, without accounting for value-based outcome improvements, such as improved depression screening and remission rates across affiliate sites.

In the second year of services, the CIBH team expanded efforts to streamline and refine care processes through data dashboard development and strengthening onboarding/training plans. Care growth continued to occur, with service reach extending to additional primary care sites (college health in August 2022 and family medicine in June 2023) and an integrated care pilot in a specialty medicine (Rheumatology, August 2022) practice.

As of November 2023, the CIBH team serves four clinical sites: one family practice clinic, one internal medicine practice, one college student health clinic, and one contracted pediatric practice within Cayuga Health System.

Projecting ahead for 2024, we plan to expand to two to three additional practice sites. In the next five years, planning will expand service reach to all ten-plus sites across the Cayuga network, focusing on primary care practices. A potential long-term goal is to offer CIBH services within specialty medicine practices such as Endocrinology, Cardiology, Pain Management, and Rheumatology.

Care Lessons And Continued Challenges

One of the features that uniquely supports the success of CIBH is its strong leadership team, dedication to the local care system and the limited accessibility of specialty mental health services. With strongly invested representation at all levels, dedicated to the integrated care mission as essential for the community, we have developed very effective local processes and robust support for administrative and clinical infrastructure vital to effective service development.

The absence of specialty mental healthcare has helped practitioners at all readiness levels to buy into utilizing CIBH services, with typical service uptake and meeting total scale-up targets within 1-3 months following service initiation. Strong support from the 3-member psychologist and psychiatrist leadership team helps with effective hiring, onboarding, and supervision for behaviorists. Investment in these non-billable clinical supports helps optimize the behaviorist team's care effectiveness, creates team cohesion despite behaviorists serving differing sites, and promotes excellent retention and career development within the currently challenging mental health-hiring environment.

While robust infrastructure supports have been critical to CIBH program success, these also make CIBH care potentially challenging to translate to health systems outside Cayuga Health. With local processes and procedures explicitly tailored for Cayuga, these may not fit as well with other care systems that differ in size, practice set-up, funding designations, and care mix. Rapid buy-in for integrated care occurred partly due to the limited accessibility to referral-based specialty care in the region, which may not be accurate for all healthcare systems. Care concepts, particularly matching the service structure to the care system needs, may be a more salient lesson learned for other health systems than strict duplication of related care processes.

Additionally, the up-front investments needed to develop administrative infrastructure for integrated care may not be within reach for all healthcare systems, particularly early in program development. While the payoffs for this structure have occurred approximately one year after service initiation, support for the leadership team early on required monetary investments in salaries and health system partnership support.

Lastly, robust clinical leadership support may only be attainable for some care systems. Cayuga has benefitted from a knowledgeable and experienced core psychiatrist/psychologist team to lead service development within the primary care department. Other health systems may need help recruiting commensurate leadership staff and may instead have to train or grow these team leads, such as through national or state-based technical consultative support. Primary care teams may also be reluctant to invest in these teams under their budget, particularly if specialty mental health services may be present.

Take-Home Points

- Cayuga Integrated Behavioral Health (CIBH) offers an example of effective and sustainable implementation of a combined integrated care model, utilizing local procedures to create cohesive service delivery.

- Investment in core integrated care leadership requires up-front costs and may only be within reach for some care systems. However, up-front investments in effective and high-quality integrated care leadership can offer health systems compounding dividends in staffing, sustainability, and financial feasibility for care.

- Support at all levels for integrated care is crucial to effective service outcomes, and this can be made easier within a care environment with limited access to specialty mental health.

About the Authors

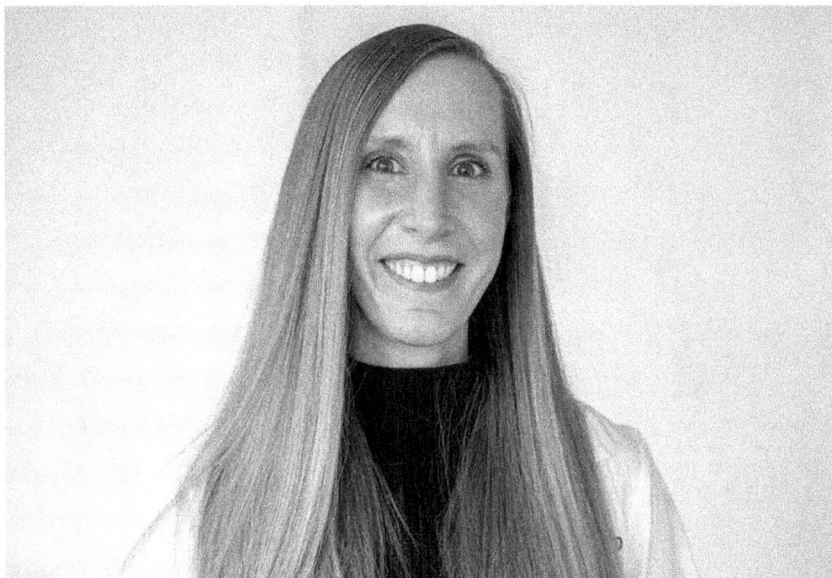

Laura Sidari, MD directs integrated behavioral health services for Cayuga Health's not-for-profit regional health system in Central NY. She is a board-certified general psychiatrist with clinical practice and leadership experience across a spectrum of different integrated care models. She began her career as an Air Force Psychiatrist, where she served in specialty mental health and integrated care roles while caring for military service members and teaching resident physicians. Prior to her role for Cayuga, she designed and implemented integrated psychiatric consultation services for Cornell University's student health center. She currently serves as a Co-Chair for the CFHA's Collaborative Care Model Special Interest Group. Outside of work, she enjoys visiting local parks and going skiing in the winters with her children and husband.

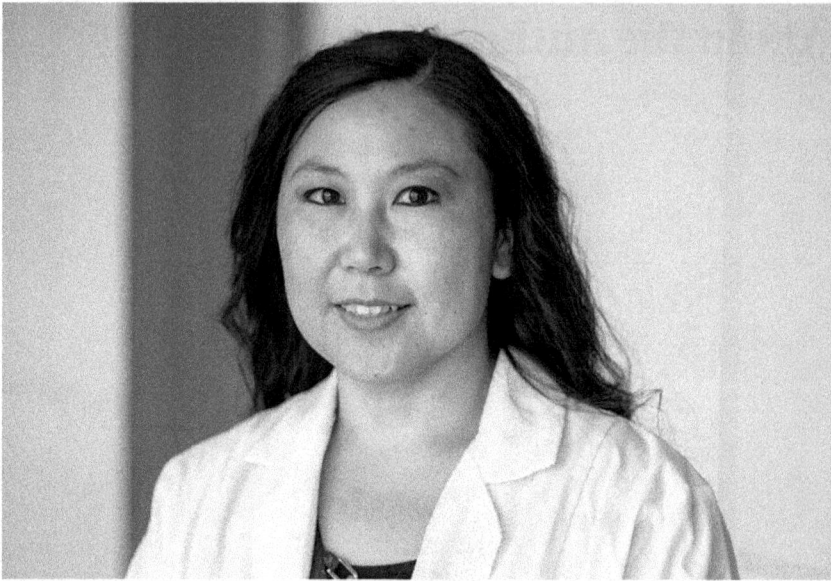

Trisha Patrician, PhD joined Cayuga Medical Associates in 2021 to assist in the development and implementation of Cayuga Integrated Behavioral Health (CIBH) in Ithaca, NY, which blends primary care behavioral health and collaborative care model in providing services to affiliated primary care practices within the health system. As one of two Assistant Directors for CIBH, Trisha trains and supervises the team of Behavioral Health Care Managers, interfaces with a variety of stakeholders both within and outside of the health system, and has held clinical roles initially as the program's first Behavioral Health Care Manager and currently as a Behavioral Health Consultant. She brings many years of experience from diverse settings and is committed to enhancing access to high quality behavioral health care.

Chapter 23: Pediatrics

By Allison Allmon Dixson Ph.D., William Leever Ph.D., Rebecca Lyren Ph.D., Destiny Singleton Ph.D., and Cody Hostutler, Ph.D.

(Allison) always knew I would work in pediatrics- how I would work with pediatrics I had no idea. I started out in graduate school thinking I wanted to merge psychology and medical care and social justice/advocacy work for children- I researched and through the guidance of mentors in my psychology graduate program was guided towards pediatric psychology. I dove in and spent my practicums and research working with children with medical concerns (Hem/Onc, Endo, Burn, Rehab, Pulm) in every capacity possible. I loved working with these patients and families and understanding the patient's context, specifically how the medical system wrapped around these patients and their families while hospitalized. I most valued having the privilege of sharing in care with patients and families who would not have otherwise received behavioral health supports. This became and still is my why. While hospitalized, we often talked with patients and families about discharge and what came next. I found myself often asking the question, "What was the context before the hospitalization?" And then, "How do I put myself in position to engage in preventative care for patients and families who would not receive behavioral health care?" The answer- Pediatric Primary Care Behavioral Health. Peds PCBH gave the how to my why. Through some generous mentors, fantastic training, and serendipitous opportunities, I became a forever learner of integrated care.

Cody Hostutler Ph.D., always had a passion for access and equity in pediatric health and started his training as a school psychologist; however, when he realized the significant inequities that existed by the time children entered kindergarten, or even preschool, he searched for a setting that would espouse a population health approach to building health, development, and well-being in a population-based and community connected context (pediatric primary care!). Cody and I met when I, as a Psychology Fellow, interviewed him for fellowship at Geisinger Medical Center. He accepted and joined the Geisinger legacy. I went off to my first independent licensed role as a Behavioral health consultant in Pediatrics and within a couple of years transitioned into a role with many hats (including BHC, Section Chair of Integrated Care, Family Medicine Residency Behavioral Medicine Faculty Member). My primary focus became growing integrated care at a mid-sized health system to expand into pediatrics, family medicine, family medicine residency, internal medicine and numerous specialty care clinics. Meanwhile, Cody shined through fellowship at Geisinger and continued to create an amazing career, including many titles, most prominently Clinical Director for Behavioral Health Integration and Psychology Co-Director of Graduate Medical Education.

With these role transitions, I am so grateful for our ever intertwined professional paths. We have lead CFHA's Special Interest Group, co-presented more times than I can count, lead workshops, co-authored papers, and most recently co-authored this chapter, which is a natural manifestation of our shared passion for Pediatric PCBH. We are often seen as an established duo in Pediatrics CFHA, which is so hard to believe as we continue to learn and grow from each other and with the brilliance of those around us every day. We are excited to be joined in writing this chapter by William Leever Ph.D., Rebecca Lyren Ph.D, and Destiny Singleton Ph.D; amazing colleagues who have each made their own significant contributions to their clinics, communities, training of others, and the field of pediatric integrated primary care. Pediatric PCBH is our foundation and CFHA's Pediatrics Special Interest Group is our home. As you continue to read our chapter and the great minds that we are humbled to be amongst, we encourage you to find your people, we found our Peds PCBH peeps, and look forward to adding you to this group!

What Is Pediatric PCBH?

The primary goal of pediatric primary care is prevention and risk reduction (NASEM, 2021). Thus, pediatric integrated primary care often focuses on a team-based approach to *keeping* kids healthy. You will notice throughout this chapter that we repeatedly emphasize that pediatric patients are not just little adult patients, and because of this, skills that you might have mastered with adults- while often effective with pediatric patients -- need to be adjusted or slightly shifted to reach maximum benefit. The major shift is that systems are uniquely critical to the pediatric population. The systems where children and adolescents grow up, such as home, school, daycare, and work, heavily affect them. Thus, there is a strong need for cross-system partnerships within pediatric PCBH models.

The GATHER (generalist, accessible, team-based, high productivity, educator, and routine) acronym is a summative way to describe the work of PCBH. This framework is largely consistent between pediatric and adult PCBH, with special consideration to pediatric patient population needs and interventions. We will use GATHER as an organizing framework for this chapter and highlight the nuances of working with pediatric primary care populations, including how to implement practical how-to skills. Throughout this chapter, we will use examples for each concept in the GATHER acronym. We acknowledge that these examples are multifaceted, and their placement in any one GATHER concept is not intended to be exclusive; instead, the opposite is true; most examples can and do fall under multiple GATHER concepts. A list of a few sample resources is at the end of this chapter, including resources that we find helpful.

GATHER: Generalist

Pediatric primary care aims to maintain the well-being of healthy children, promptly detect any potential risks in young patients, and offer prevention and early intervention services. To some, being a generalist and being pediatric-focused may seem contradictory. For those of us in pediatric settings, the incredible range of presenting concerns in pediatric populations certainly feels like a generalist approach. At any given moment, we may support a family managing difficult infant sleep habits, problem-solving toilet training troubles, dealing with separation anxiety at preschool, managing picky eating, school/learning problems, ADHD, depression, substance use... and more! Table 3 provides a more extensive list of the common presenting concerns that pediatric BHCs often support. It is worth noting that many primary care clinicians (and sometimes BHCs) initially focus on common mental health concerns (ADHD, anxiety, depression) and sometimes struggle to identify health behaviors, developmental concerns, and ways the BHCs can help infants and toddlers.

We recommend reviewing the table and reviewing these concerns with the primary care team to identify the problems that are 1) most commonly presented in the community you serve and 2) are time-consuming for the primary care team to address or are things that families struggle to implement with basic guidance. After identifying common concerns that require additional support, create a concise pathway for each problem and keep track of the number of consultations for each concern. Please refer to the routine pathways section for further guidance. Be sure that the team communicates the successes of these consults to start building an understanding of the many ways the BHC can be used to support families and physicians to keep kids healthy in primary care.

Table 3. Common Presenting Concerns for Pediatric Generalists

Sleep	Learning Problems
Toileting (including constipation, enuresis)	Pill Swallowing
Chronic Pain (Abdominal, headaches, etc)	ADHD
Neonatal Abstinence Syndrome	Abuse/Neglect
Bullying	Family Conflict
Adjustment to Life Stressors	Speech problems
Depression	Anxiety
Developmental Delays	Feeding Problems
Gender/Sexuality	Healthy Weight/Lifestyle
Disruptive Behaviors	Unexplained Physical Symptoms
School Refusal	Shot/Needle Phobia
Obsessive Compulsive Disorder	Asthma
Grief	Tics/Habits
Divorce/Custody concerns	Autism

Although there are myriad ways to support children, adolescents, and their families, a few generalist themes are fundamental when working with pediatric populations: Being comfortable with developmental expectations will be necessary. Much of the work in pediatric PCBH is helping families and PCCs differentiate what is expected and unexpected while assisting families in taking an active, evidence-based, and contextually relevant role in helping their children achieve important developmental milestones rather than waiting for problems to emerge.

Becoming comfortable with family-based, caregiver-focused interventions will go a long way across presenting concerns. Whether the presenting concern is problem-solving medication adherence, addressing picky eating, managing disruptive behaviors, or managing anxiety, it is crucial to understand caregivers' role in developing and maintaining the problem and the evidence-based intervention strategies.

You will likely need to engage in more cross-sector collaborations given the considerable involvement of schools, child protection, organized athletics, and legal systems that play a significant role in children's contexts. This chapter will explain themes such as development, families, and systems more tangibly.

The functional contextual interview is a straightforward approach commonly used with adults and can be easily adapted for use with youth. Traditionally, the contextual interview assesses love, work, play, and health behaviors. While these topics are appropriate for some youth, it is essential to adapt these domains to apply to the broader pediatric population. For example, while some youth work, the more dominant role in their life is typically school.

Thus, it is vital to incorporate school rather than work into the functional interview as the primary functional domain. Further, health behaviors also need to be developmentally appropriate. For example, health behaviors for a toddler typically require caregiver input and include specific areas such as progress in potty training, variety and quantity of food intake, and developing healthy sleep routines. Finally, development is an essential domain to assess in all youth, and we recommend adding this to the functional contextual interview for kids. We like to use family-friendly language for this domain, such as whether the parent has concerns about a child's moving, talking, thinking or understanding, emotions, or getting along with others.

In pediatrics, the contextual interview looks as follows:

Love
   Who lives at home?
   How are relationships within the family?
   How is the child's attachment to family members?

School/Work
   How is the child doing academically? Do they understand the work?
   Do they have formal educational support (504/IEP)?
   Are there disciplinary concerns at school?
   Do they get along with peers at school?

Play
   What does the child do for fun?

Are they involved in structured extracurricular activities?

Do they seek out play with family? Friends? Neighbors?

Health
Variety and quantity of food?

How much and what kinds of physical activity?

When does the child go to bed, fall asleep, and wake up? Doing it independently? Naps?

Growing/Development
Thinking - Understanding, problem-solving

Moving - Gross and fine motor skills

Talking - Understanding what others say, talking, vocabulary, articulation

Feeling - Able to calm themselves down, easily upset, difficult to calm

Getting Along- Able to make and keep relationships

GATHER: Accessible

Kids need regular care to stay healthy, and access has been a persistent problem in pediatric behavioral healthcare (Cummings et al., 2013). Healthcare resources are limited, so the available services must be delivered as effectively and efficiently as possible (Kindig & Stoddart, 2003). With an equitable distribution of care, communities benefit from targeted services delivered to more people rather than allotting extra resources to only a few patients. PCBH is well-suited for pediatric primary care settings due to its central focus on accessible, preventive care at a population level. Integrating behavioral health into primary care is one of the quickest ways to make behavioral health more available and convenient for busy families.

In the pediatric primary care clinic, BHCs are expected to make care more accessible by seeing children and families on the same day the primary care provider requests support (Reiter et al., 2018). BHCs accomplish this same-day service like their adult counterparts: warm handoffs and curbside consultations are staples of practice. However, both warm handoffs and curbside consultations take on a special significance when factoring in the ecobiodevelopmental (EBD) model. For example, capturing neurodevelopmental disorders, such as intellectual disabilities, in the earliest stages of development can significantly improve a child's life trajectory.

Patient-centered medical homes (PCMH) are at the forefront of innovation within primary care and provide a collaborative, team-based environment for BCHs to provide timely services (Asarnow et al., 2017; McDaniel & Fogarty, 2009). The PCMH model prioritizes accessible, comprehensive, patient-centered care. In general, PCMHs target interdisciplinary collaboration for physical and behavioral health problems. In a PCMH, BHCs provide direct patient care through integrated visits with the physician or separate, co-located therapy visits in the primary care office. Due to children's short attention spans, quick visits are imperative for primary care clinicians (PCCs) and BHCs. BHCs can provide brief screening and assessment services during direct care visits for various presenting concerns. These universal screening protocols often focus on routine primary care presenting problems, such as depression (PHQ-9), anxiety (GAD-7), and suicidal ideation (ASQ). However, they also involve child-specific screenings, like the M-CHAT for autism spectrum disorders.

Due to the episodic nature of treatment in primary care, BHCs often focus on the core treatment kernels (Strosahl & Robinson, 2018) of evidence-based interventions rather than providing complete treatment protocols. Standard treatment kernels in pediatric clinics come from behavior therapy and parent management training. In addition to direct care, BHCs connect higher-need patients with community organizations, such as schools, developmental disability departments, and outpatient behavioral health centers.

Keeping Kids Healthy

PCBH aims to keep children healthy rather than treat patients once a disorder has developed. To reach the best outcomes, we systematically shift resources upstream to prevent children from experiencing severe mental health impairment. Therefore, pediatric primary care relies heavily on prevention measures, such as Well Child visits and universal screenings (Wissow et al., 2013). BHCs can also implement annual behavioral health wellness visits like an annual physical in the future.

GATHER: Team-Based

Although many BHCs in medical settings operate as part of a team, this is especially relevant for clinicians in pediatric primary care settings. A team-based model is critical to ensure that behavioral health is utilized not just for acute needs (e.g., risk assessment, abuse reporting) but also for patient needs that may arise during the primary care visit. Additionally, research suggests that integrating BHCs into primary care clinics increases adherence to future well-child checks and immunizations (Ammerman et al., 2022). Many consult opportunities may be evident in the patient's stated reason for a visit; however, a well-integrated team member can support various presenting complaints, including virtually all routine well-child check components (WCC) components. Here are some examples of WCC components a BHC can be helpful with:

Current Concerns: Some patients may visit for behavioral health issues, while others may bring up concerns during their WCC, such as a child not talking.

Development: As part of a WCC, parents are typically asked about their child's developmental milestones. Firstly, BHCs provide developmental guidance and prevention strategies for young children whose development is on-track to reduce future developmental concerns. For children whose development is not progressing as expected, BHCs can determine if intervention is needed and help connect families to support. To assist eligible families, we recommend that you become familiar with your state's early intervention program, such as Help Me Grow, and the application process for special needs preschools. These resources can be pretty helpful.

Nutrition/Elimination/Sleep: Depending on the age and developmental level of the patient, concerns in eating, toileting, or sleeping may be behavioral or a symptom of a mental health diagnosis (e.g., sleep difficulties in the context of depression). Although some of these concerns may benefit from medical intervention (e.g., sleep apnea), collaboration with behavioral health may lead to improved outcomes and lasting changes. Further, BHCs can ask clarifying questions to determine the potential root cause of these concerns, as these concerns may not be fully assessed as part of a WCC.

School: Many parents bring up academic concerns during the WCC. As poor school performance can be a symptom of various mental health concerns, integrating BHCs can aid in understanding the issue (e.g., are academic difficulties a symptom of anxiety or related to a learning concern?) and point families in the right direction. Behavioral health clinicians can also help families navigate the Individualized Education Plan (IEP) process. A letter to provide parents to request an IEP evaluation is an excellent resource in your clinical toolkit. Be sure that school-based resources are written with a tone of collaboration (e.g., we recommend that family and school work together to determine if a 504 plan is needed) rather than prescriptive (e.g., this patient needs a 504 plan) as family-school relationships are a significant predictor of a child's success in school. We should not assume we have all the information to decide what a child needs.

Medication: Behavioral health clinicians can also provide support regarding medication adherence.

Clinicians can work with children and their parents to learn more about why the child has not been taking medication. Clinical strategies and tools such as motivational interviewing or a clinic pill-swallowing practice kit can be valuable tools to help promote behavior change. Helpful resources for starting a pill-swallowing kit are found later in this chapter.

Immunizations: As part of many WCCs, children may need to complete a blood draw or receive immunizations. Behavioral health clinicians can support the child with a deep breathing exercise or a distraction technique or utilize the tools in their immunization kit (more information is provided later in this chapter).

It can be challenging to educate your medical providers about all the elements a BHC can be helpful with. Below are a few tips to get the process started:

Scope: You must understand the scope of your practice and communicate that clearly to providers. Frequently the role of the BHC and clinical social worker may have some overlapping components (e.g., both may complete risk assessments or reports of child abuse). If you have a social worker on the team, it may be helpful to talk with them about their role in the clinic and how you can support each other in patient care (e.g., you can also complete risk assessments but may rely on social work for assisting with transportation needs).

Clinic Space: Depending on the setup of your clinic, you may have your own office space. Although this provides many benefits, it may make it harder to connect with your team, at least initially. Consider sitting by the providers in a clinic to catch consults and provide curbside consultations as needed.

Observe: When applicable, observing a few WCCs (i.e., one early childhood and one teen) may be helpful; this allows you to see the types of questions the provider asks and can help you develop rapport with medical providers.

Warm Handoff: Use warm handoffs whenever possible, especially when starting. For many families, you may be their first contact with behavioral health. Having the medical provider introduce you to families normalizes your presence in the clinic and establishes you as another trusted healthcare provider.

Clinic Flow: While meeting with a family on a PCP schedule, keep clinic flow in mind. As a consultant, you provide services for patients scheduled with their medical provider. It is essential to keep this in mind and provide targeted, focused services to ensure clinic flow is not disrupted. Due to many factors, including children's shorter attention spans, difficulty transitioning to the exam room, and non-compliance during immunizations, pediatric visits can take longer than adult primary care visits. It is crucial to balance providing high-quality care with efficiency.

Telehealth practice: First, ensuring the family can connect to telehealth services is essential. When getting to know your team, it is helpful to know whom to refer families to if they are having trouble connecting to telehealth services. Telehealth can be a very effective tool in increasing access to services for families with scheduling or transportation barriers and creating opportunities for you to view behavioral concerns in the home setting. You can also use this to your advantage in appointments. During telehealth appointments, provide small breaks during a session if your patient has difficulty focusing. These breaks can be a reward and an opportunity for the child to show you something at home that interests them (e.g., a favorite book or pet). You can also use a sticker chart (virtual or something you show the child during the session). However, it is vital to work with the family to ensure that the child can access a reward for maintaining appropriate behavior during the session. The child's family can provide a tangible reward, or you can save some time at the end of the session to listen to a favorite song, complete a show-and-tell, or play a brief game.

Screening Flow Integration: As part of the primary care team, BHCs can also play an essential role in early identifying children with developmental concerns. For example, routine screening in primary care can reduce the age of autism spectrum disorder diagnosis (Carbone et al., 2020), which is critical for children to receive early intervention. However, research suggests that pediatricians encounter many obstacles in implementing screening, including limited time and a lack of knowledge about autism (Morelli et al., 2014; Mazurek et al., 2019). Introducing behavioral health into WCCs and noting developmental concerns can help address these issues and promote the BHC service to medical providers.

GATHER: High Productivity

As mentioned previously, a primary goal of pediatric primary care is to keep children healthy. In a very literal sense, every child would benefit from a consult with a BHC to promote healthy development. In addition, pediatric mental health needs are highly prevalent, with approximately 50% of youth meeting the criteria for a mental health disorder at some point prior to age 18, and 75% of all mental health disorders start by age 24 (Merikangas et al., 2010). There are also significant physical health and educational disparities across all age ranges. Pediatric practices have plenty of clinical work to handle, making them a perfect fit for high-productivity population health approaches that define the PCBH model.

Pediatric approaches to PBCH vary in how they spend this high productivity time. Programs like Healthy Steps focus exclusively on using BHCs to screen and support youth development during every well-visit from birth to five (Briggs, 2016). Some programs (like Nationwide Children's Hospital in Ohio) use a more traditional PCBH model and fill in empty spaces in our day with prevention work (Snider et al., 2020), while others focus exclusively on a more traditional PCBH model and only get involved once a concern has been identified. When determining the appropriate approach to implement, factors such as the skills and training of the Behavioral Health Clinician (BHC), productivity expectations, the extent to which prevention services can be billed or supported, clinic volume, and the workforce's availability should be considered. Regardless of your approach, consider the needs of the population and the best ways to maximize the use of the BHC team. It can be tempting to revert to a specialty model for some pediatric BHCs since care in the community can be scarce, resulting in low productivity and population penetrance.

GATHER: Educator

As educators in pediatric primary care, BHCs can provide interventions to more patients than they can individually serve. In pediatrics, this educator's role and responsibilities, such as providing curbside consultation and presentations to medical providers, may look similar to those in the adult world, but the content is vastly different.

It is essential as the pediatric BHC to identify common needs in your clinic and then educate your whole team (e.g., primary care providers, RN, MA staff). Some common needs and the questions that they often answer include behavioral management in the clinic (e.g., "How do we help kids have a positive experience in their visit and get all their medical needs met- height, weight, BP, hearing test, physical?"), immunization support (e.g., "How do we help this patient get their immunization with minimal trauma?"), and adherence to new medication regimens (e.g., "What if they cannot swallow a pill?").

It is crucial to understand what staffing supports are available in your clinic to implement these routine interventions (e.g., can our nursing staff, with their other responsibilities, take on this initiative). We recommend talking with your clinical manager to understand if the intervention would fit into a standard workflow and how best to provide the education. If you can join an already scheduled meeting, that is best. Outlined below are three everyday needs that we often provide education on/ support for in our clinics:

Behavioral Management

As behavioral health providers, we are behavior experts; as pediatric BHCs, we turn those skills into behavioral support across our entire clinic population by educating our teams. For example, we all know about the power of positive reinforcement; using that same principle, we encourage creating a positive reinforcement system for all pediatric patients. We call ours a "clinic behavior passport." A clinic behavior passport lists all desired behaviors by the patient during an appointment (e.g., using walking feet) and an agenda of what to expect (e.g., getting your height). Once the desired behaviors are identified and completed, caregivers and staff can mark them as complete on the patient's behavior passport by checking them off or drawing a star. Patients can then show their behavior passports at check-out and get a prize from the clinic prize box. Naturally, that means we also recommend a clinic prize box; this can contain stickers, small bubbles, small fidgets, etc.

Adherence to Medical Regimen Recommendations:
Immunization, Procedure Support, Pill Swallowing

Imagine the following: A child coming in for a wellness visit and doing great with their exam. At the end of the exam, the provider discusses immunization; the child begins to cry and becomes upset; the caregiver tries to soothe the child, who becomes upset, saying let's get this done, the staff comes in and tries to soothe the child, but he ends up restraining the child for the immunization.

The above scenario often occurs in clinics, not because staff or caregivers don't want to do something different but because they do not know what to do. Teaching staff immunization/procedure support can improve the experience with the clinic visit for the family and staff. We recommend training all staff to recognize the difference between normative anticipatory anxiety for immunizations/procedures that is transitory and needle phobia, which is a reaction out of proportion for development, where a child cannot be calmed/soothed/distracted following the immunization or procedure and comes with perseveration and avoidance/distress when immunization is broached. With this knowledge, staff can save needle phobia for the BHC, who can use exposure to manage the phobia and reduce the trauma children can experience during a visit.

We encourage teaching staff the following steps:
> **Preparation:**
> When to Introduce: Encourage preparation by caregivers before the appointment; the adult/parent/caregiver can inform the child the morning or day of

the visit; if the patient is unaware, tell at the start of the visit.

What to say: Provide information with procedure expectations (e.g., "First, the nurse will clean your arm with the alcohol pad, next"). Describe the procedure in concrete, specific and simple language (e.g., "the procedure will be shorter than XX TV program). Encourage coping (e.g., "When I count to 3, blow the feeling away from your body"). Praise the child (e.g., "You did a great job at deep breathing, holding still; that was hard. I am proud of you.")

What not to say: Avoid emotive language or focusing on the negative (e.g., "This is going to hurt."), giving too much control (e.g., "Tell me when you are ready."), over-reassurance (e.g., "There is nothing to worry about."), criticism (e.g., "You are acting like a baby."), and vague information (e.g., "The nurse will draw your blood.").

Procedure:

During the procedure, we recommend the following: only take the needle out at the time of the immunization, proceed quickly, encourage bringing familiar, comfortable, or distracting items to the visits, and have some available in an immunization kit (see immunization kit ideas below), educate families about effective coping strategies to practice at home (e.g., deep breathing with bubbles or pinwheels, guided imagery, normalization through medical play), and enlist caregivers as coaches (e.g., have them hold the child in a comfortable position, use of coping skills).

Consider the following for your immunization kits:

Buzz bee: small vibrating bee with ice pack wings that help block pain and provide a distraction (see link below)

Distraction items that encourage coping skills, such as pinwheels or bubbles for breathing

Reinforcement: stickers, prizes

Note: There are many other procedural supports for which BHCs can provide education. Remember pill swallowing? If staffing resources permit, this could be an excellent educational opportunity.

Share Resources

BHCs have a ton of great resources. Sharing these resources with staff in a way that makes them accessible, user-friendly, and easy to remember means staff can disseminate these, and BHCs can spend time seeing more patients! We recommend gathering resources (locations, phone numbers, websites, etc.) and creating family resource lists. Consider key social determinants of health to guide what should be included on your lists. Ask yourself, "What is it that I look up repeatedly?" Answers will likely vary based on your clinic population and their needs (e.g., housing resources, food pantry locations, and daycare openings). If available, leverage social work support to aid in providing those resources on a broader, more systemic level. Once you have your list of resources, make them accessible. How does your team typically share information with families (in the electronic medical record, patient instructions, printed handout)?

We recommend using your electronic health record whenever possible; create handouts that are easy to find and put into patient instructions so that staff can quickly put them into practice. Once created, do not forget to spread the word; use your team's preferred method of communication and layer this in staff meetings, email blasts, and instant messages.

Finally, follow up: communication to staff should be repetitive and reflective (e.g., is the document helpful, what is missing, how should it be altered to improve). These are living documents that will require editing over time. We have check-ins on resources every three months in staff meetings and a central location where any staff member can include suggested edits or updates to materials.

GATHER: Routine Pathways

While we practice from a generalist model, there will be high-yield conditions that you will encounter in the clinic that deserve the creation of a specific pathway. Many of these families would benefit from services your primary care team can initiate. These may include comprehensive psychological evaluations, lethality intervention, school-based accommodations or interventions, child welfare services, legal support, and financial assistance with medical care, food, housing, and utilities. Without proper planning, hearing these concerns during a medical appointment can cause discomfort as your team tries to balance the desire to help but a limited understanding of how you can support them and the patient.

High-yield conditions you can anticipate witnessing in primary care include lethality, depression, ADHD, and an autism spectrum disorder. Developing routine pathways to address each presenting concern can set your team up for success. These pathways can help determine how to access, treat, and follow up with children endorsing these conditions within the capacity of your clinic. The following displays examples of different pathways that can be implemented to address high-yield conditions. For each pathway, you will need to consider a process for patient identification (screening) and the treatment pathway you will offer.

> **Screening:** Your clinic could benefit from implementing a formal process for identifying children at risk for high-yield conditions. As you work with your primary care team, consider these questions:
> Who will be receiving the screener?
>
> What is a reliable, validated, and affordable screener your clinic can use to identify children at risk for a high-yield condition?
>
> When is an appropriate time to administer the screener - will you give it during all medical visits? Sick visits? WCC?
>
> Where will data be collected and stored?
>
> How will your team integrate the screener within the flow of your clinic?
>
> **Treatment:** Upon determining screening practices for high-yield conditions, becoming familiar with the pediatric guidelines for treating these conditions can be valuable. These guidelines have been extensively

researched and were developed by leading organizations such as the American Psychological Association and the American Academy of Pediatrics. Sprinkled into the proceeding sections will be treatment recommendations based on the guidelines. As you continue reading, some of the guidelines may seem overwhelming. As you work with your team to build a practice, it is important to consider practices that will be sustainable, which involves making a realistic plan. A part of the process of implementing PCBH is recognizing how you can incorporate evidence-based practices to fit the resources of your clinic. As a result, keep reading, take some deep breaths, and remember that building a system is a process.

Pathways for high yield-conditions:

Lethality:

Screening Age Group: 12 years and older

Tools: Ask Suicide-Screening Questions and Columbia Suicide Severity Rating Scale

Treatment:

Risk Assessment: All children who endorse past or current suicidal ideation or behaviors during a visit (e.g., verbally or on a screener) would benefit from completing a risk assessment. The assessment can further explore the severity of the thoughts and behaviors. Additionally, a thorough assessment can help the team understand the appropriate next steps for treatment, including safety planning therapy and hospitalization.

Safety Plan: If ideation or behaviors are endorsed, a clinician can guide a child and their family through developing a safety plan. This plan can include identifying values, warning signs, adaptive coping strategies, people the child can call for a distraction or crisis management, professional crisis agencies, and environmental strategies to prevent or reduce harm.

Follow-up plan: Work with your team to craft your follow-up plan upon completing a risk assessment and safety plan. While developing your plan, consider when the child will return to the clinic. Who will be involved in the visit? What will be the focus of the appointment? Examples of a follow-up plan include:

Joint medical and behavioral health visits to reassess safety, update safety plans, and provide strategies to address co-existing conditions.

If a child expresses serious concerns, they may be referred to a higher level of service. Safety check-ins can also be conducted in primary care until the family is connected with their regular provider.

Targeted interventions for teaching, practicing, and reinforcing skills.

If a child is not responding to targeted services, consider an external referral to provide more frequent teaching, modeling, and reinforcing skills.

Depression:

Screening Age Group: 12 years and older

Tools: Patient Health Questionnaire-9

Pediatric Guidelines: The American Psychological Association (2019) describes the following pathways for treating different levels of depression:

Mild: nondirective supportive therapy, group cognitive-behavioral therapy, or guided self-help.

Moderate to severe: brief psychological therapy (individual cognitive behavioral therapy, interpersonal psychotherapy, family therapy, or psychodynamic psychotherapy) with or without fluoxetine.

Depression that is severe, recurrent, unresponsive to treatment, or psychotic: intensive psychological therapy of an alternative therapy than what was already tried, systemic family therapy, or 30 weekly sessions of individual child psychotherapy. The treatment can be administered with or without the use of fluoxetine.

If a child does not respond to fluoxetine: sertraline, or citalopram

Follow-up Plan:

If medication is being prescribed, joint medical and behavioral health visits to monitor response to medication and provide brief psychological interventions during medical visits. Interventions include safety planning, behavioral activation, sleep hygiene, healthy nutrition, and cognitive reframing.

Targeted series of visits to provide opportunities to teach and practice evidence-based strategies.

If a child is not responding to targeted services, consider an external referral to provide more frequent and intensive psychological interventions.

Bridge services in primary care until the family is linked with their ongoing provider.

For additional treatment guidelines for supporting this sub-population, refer to the American Psychological Association (2019) and Zuckerbrot, Cheung, Jensen, Stein, and Laraque (2018) from the American Academy of Pediatrics.

Attention Deficit Hyperactivity Disorder:

Screening Age Group: children four years or older demonstrating significant concerns with inattention or hyperactivity in two primary settings.

Tools: Vanderbilt Assessment Scale - Teacher and Parent form

Pediatric Guidelines: Once you have determined that a child meets the criteria for ADHD, your team can offer different treatment options to help manage their symptoms. The Subcommittee on Attention-Deficit/Hyperactivity Disorder, Steering Committee on Quality Improvement and Management (2011)

from the American Academy of Pediatrics published the following pediatric guidelines:

Preschool-aged children (4-5 years of age): Behavior therapy administered to relevant stakeholders (e.g., parents, teachers). If therapy does not significantly improve a child's functioning and they continue to demonstrate moderate to severe impairment, methylphenidate can be considered.

Elementary school-aged children (6-11 years of age): US Food and Drug Administration-approved medications for ADHD and behavioral therapy.

Adolescents (12-18 years of age): US Food and Drug Administration-approved medications for ADHD and behavioral therapy.

Follow-up Plan:

If medication is being prescribed, joint medical and behavioral health visits to monitor response to medication and provide family behavioral management strategies on setting routines, rewards, effective commands, time-out, or job cards. Suppose you want to improve a child's performance in school. In that case, educating them about school-based services such as daily behavior report cards and individualized education plans can be beneficial.

Targeted series of visits to provide opportunities to teach, model, and coach evidence-based behavioral management strategies.

If a child is not responding to targeted services, consider external referral to provide more frequent teaching, modeling, and coaching on behavioral management strategies.

Bridge care in primary care until the family is linked with their ongoing provider.

Autism Spectrum Disorder:

Screening Age Group: 18 and 24 months

Tools: Modified Checklist for Autism in Toddlers, Autism Diagnostic Observation Schedule, Second Edition, Childhood Autism Rating Scale, Second Edition

Pediatric Recommendations: If signs of autism are evident through your screening, Hyman et al. (2020) from the American Academy of Pediatrics published the following pediatric guidelines:

Evaluation: Completing a comprehensive multidisciplinary evaluation can help identify the child's strengths and areas that warrant improvement. An evaluation includes assessing language, cognitive, adaptive abilities, motor skills, hearing, vision, sensory processing, and genetics. Completing a comprehensive evaluation entails building awareness and relationships with specialty providers across disciplines. As a clinic, building a referral toolkit that includes local speech-language pathologists, occupational therapists, physical therapists, developmental-behavioral pediatricians, and applied behavioral analysts in your area could be helpful.

Collaboration across systems: It is important to remember that symptoms of ASD can impact a child's academic, social-emotional, and behavioral skills. As a result, while working with families, it is recommended to advocate for implementing evidence-based practices that holistically address the diverse needs of these children. Helpful strategies can include consulting with schools to assist with developing individualized education plans, linking the child to mental health care services, identifying appropriate respite services, and exploring fun extracurricular activities for the child.

Planning for adolescence and adult care: As children with autism grow older, families may continue to have questions about their child's development. For optimal support of children throughout their lifespan, it is advisable to offer family education regarding transitional stages, link them with support organizations, and guide families toward ongoing clinical research opportunities.

Follow-up Plan:

Joint medical and behavioral health visits to provide contact information for relevant referrals, including speech therapy, occupational therapy, physical therapy, special needs preschool, early head start, or the state developmental disability board. Providing behavioral strategies to address various concerns can also be helpful, including sleep hygiene, picky eating, social communication, temper tantrums, and safety.

Targeted series of visits to provide opportunities to teach, model, and coach evidence-based behavioral management strategies.

If a child is not responding to targeted services, consider an external referral to provide more frequent teaching, modeling, and coaching on behavioral management strategies.

Bridge services in primary care until the family is linked with their ongoing provider.

Local School System Engagement

One additional routine pathway to consider is how to broadly engage with the local school systems and community organizations serving your pediatric population. Here are some ways to consider collaborating effectively with schools and other organizations. Note that even though your primary care team will likely have limited control over the services delivered at school, you can provide a crucial service as an educator to parents and the care team on available resources to prepare them to advocate for their children/ patients as they navigate the educational system. Resources you can start familiarizing your team with include:

List of early childhood resources

Handouts on some interventions that can be implemented at school (e.g., daily behavior report card).

Federal definitions of 504 plans and IEPs

Process for initiating special education services in your nearby districts

A standardized template you can use to document a child's diagnosis, endorse your support for the family and school to collaborate to determine if special education services are warranted, provide an invitation for further collaboration, and provide your preferred contact information.

Local resources that can help with tutoring, homework support, and extracurricular activities.

Besides becoming familiar with supports that address school-based concerns, exploring community organizations that can help advance the overall well-being of the families you serve will be helpful. These include:

Mental health organizations

Child protective services

Free legal advice for families

Support with housing, utilities, food, clothing, and transportation

Local crisis numbers

In conclusion, encountering a complex pediatric condition during a primary care visit can feel daunting. However, with the proper preparation, your team can build routine pathways to address the concerns you will likely face in your clinic. The key is preparation and proper engagement of the care teams in building solutions that work for patients and care providers.

Ethics

There are many ethical considerations and nuances when working in pediatric primary care. We will not address these in detail here, but you should be aware of the following areas of concern.

- We recommend exploring your local institution, state laws, resources, and planning before an issue arises. For example, considerations for consent and assent are imperative when working in pediatrics. Consider at what age you will see a child without a parent/legal guardian in person and via telehealth and how to manage custody/divorce and foster placement.
- Know your mandatory reporting laws and incorporate an understanding of these into your informed consent process.
- Understand the impact of open notes on minors in your institution, including who has access to patient notes and how that might impact your documentation. Many EHRs offer a do not share option; it is vital to understand that option's requirements and limits.
- Finally, while PCBH often requires navigating multiple relationships, consider how to set healthy boundaries in

situations involving a staff member's child as the identified patient.

References

American Psychological Association. (2019). Clinical practice guidelines for the treatment of depression across three age cohorts. Retrieved from https://www.apa.org/depression-guideline

Ammerman, R. T., Herbst, R., Mara, C. A., Taylor, S., McClure, J. M., Burkhardt, M. C., & Stark, L. J. (2022). Integrated Behavioral Health Increases Well-Child Visits and Immunizations in the First Year. *Journal of Pediatric Psychology*, 47(3), 360-369. https://doi.org/10.1093/jpepsy/jsab104

Asarnow, J. R., Kolko, D. J., Miranda, J., & Kazak, A. E. (2017). The Pediatric Patient-Centered Medical Home: Innovative models for improving behavioral health. *American Psychologist*, 72(1), 13-27. https://doi.org/10.1037/a0040411

Briggs, R. D. (Ed.). (2016). *Integrated early childhood behavioral health in primary care: A guide to implementation and evaluation.* Springer.

Cummings, J. R., Wen, H., & Druss, B. G. (2013). Improving access to mental health services for youth in the United States. *Journal of the American Medical Association,* 309(6), 553-554.

Garner, A. S. (2016). Thinking developmentally: The next evolution in models of health. *Journal of Developmental and*

Behavioral Pediatrics, 37(7), 579-584. https://Doi.org/
10.1097/DBP.0000000000000326

Hyman, S. L., Levy, S. E., & Myers, S. M. (2020).
Identification, evaluation, and management of children
with autism spectrum disorder. *Pediatrics,* 145(1), Article
e20193447. https://doi.org/10.1542/peds.2019-3447

Kindig, D., & Stoddart, G. (2003). What is population
health? A*merican Journal of Public Health,* 93(3), 380-383.

Masten, A., & Cicchetti, D. (2010). Developmental cascades.
Development and Psychopathology, 22(3), 491-495. https://
doi:10.1017/S0954579410000222

Masten, A. S., Lucke, C. M., Nelson, K. M., & Stallworthy, I.
C. (2021). Resilience in development and psychopathology:
Multisystem perspectives. *Annual Review of Clinical
Psychology,* pp. 17, 521-549. *doi.org/10.1146/annurev-
clinpsy-081219-120307*

Mazurek, M. O., Harkins, C., Menezes, M., Chan, J., Parker,
R. A., Kuhlthau, K., & Sohl, K. (2020). Primary care
providers' perceived barriers and needs for support in
caring for children with autism. *The Journal of Pediatrics,*
221, 240-245. https://doi.org/10.1016/j.jpeds.2020.01.014

McDaniel, S. H., & Fogarty, C. T. (2009). What primary care
psychology has to offer the patient-centered medical
home. *Professional Psychology: Research and Practice,* 40(5),
483-492. https://doi.org/10.1037/a0016751

Merikangas, K. R., He, J. P., Burstein, M., Swanson, S. A.,
Avenevoli, S., Cui, L., ... & Swendsen, J. (2010). Lifetime
prevalence of mental disorders in US adolescents: results

from the National Comorbidity Survey Replication-Adolescent Supplement (NCS-A). *Journal of the American Academy of Child & Adolescent Psychiatry*, 49(10), 980-989.

Morelli, D. L., Pati, S., Butler, A., Blum, N. J., Gerdes, M., Pinto-Martin, J., & Guevara, J. P. (2014). Challenges to implementation of developmental screening in urban primary care: a mixed methods study. *BMC Pediatrics*, 14(1), 1-11. https://doi.org/10.1186/1471-2431-14-16

National Academies of Sciences, Engineering, and Medicine 2021. Implementing High-Quality Primary Care: Rebuilding the Foundation of Health Care. Washington, DC: The National Academies Press. https://doi.org/10.17226/25983.

Reiter, J. T., Dobmeyer, A. C., & Hunter, C. L. (2018). The primary care behavioral health (PCBH) model: An overview and operational definition. *Journal of Clinical Psychology in Medical Settings*, 25(2), 109-126. https://doi: 10.1007/s10880-017-9531-x

Shahidullah, J. D., Lee, E., Shafrir, R., & Pincus, L. (2018). Systems of Pediatric Healthcare Delivery and the Social-Ecological Framework. In *Handbook of Pediatric Behavioral Healthcare*, (pp. 3-15). Springer, Cham.

Strosahl, K. D., & Robinson, P. J. (2018). Adapting empirically supported treatments in the era of integrated care: A roadmap for success. *Clinical Psychology: Science and Practice*, 25(3), 20.

Wissow, L. S., Brown, J., Fothergill, K. E., Gadomski, A., Hacker, K., Salmon, P., & Zelkowitz, R. (2013). Universal mental health screening in pediatric primary care: a systematic review. *Journal of the American Academy of Child & Adolescent Psychiatry, 52*(11), 1134-1147.

Zuckerbrot R. A, Cheung A, Jensen P. S, Stein R.K, Laraque D., & the members of the Guidelines for Adolescent Depression in Primary Care Steering Group. (2018). Part I. Practice preparation, identification, assessment, and initial management. *Pediatrics, 141*(3), e20174081. https://doi.org/10.1542/peds.2017-4081

Sample Resources

- Collaborative Family Healthcare Association Pediatrics Special Interest Group: https://members.cfha.net/page/PedsSIG

- Division 54 Pediatric IPC Special Interest Group (Bibliography and Training program resource): https://pedpsych.org/

- GATHER Resource/Handout: https://www.aafp.org/pubs/fpm/issues/2021/0500/p3.html

  - https://www.behavioralconsultationandprimarycare.com/wp-content/uploads/2015/07/10.F.3-Figure-10.3-GATHER-An-example-of-a-BHC-educational-handout.pdf

- Immunization resources:

  - https://itdoesnthavetohurt.ca/

  - Sid, the Science Kid: Getting a Shot, You Can Do It! https://youtu.be/nemlAvrOzTA

- https://www.buzzy4shots.com.au/
- Pill Swallowing:
  - https://kidshealth.org/en/parents/swallowing-pills.html
  - https://copingclub.com/clay-works-on-pill-swallowing-using-candy/
  - https://www.cincinnatichildrens.org/-/media/cincinnati%20childrens/home/research/divisions/c/adherence/parents/helping-article1-pdf-strategies%20to%20help%20kids%20swallow%20pills
- Milestones:
  - https://www.cdc.gov/ncbddd/actearly/milestones/index.html
  - https://www.cdc.gov/ncbddd/actearly/pdf/parents_pdfs/milestonemomentseng508.pdf
  - https://brightfutures.aap.org/Bright%20Futures%20Documents/BF4_POCKETGUIDE.pdf
- School:
  - Sample letter for IEP: https://www.med.umich.edu/1libr/PedPsych/IEPLetter.pdf
- Screening:
  - https://www.cdc.gov/ncbddd/childdevelopment/screening.html

- https://brightfutures.aap.org/families/Pages/default.aspx

- https://www.parentcenterhub.org/ei-overview/

- https://www.tuftschildrenshospital.org/The-Survey-of-Wellbeing-of-Young-Children/Overview

- ASQ- 3: https://brookespublishing.com/product/asq-3/

- MCHAT: https://mchatscreen.com/mchat-rf/

- Sleep:

  - Pediatric Sleep Problems: A Clinician's Guide to Behavioral Interventions supplemental site by Lisa J. Meltzer, Ph.D., CBSM, and Valerie McLaughlin Crabtree, Ph.D., CBSM. http://pubs.apa.org/books/supp/meltzer/?_ga=2.224043739.114980277.1600982036-426019459.1595006617

  - babysleep.com

  - American Academy of Sleep Medicine - http://www.aasmnet.org/

  - American Sleep Apnea Association - http://www.sleepapnea.org/asaa.html

- ADHD/Behavioral Interventions:

  - Wolraich, M. L., Hagan, J. F., Allan, C., Chan, E., Davison, D., Earls, M., ... & Zurhellen, W. (2019). Clinical practice guideline for the diagnosis, evaluation, and treatment of attention-deficit/

hyperactivity disorder in children and adolescents. *Pediatrics*, 144(4).

- Parenting with Love & Logic (https://www.loveandlogic.com/parents/what-is-love-and-logic-for-parents?campaignid=118209153&adgroupid=40756213599&creative=252966543819&keyword=love%20and%20logic%20parenting&gclid=EAIaIQobChMIut6P-6_J3AIVUrjACh3jygiJEAAYASAAEgIK7_D_BwE)

- Patterson's Parent Management Training (Oregon Model) https://www.cebc4cw.org/program/the-oregon-model-parent-management-training-pmto/detailed

- Helping the Noncompliant Child: Family-Based Treatment For Oppositional Behaviour (Second Edition) by McMahon and Forehand 2003.

- Eyberg's Parent-Child Interaction Therapy (http://www.pcit.org/)

- Russell Barkleys' parent training for the defiant/ADHD child (https://www.researchgate.net/publication/232552340_Defiant_Children_A_Clinician's_Manual_for_Parent_Training)

- Webster-Stratton's Incredible Years (http://www.incredibleyears.com/team-view/carolyn-webster-stratton/)

- Zero to Five: 70 Essential Parenting Tips Based on Science. https://www.amazon.com/Zero-Five-Essential-Parenting-Science/dp/0983263361

- First the broccoli, then the ice cream: A parent's guide to deliberate discipline by Tim Riley. https://www.amazon.com/First-Broccoli-Then-Ice-Cream/dp/0984142312

- http://alankazdin.com/everyday-parenting-the-abcs-of-child-rearing/, Everyday parenting, the ABCs of child rearing: free online parenting course by Alan Kazdin; 20 how to videos addressing problems in school and home

- apa.org/act: APA's Violence Prevention office discusses 8-week class curriculum

- http://www.apa.org/topics/parenting/resilience-tip-tool.aspx, Resilience booster: parent tip toolkit

- http://depts.washington.edu/hcsats/PDF/TF-%20CBT/pages/positive_parenting.html

- healthychildren.org: a guided development resource for parents by age

- ACT raising safe kids

- "Parenting the Strong-Willed Child" by Rex Forehand

- 1-2-3 Magic! series. There are some YouTube videos demonstrating the skills in addition to the written materials

- http://csefel.vanderbilt.edu/: Social and emotional development

- Depression:

  - Guidelines for Adolescent Depression in Primary Care (GLAD-PC): Part I. Practice Preparation, Identification, Assessment, and Initial Management. http://pediatrics.aappublications.org/content/early/2018/02/22/peds.2017-4081

  - Guidelines for Adolescent Depression in Primary Care (GLAD-PC): Part II. Treatment and Ongoing Management. http://pediatrics.aappublications.org/content/early/2018/02/22/peds.2017-4082

About the Authors

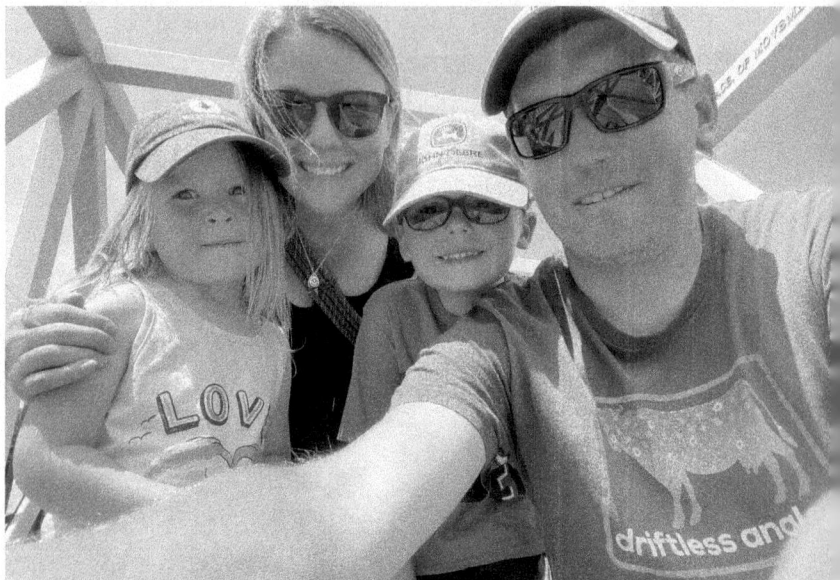

Alli Allmon Dixson, Ph.D. (she/her) is the Section Chair of
Integrated Care, Behavioral Health Consultant in Pediatrics,
and Behavioral Medicine Faculty at a Family Medicine
Residency. She practices psychology in pediatrics
integrated primary care and supports behavioral health
consultants across a midwestern health system integrating
behavioral medicine into primary and specialty care clinics.
In family medicine she precepts, teaches, and supports
family medicine residents. Alli has a passion for primary
care behavioral health, social justice, and serving children,
adolescents, and families who might not otherwise receive
behavioral medicine services. Alli was an Army brat and
moved almost every year growing up, mostly in Europe and
the United States. While she still loves to travel, she is
enjoying growing roots for her family and work. She finds
joy in having a front row seat to her children's passions

(currently unicorns and semi-trucks), hiking and all things nature, reading, music, and learning from all those around her.

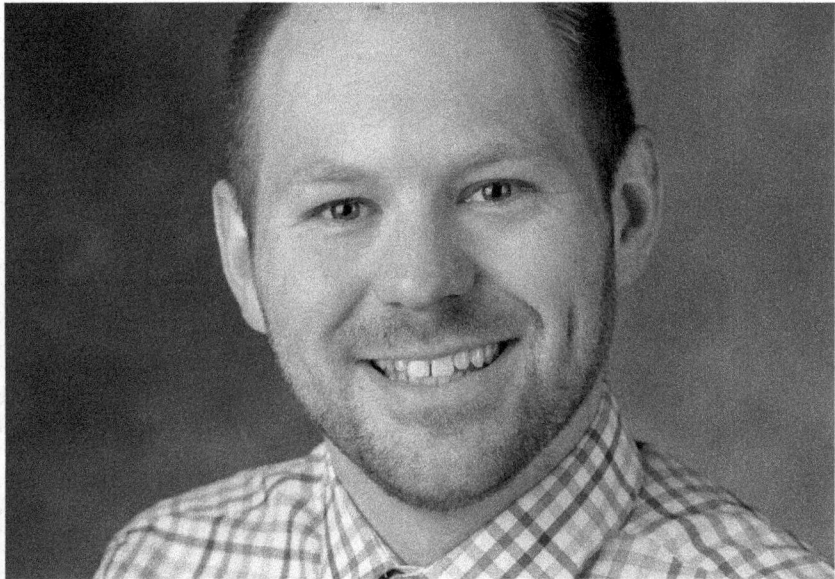

Cody Hostutler, PhD, is the clinical director for behavioral health integration at Nationwide Children's Hospital and Assistant Professor of Pediatrics at The Ohio State University. He is passionate about increasing access to quality, accessible, and equitable behavioral healthcare for families within their primary care medical home through clinical work, consultation, research, and advocacy. He also enjoys cooking, playing music, and spending time outdoors with his family.

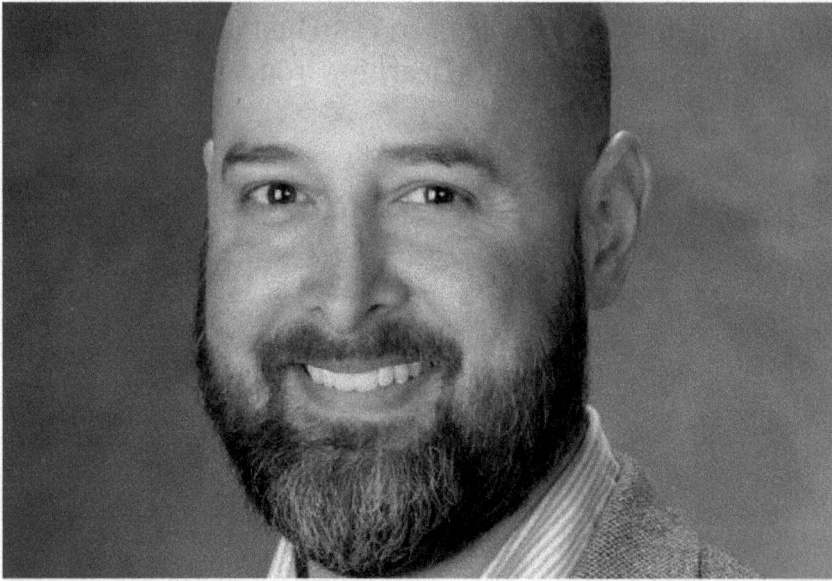

William Leever, PsyD, is an Assistant Professor of Pediatrics in the Division of Pediatric Psychology and Neuropsychology at Nationwide Children's Hospital and the Ohio State University College of Medicine. Dr. Leever currently leads a new program that focuses on increasing access to pediatric behavioral health care using brief transdiagnostic therapy, digital technology, and task sharing with non-specialist providers. Dr. Leever received his Bachelor of Arts in Psychology from the College of Wooster, and his Doctorate of Psychology from Xavier University. In addition to clinical care, Dr. Leever engages in stigma-reducing educational efforts to increase awareness around the importance of social connection and belonging for youth mental health.

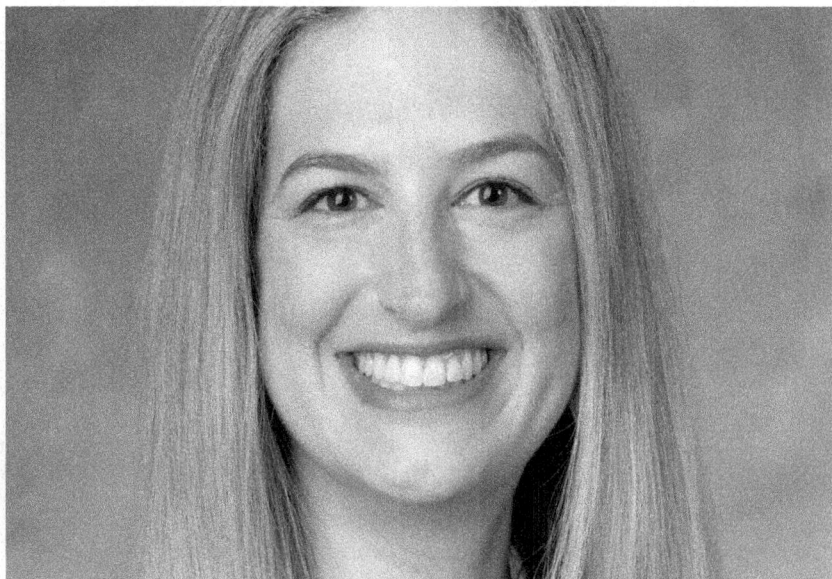

Dr. Rebecca (Becca) Lyren, PhD is a pediatric psychologist at Nationwide Children's Hospital, where she works in integrated primary care and serves as co-director of the Williams syndrome clinic. She is passionate about increasing access to care for all children and has a special interest in improving outcomes for patients with disabilities through integrated care. Outside of work, you can find her cheering on The Ohio State Buckeyes, checking out new restaurants, or reading a good book.

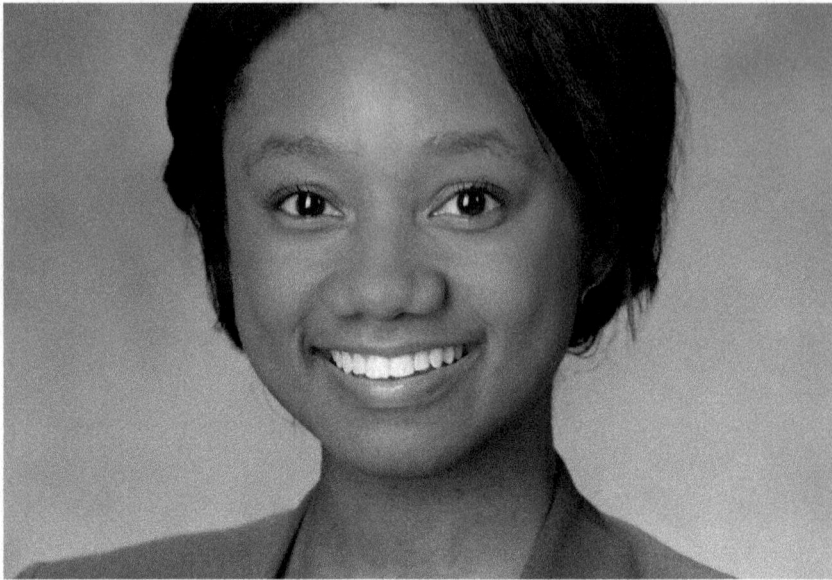

Destiny Singleton, PhD, is a pediatric psychologist at Nationwide Children's Hospital and an Associate Professor at Ohio State University. Dr. Singleton spends most of her career providing prevention, intervention, and consultation services in an integrated primary care setting. She is passionate about collaborating with families and professionals across the home, medical, and school systems to help promote the development of the children she serves. Before settling in Ohio, Dr. Singleton worked in schools, outpatient behavioral health clinics, and hospitals across Florida and Nebraska. Alongside work, Dr. Singleton enjoys watching horror movies and traveling. Her favorite vacation spot is Serbia!

Chapter 24: Quality Monitoring

By Meghan Fondow, PhD

ince the original publication of this book, my role on the team has shifted from staff BHC to now Director of Behavioral Health. As I have taken on more leadership and administrative duties, my time has shifted away from data and metrics, with less time for research activities. Currently, my use of metrics is more directed to our BHC team's day-to-day operations and staffing.

In recent years, there has been a lot of discussion about measurement-based care and metrics. There are more resources about what measures and metrics to use, how to use them, and how to track them (check out CFHA Learns for continuing education videos, and Drs Beachy and Bauman's PCBH Corner video series).

PCBH has continued to evolve, as models do, with more sites nationwide utilizing PCBH or some version of the model. Most sites have blended integrated care programs, with parts of PCBH, parts of CoCM, and perhaps some co-located care. Deciding what measures and metrics to use and track will depend on your site.

It can be helpful to think about measures and metrics, including organizational/program and patient care measures. Patient care measures can include screening and outcome measures to move clinical care forward. These measures can also be a source of information for understanding your patient population. They may be part of what needs to be reported to agencies like HRSA or others overseeing your organization.

Much of my focus in the past years, particularly around the challenges of COVID, has been on organizational or practice-level measures. Tracking adherence to the integrated care model or its specific components can be achieved using certain benchmarks or metrics. For example, tracking the average number of visits per year for unique patients can help assess whether the program is adhering to PCBH or experiencing drift, with fewer patients being seen more often; this can help lead to conversations between directors and BHCs on any potential mismatch between model goals of population-based care and the day-to-day experience of the BHCs carrying out the work.

I have also found tracking of metrics related to follow-up visit frequency to be helpful to track, as the data assisted in confirming the subjective experience of my team that we saw a significant increase in demand for more follow-up visits starting in 2020; this appears to be due to a combination of factors, including decreased availability of outpatient behavioral health resources in our local community and increased demand for services with the COVID pandemic.

Bringing these data back to my BHC team led to valuable and productive conversations about how to approach individual visits and navigate the new reality that we were scheduling out several weeks instead of a few days to one week; this was a significant downstream impact of increased demand that we saw operationally across all clinic sites. Generally speaking PCBH calls for a diverse distribution of follow-up rates with more than 50% of follow-ups occurring between two and four weeks from an initial visit, a minority of patients seen in a one week window (perhaps 10% or less) and the remaining 30-40% of patients seen in 5 or more weeks. There are no hard and fast rules here, but these can serve as general guardrails for programs to follow.

Several other metrics that can be good to track, include penetration into the medical population, rates of follow-up visits, and team and individual provider productivity. Penetration into the medical population can be parsed out by specific groups as desired, such as pediatrics vs. adults, to explore trends and utilization. These numbers can help understand the population-based care approach of the BHC team. Generally speaking a robust PCBH program will have a penetration rate into the overall patient population of 20%. A newer program is likely to start with goals of 10 to 15% penetration (as defined as a numerator of all unique patients seen by BHCs in a given year over a denominator of all unique patients seen by the PCPs in a year).

For follow-up visits, I am generally looking at how our team is performing related to recommendations for the PCBH model. What is our median number of visits, and what percentage of patients meet with BHCs 4 times or less in a given year, and conversely, four times or more? Our team does not have rigid rules or policies on the number of visits available to patients. Instead, we follow patients as needed for an episode of care. I have been working for Access for 15 years, and there are patients I have seen on and off for those years. They reach out for support as their own needs arise, just as patients reach out for primary medical care as needs arise. Generally speaking PCBH calls for most episodes of care to fall between one and three visits per patient per 6-12 month period, therefore your mean visit per patient metric is likely around two in a PCBH program. Your mode is one visit per patient per year. And a minority of your patients are seen four or more times per year, perhaps up to 10-15% of your overall population of patients seen by BHCs.

Team and individual productivity can be helpful to track, though it should not be the sole measure of the worth of a BHC. Much of the work of a BHC will not be captured by visit numbers, given our other tasks of curbside consults, coordination of care, and education to the overall healthcare team. Team and individual productivity are, however, frequently considered when creating budgets and assessing staffing needs. Our team has grown from 1 part-time BHC covering two sites to 12 BHCs, one consulting psychiatrist, and 2 Behavioral Health Care Coordinators (BHCCs) covering three sites. Sharing data with our BHC team for transparent communication has been constructive.

Tracking this data has also helped me to move staff across clinics to match better the demand we experience. Individual data can help with staff development conversations and validate the subjective experience of busyness we all feel. Our team growth has supported team wellness and sustainability, as we can take time off without leaving clinics unattended, allowing staff to truly take time away.

One tip is to become good friends with whoever helps handle data in your organization. Over the years, my team has developed a strong working relationship with our accounting team, and this has helped create a partnership to be able to establish a routine for regular reports from accounting to the BHC team regarding provider productivity, team productivity, and productivity by site by day of the week. These reports assist in ongoing conversations with BHC staff regarding our work and help identify trends in performance. The productivity by site by day of the week assists in our staffing allocations, allowing us to respond to changes in which sites are busier on particular days rather than relying only on subjective reports. We have used the data for team awards for high productivity, and for some, this creates a friendly competitive spirit.

There are some metrics I wish I had access to that I have seen other sites discuss in various email threads via the CFHA list serve, including tracking new BHC patients and handoffs. Our sites use EPIC, and our build of EPIC has not had a discreet field to track whether a patient is new to BHC or if they are a same-day handoff in an easy-to-retrieve field. Thanks to some creative thinking from our data/QI department, we will have access to these measures soon. I have done some tracking by hand, which is helpful, but not sustainable, over time. And this is one of the other key tips with respect to metrics - they must be sustainably collected and digested for them to be helpful. Choose only the most helpful metrics and stick with them only as long as they retain their usefulness.

An exemplar dashboard is included below to illustrate how you could put together the metrics you select into a document to share with leadership and your team. Note the three main areas, Clinical, Operational, and Financial. Note also the use of the color code to quickly identify areas to work on and areas to celebrate. In the exemplar dashboard, the Service Delivery Rating refers to a clinical outcome metric, in this case, the Outcome Rating Scale.

Table 4. PCBH Dashboard, All Clinics

	Q3 2024	Q4 2024	Definitions
Clinical			
Service Delivery Rating	15%	23%	Percent mean change in ORS score in sampled patients
Diversity Impact	52%	51%	Percent of all patients seen in qualifying diversity and/or vulnerable populations categories
Complexity Ratio	80%	88%	Percent of patients seen with at least one chronic medical and behavioral health condition on problem list (ideal vs all clinic mean)
Provider Impact	40%	39%	Percent of providers referring more than XX patients
Operational			
Accessibility 1	22 Days	19 Days	Average time to third next available f/u appointment as measured at end of quarter

	Q3 2024	Q4 2024	Definitions
Accessibility 2	2 Weeks	1.5 Weeks	Average duration between visits
Consult Length	40% | 6%	36% | 8%	Percent of 90832 | 96158 (H&B Codes)/ All Codes
Population Penetrance	12%	11.5%	Raw number of patients seen/ Total primary care patients
Patient Visits | # Sessions	219 | 28	199 | 32	Raw number of patients seen | Raw Sessions (Half Days)
Visits Per Patient	3.8	4	Raw number of visits/ Raw Unique patients seen
Warm Handoff Ratio	28%	22%	Percent of same-day visits (warm handoffs/total raw)
Financial			
Charges Generated	$109,500.00	$106,000.00	Total charges generated for clinical care
Other Funds	$60,000.00	$60,000.00	Other funds feeding into program
Program Costs	-$190,000.00	-$190,000.00	Salary costs and incidental costs
Net	-$20,500.00	-$24,000.00	Sum of above
Color Code:	Improved or Meets Standards	Steady (or insignificant)	Decreased or Below Standards

About the Author

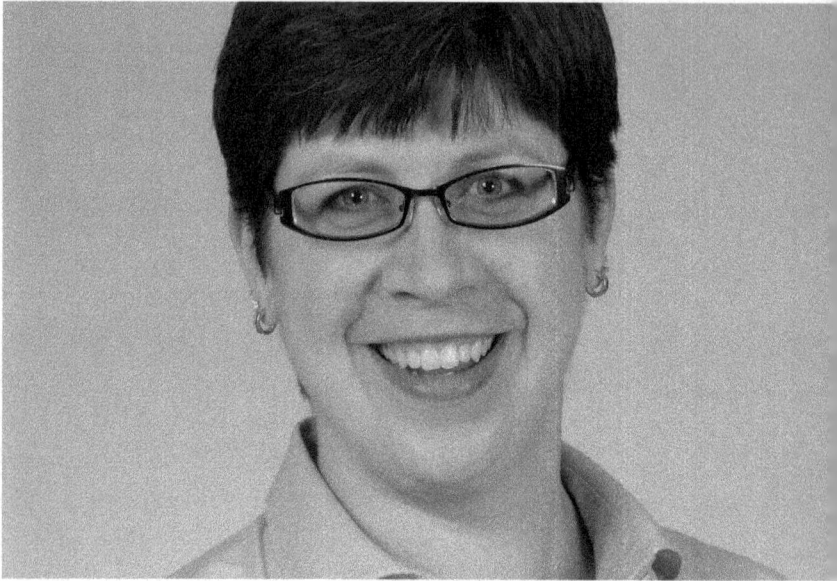

Meghan Fondow, PhD, is the Director of Behavioral Health at Access Community Health Centers in Madison, WI. She has worked as a Behavioral Health Consultant within the Primary Care Behavioral Health model for over 15 years. Meghan serves as the Clinical Training Director at Access, providing oversight and supervision for fellows and other trainees. Part of her role as Director of Behavioral Health has included organizational trainings on communication, teamwork, wellness and resiliency. Meghan enjoys the variety and diversity of clinical work within the PCBH model in the context of an underserved population, working with students and fellows from interdisciplinary training backgrounds within the PCBH model, and supporting the overall organization.

Chapter 25: Care Coordination

By Ashley Grosshans, PsyD

How did we do this job before we had our BHCCs?!"
I've heard this exclaimed many times since
implementing the Behavioral Health Care
Coordination (BHCC) role. Adding the BHCC position to our
practice has been a game-changer. BHCs, PCPs, and our
patients have benefited from the additional support this
role provides within the clinic and with connection to
services beyond our walls. The BHCC position has shifted
the division of work to support the sustainability of the
BHC workload and has allowed us to expand the services
we offer.

The Primary Care Behavioral Health model teaches us to be
generalists, "lead with yes," and fill a mental health gap.
BHCs provide an essential service to the patients and staff
of our primary care clinics. Our goal, however, is not to
replace specialty mental health and substance use disorder
services. Some patients' needs exceed what can be safely
and adequately addressed within the primary care setting.

Some patients request connection to a consistent therapy provider or a targeted therapy approach that doesn't fit within the scope of the BHC model. Other patients need specialty psychiatry or case management services. These are examples of patients who would benefit from establishing with specialty services in the community.

Historically, our BHC team kept all knowledge of specialty mental health and substance use disorder resources available to our patients. We knew the names of most mental health clinics in our community and which types of insurance were accepted by each resource. I could dial up various arms of our county mental health clinic by memory to assist a patient with connection to services. A significant chunk of BHC time was spent on care coordination efforts - getting patients connected to care outside of our walls, making calls to gather information about the services a patient is already established with, or advocating for connection to additional resources. Having clinicians spend significant time on care coordination work was not the best use of training and talent. Because of clinical demands and time constraints, BHCs couldn't thoroughly provide care coordination support.

For years, we had thrown around ideas about freeing up our BHCs to see more patients for clinical care while maintaining workload sustainability. "Wouldn't it be nice if we had BHC support staff?" Fortunately, the BHC team is genuinely valued on an organizational level at Access, and our PCPs have consistently provided positive feedback about the support BHC delivers to them. This foundational belief in integrated care by leadership has allowed us to continue to grow, expand, and explore creative solutions such as creating the BHCC role.

We defined the role once we received organizational approval to develop and hire for the BHCC position. Our primary goals for the position included:

- Providing generalized support to BHCs (e.g., admin, calls, logistics)
- Supporting referrals to mental health and substance use disorder treatment in the community
- Care coordination for high-risk and vulnerable patients

We had an existing Patient Services team who assisted with specialty health referrals and insurance navigation and provided resources to address concerns related to social determinants of health. Thus, we needed to define the role and scope of the BHCC position to clarify how this new role would fit into the services provided in the clinic.

As we prepared to recruit for the BHCC position, we worked closely with Human Resources to create a job description and outline the skill set we were looking to hire for. We initially recruited masters-level social workers, knowing this cohort of prospective BHCCs would come to us with prior knowledge and training that would match our needs. We prioritized hiring candidates comfortable working with a high-risk patient population, felt confident with advocacy work, had strong verbal and written communication skills, and valued teamwork. We were thrilled to hire and begin onboarding our first BHCC team member in December 2019.

When the Covid-19 pandemic hit, our BHC encounters skyrocketed. There was an exponential increase in the demand for mental health services. Like everyone else, we scrambled to adjust to remote work while continuing to meet the needs of our community amid a global pandemic. We were so grateful to have our BHCC position to help support the team, and our patients navigate the mental health system during this time. Among many roles offered, our BHCC helped keep us updated on what other community mental health agencies were doing, who was going remote, and who was suspending services. The chaos of the pandemic highlighted the value of the BHCC's position in supporting the sustainability of BHC work and enhancing excellent patient care.

Although recruitment was slow, we filled our two BHCC positions with strong candidates. To promote retention of our masters-level BHCCs, we also began offering an opportunity for clinical training hours. Many masters level social workers seek clinical licensure, and we wanted to support career growth. To balance care coordination needs and professional development, we offered one full day each week of clinical training to our BHCCs. While our masters-level BHCCs valued the organizational mission, the team-based care, and the opportunity to work with our patients, they eventually sought other opportunities that offered further clinical training.

Through recruitment for the BHCC role and having staff in the role, we've learned a lot about how to make this a fulfilling position. We decided that to reinvigorate the job, it would be essential to shift our minimum requirement to a bachelor's level degree in a human services field (psychology, social work, sociology, etc.). We again worked with Human Resources to rewrite our position description and begin recruitment. Almost immediately, applications for the position started pouring in. Many applicants were pursuing a master's degree in social work and were interested in learning about integrated care.

Hiring bachelor's level BHCCs has required intentional shifts in our onboarding process to ensure we offer adequate training. It has also created opportunities for career pathways that we are very proud of. Bachelors-level BHCCs in a social work master (MSW) program can potentially complete their practicum/internship hours with the BHC team. Upon graduation from the MSW program, they can apply for our Social Work Training Fellowship, which provides supervised hours toward clinical licensure (LCSW in Wisconsin); this opens the door to being hired as a BHC with years of training in integrated care. This pathway creates valuable opportunities for employees and helps to address workforce shortage issues that plague the mental health system.

Considerations for Onboarding BHCCs:

- Adequate opportunities to shadow BHC to gain a strong understanding of the model, including the scope and limitations of BHC services
- Providing readings about PCBH work and other integrated care models
- Opportunities to shadow other care team members (PCPs, Consulting Psychiatry, Nursing Teams, Registration, etc.) to gain a strong understanding of the culture of primary care and who does what in the clinic

- Training on the electronic health record
- HIPAA training
- Providing education about local mental health resources and the larger mental health system
- Communication skills and de-escalation training

While a connection to specialty mental health and substance use disorder services remains the foundation of the BHCC position, we've continued to develop the role. The scope of the position has grown to include various other tasks under the umbrella of behavioral health care coordination.

Examples of BHCC referrals include:

- Requests to coordinate care with schools to gather teacher impressions and understand what services are being provided in the school setting, request IEPs, and advocate for support with resource connection
- Coordination with other mental health providers
- Coordination with social workers in hospitals and inpatient programs to advocate for connection to a higher level of care upon discharge
- Summarizing mental health records in the chart
- Educating community agencies about BHC services and what can be provided in the primary care setting

Care coordination requests are often sent through the electronic health record by PCPs or BHCs. We created a BHCC in-basket pool within our EHR (Epic) so requests could be sent to our BHCCs as a group, and then work could be divided equitably. PCPs and BHCs are now doing a significant amount of remote work, which means many of the requests our BHCCs receive are for outreach by phone or MyChart to provide resources.

Our BHCCs also take handoffs in the clinic following PCP or BHC visits. These handoffs often involve providing resource lists, assisting patients with making calls to community agencies, completing online referrals to services, and gathering additional information about resources that a patient may already be connected to. BHCCs document all work in the electronic health record. We've developed standard templates for phone and in-person contacts for ease of charting.

Workflow Considerations:

- How and where to document BHCC work
- Limits on attempts made when performing outreach to patients and community agencies
- Processes for communication back to staff who made the initial BHCC request
- How quickly requests are addressed (initial attempt within 48 hours?)

Much work has gone into developing community resource lists housed within our EHR. In Epic, these are smartphrases that can quickly be dropped into an After Visit Summer (AVS), sent via Mychart, or put into a letter to be mailed to a patient. Most of our resource lists are organized by type of insurance. Insurance status typically guides where a patient can go in the community for mental health and substance use treatment. We have found it crucial to be able to update resource lists quickly and often because resource availability is frequently changing. We also keep lists of support groups, agencies that provide community advocacy, providers who offer specific therapy modalities (DBT, EMDR, Couples Counseling, etc.), and other areas of expertise (gender-affirming care, ADHD assessment, court-mandated treatment, etc.).

To promote visibility and communication with various care team members, our BHCCs sit in the care team space alongside PCP, BHC, and nursing colleagues; this has supported utilizing the BHCC team and encouraged direct handoffs for care coordination support.

Our BHCCs do not have their own schedule; however, we continue to discuss and consider it. If we create a BHCC schedule template, we plan that only BHCCs can schedule patients. If a patient requests a call at a specific time, the schedule could be used to organize the day. The BHCC can schedule a patient when handed off in person, which may help track work and BHCC metrics. Again, this is something we may explore further in the future.

Development of the Behavioral Health Care Coordination position has proven to be vital for the continued growth of our Primary Care Behavioral Health program at Access. This role's support to our BHCs, PCPs, patients, and the larger care team has become essential to our work. Our BHCCs are the keepers and organizers of resource knowledge. They help to bridge communication between agencies, advocate for our patients, and avoid gaps in care. They help us better understand the larger scope of support our patients have access to, and they compassionately support our patients in making connections to community partners. Creating this role has been a learning process, and we continue to learn as we go. Approaching it with a goal, direction, flexibility, and organizational support has helped us succeed. I don't know how we did our work before implementing the BHCC role, but I'm grateful we have their support moving forward.

About the Author

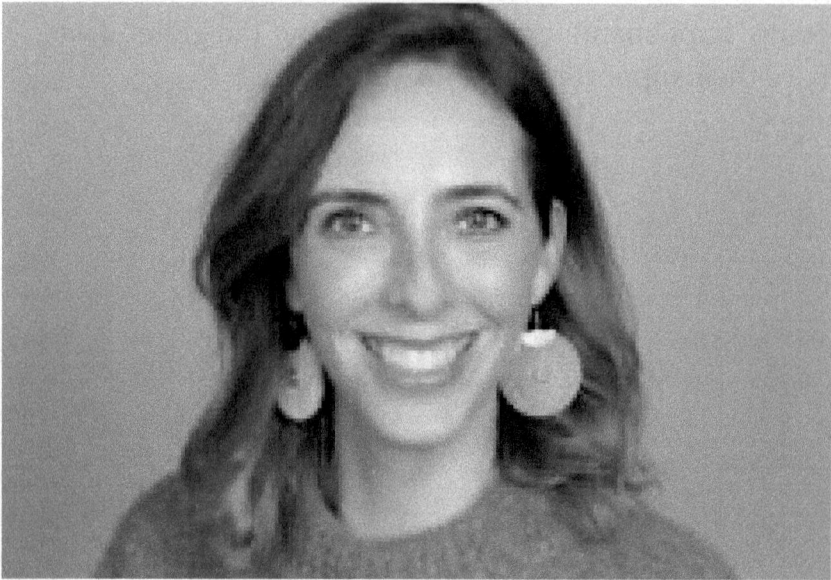

Ashley Grosshans, LCSW is a Behavioral Health Manager at Access and leads the Care Coordination team. She has been with Access since 2011 and has been instrumental in developing care management strategies to support PCBH work. She loves camping and spending time with her husband Austin and son Cedar.

Chapter 26: Leveraging Technology

By Neftali Serrano, PsyD with Alex D. Smith, PsyD &
Meghan Fondow, PhD

uch has changed since the first edition of this
book in the area of technology, yet much has
stayed the same. We continue to have challenges
with electronic health record (EHR) systems, but those
tools have also demonstrated improvements specific to
team-based care. We also continue to experience issues
with team communication, which require specific solutions
based on clinic characteristics. And we have ongoing needs
for care management and registry functions that are
sometimes difficult to solve technologically. This chapter
will give you a taste of where Access is as a clinic. I hope
you can extrapolate from Access' experience and devise
your approaches for your setting.

Electronic Health Records

Access is privileged to use medical record software by Epic
Systems (Epic), one of the most widely used EHR systems.

Small clinics, like ours, do not usually use this software since most of their implementation is in large hospitals. However, our relationship with the University of Wisconsin Medical Foundation (UWMF) comes with the privilege of piggybacking off their network. Like most EHR systems, Epic's software does an excellent job of providing a systematic approach to documenting patient encounters and a good job of allowing for coordination between providers. However, like most electronic health records, this software has limitations. Let's start by reviewing how we have found this technology helpful and then get to our gripes.

Epic's EHR system makes documentation easy for us. We use the same section primary care clinicians use to chart, so some areas within that template do not apply to us (like allergies, vitals, etc.); however, we skip these sections. Too often, I have seen new primary care behavioral health programs start by creating their own templates, requiring adjustments in the EHR. Consistent with program philosophy, you should make as few changes or differentiate your program as little as possible. If there is a free text area somewhere in the basic note module, use it. With time, as you get to know your program needs, you can become more sophisticated and make adjustments. At the outset, people put too much effort into modifying EHR systems and end up not using (or not effectively using) the tools and templates they create.

One of the standard features of the EHR is the ability to create drop-in text snippets. In Epic's EHR system, these are called Smartphrases. In our case, we developed (typed, to be precise) a SOAP note template (actually APSO), which is called into the free text portion of the visit encounter when the user types in ".2AAVISITFULL", ".2ABVISITBRIEF", or ".2ACTELEPHONE". These are arbitrary names of convenience. For example, putting the number at the beginning of the dot phrase helps it to appear higher in the list of phrases that pop up. With time, Access staff also created many other Smartphrases for different kinds of information or note sections. For example, Access has Smartphrases for community resources (they drop them in and then print them for patients), medication information (with dosage, titration, and lab monitoring information), and others. Again, creating a bunch of Smartphrases initially is unnecessary. You and your team will figure out in time what you will need.

Many EHR systems also have basic tracking sections that mimic the tracking typically done for height, weight, and other vitals. In Epic's EHR system, our behavioral health providers enter information in a variety of sections including the Mental Health Activity (e.g., PHQ-9, PHQ-A, GAD-7, C-SSRS, Vanderbilt Assessment Scales, SLUMS), Alcohol, Drugs, & Tobacco Activity (e.g., AUDIT, DAST-10), and SBIRT Activity (e.g., PHQ/2, ADUIT-C, NIDA) tabs. These "Activity" tabs are created by the organization and not the individual provider. Other EHR systems I have seen provide more flexibility in tracking than Epic's, for example, allowing you to input whatever data you want without requiring a template. Again, in line with program philosophy, simplicity demands tracking only what you need and what is truly relevant. It is often true that programs will start tracking things and stop tracking them when they become irrelevant. Particularly in an environment where you have to ask someone else to create templates or program changes, it pays to be sure about tracking a particular piece of data.

The other main benefit of EHR systems is the messaging system often built in. In Epic's EHR system, this is called your in-basket, which is comparable to an email inbox. This in-basket is where messages of different kinds are relayed from user to user; this becomes an essential tool for the primary care team in managing patient care outside of the clinic visit. This system sends messages regarding medication recommendations or patient forms that require completion. You can also send your notes to the primary care clinician following each visit to ensure you are all current on what is happening with a patient.

Additionally, Epic's software allows for instant messaging through Secure Chat. This feature lets you send direct messages to users within the EHR system. Unlike in-basket messages, users are notified in real-time when they receive a message through a pop-up notification; this is a valuable means of communicating when there is an immediate ask. For example, Access' behavioral health team will send a Secure Chat message to our on-site interpreters when we require their service for a visit.

A critical and nuanced skill concerning this kind of messaging is knowing how and when to use it and when not to use it. Much like email, certain etiquette is required to ensure that communication occurs effectively; this means avoiding spamming other primary care clinicians with unnecessary messages or concerns or sending concerns using the internal messaging system, which is better communicated using other means such as a conversation or regular email. If you misuse the EHR email system, you will find that primary care clinicians will no longer read your messages after a while.

Another critical use of the in-basket messaging system is the work organization between the primary care team for task management. At Access, the responsible team member self-assigns an in-basket message when it requires additional action by using the "Take" feature. The team has developed rules to ensure the tasks are completed on time. For example, a generic patient request that may not belong to one team member is automatically handled by the team that is at the clinic that day. Over time, your team will determine the rules necessary to organize its online work.

A final standard function of an EHR is the creation of patient lists. Various team members can add to these lists and may help track patients with certain conditions. An example of a patient list would be patients who have recently visited an emergency department. Patient lists in Epic's EHR system have some utility when more robust tracking systems are unavailable. The functionality is limited and allows users to add and subtract patients from the list. The main shortcoming of modern EHR systems is the inability to track patients robustly. This function is called care management and includes the ability to identify patients with specific characteristics, obtain certain information about those patients, and then record actions necessary to the patient's care based on a review, whether automated or done by a care manager or provider.

For example, a good care management function would allow a provider to create a list of patients with a diagnosis of depression in a given time frame and then, in the list, see specific details about the patient, such as the dates of the last two visits, current medications, date of the last medication adjustment and the last two PHQ9 scores. Hopefully, it is obvious how this could be helpful; this would allow for proactive management of patients who may need more aggressive medication management, more frequent follow-up, or phone contact. This function would also allow for recording actions, such as noting when a patient was called or what needs to be done, along with reminder functions, such as alerts to contact the patient or do a chart review.

Most EHR systems do not have such a function or have parts of such functions dispersed throughout their software. In most cases, organizations must piece together their own system or buy a software package that may interface on some level with their EHR. More recently, EPIC has made care management functions available (depending on your version of EPIC) under its reporting workbench feature. You usually have to work with the IT department and a superuser to get this to work well. So, it is an advancement in capability, but it still requires customization.

We have undergone various iterations of care management approaches (see Serrano, et al article); these included using an Excel spreadsheet to track PHQ9 scores and iPod-based databases (yup, iPods). We then transitioned to a process that exported PHQ9 scores from EPIC into a separate custom database. None of these were ideal, but each improved the previous version. Currently, most care management occurs within EPIC, using the reporting workbench feature. So, one of the critical points about technology is that there is no holy grail, no perfect solution. There are only approximations; this means that you will always be working on a better solution to your data management needs (or at least you should be). That's okay. The important thing is to keep in mind the simplicity mantra so that our approximations do not become powerful and less usable all at once. Better should not always mean more complicated. A good rule of thumb is to start with what is called an MVP in the software development world, a minimum viable product. Start with something that works without bells and whistles, then iterate to find your best improvements.

One of the things I have found as the key person on our team for technology is that if I am too removed from using the solutions I create, I often miss out on the actual usefulness of the tool. For example, I created an iPod database for my staff that I thought was easy to use. Since I tend to see fewer patients than they do with my administrative time, I missed out on how hard it was to remember to use the database since it was beyond the usual workflow and served no immediate purpose for the behavioral health consultants; it was also a burden to sync, requiring specific steps that, for me were easy as an avid techie, but for them was, often fraught with frustration and error. The bottom line was that it needed to be a more sustainable practice, and fortunately, we were able to find a better solution. To do so, though, I needed to listen to my staff's complaints and take them seriously, as well as manage my frustration at the failure of my solution. Too often, the end-user gets blamed for not using technology well when technology should bend to the whims of the end user.

Previously, another need at one of our clinics with two floors was a communication system for providers to reach behavioral health consultants and for behavioral health consultants to talk to each other. Once again, we went through various iterations. The specific needs were to find a way for providers in exam rooms to text a request to a behavioral health consultant since two floors meant that behavioral health consultants could be in any number of rooms (as opposed to our other clinics where it is relatively easy to see where a behavioral health consultant was located). In addition, we needed a way for the behavioral health consultant to coordinate with other behavioral health consultants to decide who would get to that consult first and in what time frame.

I rejected pager systems immediately since I had seen these fail at other clinics and hated the idea of a pager. Cumbersome walkie-talkie solutions were also not helpful and, frankly, looked bad. So, we tried a solution that repurposed those iPods we had purchased for the database solution after that no longer worked for us. Providers would send a message to us through a webpage, which would appear on the iPod. Things as simple as getting the notification system to work well took a lot of work, research, and testing. And then, of course, technology shifted on us. iPods became obsolete, and EPIC developed the Secure Chat system that filled the void of quick team communication; this, along with Webex, is what Access currently uses.

Nothing Replaces Good Communication Skills

One of the unfortunate side effects of technology is that it can make people lazy regarding solid communication skills and etiquette. My high school, a humanities-based school in New York City, taught me key, classic communication skills. For example, we were not allowed to begin a sentence with "because" even verbally. We were instructed to speak and write in complete sentences. And because we took Latin and one additional language, we became familiar with the basic structure of language and the nuances of communication. In short, words, whether spoken or written, are powerful.

Each time I write a simple in-basket message, I consider the impact of the communication I deliver. I could leave a word misspelled or use partial sentences; most of the time, it would not make a difference. And yet, the cumulative impact of this kind of communication is potentially damaging to relationships in the team. If all I write to the triage nurse is something like, "Call PT. Contact PCP re: refill ASAP," eventually, that person might disconnect relationally since all I am doing is issuing commands. And frankly, it is hard to respect someone whose communications are akin to a teenager's texts.

This does not mean that communications need to be lengthy or convoluted, but simply that they should be respectful and written with the notion that the communication is more than just its content. I prefer to write something like: "Cindy: Thanks for your work on this issue. Please call the patient after consulting Sarah regarding the refill. Sooner would be better for the patient since withdrawal effects are likely to ensue within the next day or so. Let me know if you need anything else from me."

Similarly, with SOAP notes, exemplary grammar and writing skills communicate a great deal about the level of professionalism of the behavioral health team. Clinicians are more likely to respect someone whose writing reflects thoughtfulness and education. So, set reasonable standards for your team regarding communication, and you will have a team whose language advertises its commitment to excellence. Additionally, given that chart notes, as well as most of the in-basket messages, are available for patients to see related to Open Notes, it is good to practice professional and patient-friendly language across areas within EPIC, from in-basket messages to telephone calls to visit notes.

One of the first things I learned in managing teams, particularly larger teams across different sites, was the need for multiple communication layers. These layers needed to be flexible enough to work well for the different styles of team members and coherent enough that there was some consistency in group expectations. Here, we will discuss some of our implementation of tools on both the macro and micro level.

Macro-Communication

Macro-communication relates to the function of systems as a whole. This kind of communication necessitates depth, time, and multiple individuals. Often, email is used for this kind of communication. Still, email is often a poor tool in these instances because emails are difficult to keep track of and sometimes difficult to organize into coherent conversations (especially when email threads get long, or someone changes the subject line!).

Meetings are another typical venue for macro-communication, which can be effective but have some significant drawbacks. For example, an in-depth discussion on a topic to which team members are just reacting in a meeting (no pre-work has been done) often results in much discussion and groundwork exploration but little progress. So, this is how one meeting turns into another and so on. Meetings are also time-consuming and inconsistent with the frontline "on-the-field" culture of primary care (most providers hate meetings).

To solve this need for macro-communication, we tested and developed various tools that would help us track conversations easily, reduce our reliance on face-to-face meetings, and help everyone feel involved and invested in various larger topic areas. Below are the tools Access used and their characteristics.

In the past, Access used Yammer, a Microsoft product that was essentially Facebook for work. We replaced Yahoo groups with Yammer because Yammer allowed for a variety of communication, had an easy-to-use web interface, and did a decent job of allowing for collaboration on documents. Just like Facebook, Yammer allowed for posting brief comments or updates but also allowed for conversations in a thread-like format. Another tool with similar functionality is called Basecamp. This tool is excellent for project management, including task assignments and sharing resources and progress updates.

More recently, Yammer has been replaced by Webex with customized "rooms" by work area and across multiple work areas. For example, Access' BHC Team has a shared room with nurse triage to coordinate on the phone with a patient in real-time. Currently, most staff communications occur over Webex. This platform allows users to communicate 1:1 or establish groups to discuss specific topics. Organizational information is typically posted on ADP, and training is offered through Access' Learning Management System.

Google Docs is another system Access uses heavily. For documents with lasting value, such as the Intern Trainee Manual, Access uses Google Docs as a storage and collaboration center. Within Google Docs, you can create documents, spreadsheets, and forms and work on them with others on the team. An additional important use is the forms feature. Access placed its intern self-evaluation forms online, which allowed the team to track their completion and automatically store them. This central repository is a great way to organize and share critical documents.

Another sub-feature of Google is Google Calendar, where the BHC team houses its behavioral health consultant schedules for all clinics. The main team scheduler handles the scheduling component; all the team has to do is check to see where they work that day.

Micro-Communication

Communication that is brief and often task-oriented in nature is what we are calling micro-communication. This form of communication is often the most important. It forms the granules of our trust and connection between team members. Good micro-communication can lead to a sense of efficacy because team members feel they can get things done now.

You don't get more micro than texts. Texting between our smartphones is a quick and easy way of communicating critical, brief information, and we do it all the time. If someone is sick, they will text our scheduler, and that person will text any scheduling changes immediately to the team. If I have a quick question about an issue, I will text the individual for a yes/no type response. In other words, texting is not for long conversations but is excellent for getting critical information in a timely fashion. Of course, occasionally, a good old-fashioned phone call is also indicated, but Access uses this option far less than our other tools.

The key, of course, is training staff to keep all patient data and identifiers off communications. To this end, Access uses Secure Chat, a function of WebEx, to communicate between team members around various issues; this has become the primary strategy for micro-communication, given its security and ubiquity across the organization.

Managing Tool Overload

Of course, with all of these tools, it can be easy for team members to get tired of managing all the passwords and communication strategies. So, it is crucial to add tools when the time is right for their implementation and provide as much support as possible to foster the use of the tools. In our case, I tested tools out, sometimes by myself and sometimes with one other team member initially to evaluate the tool. A simple Plan-Do-Study-Act (PDSA)-type approach can be helpful in this regard.

The point is that there will always be resistance to any change in workflow or the introduction of anything new. You want to work patiently through this resistance, but also make sure that if you sell a tool to your team, you have a good one to sell. My team rolled their eyes at me more than once about a tool I was proposing, and sometimes they were right, but in the end, they knew that only the tools that were genuinely going to help them and us work well would survive. They grew in appreciation of most of the tools because they facilitated the connection with the lifeblood of our team, clinic, and mission.

It is also important to note that different team members will react differently to various tools. That is okay. Some team members will use one tool more than another. That is one of the benefits of having multiple tools. For example, some team members feel a need to communicate frequently to feel connected. The micro tools work for them well. Other team members like the macro tools most since they like longer, infrequent conversations. Nonetheless, the variety of communication strategies creates enough variety for everyone's style.

The Cycle of Technology

One harsh reality of technology is that it is ever-changing. Companies come and go, and software and hardware evolve. It is truly a Darwinian enterprise. So, it is crucial to consider this when selecting software solutions. First, don't put all your eggs in one basket unless you are sure the company is not likely to go away, and always keep on the lookout for new tools. Your needs will change, and so will the tools. You certainly want as much stability as possible so that tool fatigue does not set in among team members, but don't be surprised at the changes and updates required for managing tools. You will not be using the same tools in 10 years, so I imagine a 3-5-year window when a tool (other than your EHR) will likely remain in use.

For this reason, one-trick ponies are often really good solutions. For example, there are a slew of project management tools out there that are great for task management but horrible for communication. There are some that are good at document sharing and terrible at task management. Instead, I have often found that tools dedicated to the one function of project management and tools good at document sharing are best. What works nicely is when the tools coordinate well, which is increasingly the case with web-based tools.

Another factor to consider with technology is cost. We have gone through times when we paid for certain services, such as a video conference tool. It worked for the time and was feasible. But you likely want to rely on free or low-cost tools when possible. Save money for significant tools such as databases or specialized software. That said, if you have a really essential function, say a communication tool between behavioral health consultants at a large clinic or between behavioral health consultants and primary care clinicians at that site, it may be that a paid tool works best. Technology is an investment. Choose wisely.

Working With Your IT Department

Writing this section is difficult without sounding overly negative about all information technology (IT) professionals. The reality is that for all the promise of technology, IT departments have generally organized themselves around maintaining hardware and software and providing security; this is like having a policeman in charge of the creativity division of your organization. For this reason, it is not uncommon for healthcare providers to encounter barriers whenever they attempt to implement a technology-based solution within an organization without much flexible IT support. I completely understand the need for security, especially in healthcare, where sensitive data is the heart and soul of the work. However, I find it frustrating when a free, publicly available piece of software meets the resistant, glaring stare of an IT professional whose first thought is not about how great it would be to make your team function better but rather how this will either cause more management headaches or a very theoretical security concern.

You must consider security and sustainability when choosing your software and hardware products. On the security side, it is crucial, for example, to train your behavioral health consultants to send information securely and to remember which tool they are using when they communicate. For example, sending a text to another team member with confidential patient information is not a good idea. It is okay to send a generic query, but nothing that would compromise the privacy of the patient's health data. Another example of a common security breach is when someone sends a spreadsheet with confidential patient information to a nonsecure email account. So, be mindful of the data being transferred and the vehicle by which it is shared. The reality is that there is always a risk of HIPAA breaches in any form of communication, including the EHR itself. The issue is a matter of level of risk. It is theoretically pretty difficult for someone to hack into a server housing an EHR because of the protections in place. It is much less complicated for someone to hack into a personal email account.

Sustainability is another concern of IT departments; this is a reasonable concern on their part since every new tool and new piece of hardware introduces more work for them to maintain. So, it behooves you to make choices that respect the need for sustainability. Access does not have an IT department at present. Its IT is provided for by the local university, the University of Wisconsin; this presents certain advantages, such as our ability to use Epic's software and the suite of Microsoft Office products. However, it also presents a disadvantage since all major software decisions are out of our hands.

This being the case, one of the things that I asked the organization to do for our team was purchase and allow us to use Apple computers on the university's network. As you can imagine, this took a lot of effort and persistence with our administration and the University. In making this decision, which did not come about until several years after initiating the primary care behavioral health service, I had to factor in whether this would be a sustainable strategy for me and the organization. The benefits of this strategy would be that we could purchase our own software whenever we wanted to and develop unique solutions for our team. However, this also meant that I needed to be able to maintain all of the hardware and software.

In a pro/con analysis, I determined that the benefits outweighed the costs of maintaining the strategy; this has fortunately been borne out throughout our program's development. It did mean, however, that I had to devise strategies for things like keeping our computers updated, disseminating software, and occasionally making additional purchases. I doubt this would be a wise solution for most of our readers at this point, but in the late 2000s, this made sense. The Apple desktop computers served their role well for many years, allowing our team to innovate in ways we could not with locked-down PCs. Over the last few years, that has changed as the need for flexibility decreased, so Access has retired all the Macs.

The moral is two-fold: a. if a tech decision will serve you well for more than 3-4 years, it may be worth the effort, & b. there are some decisions you'll find unsustainable, no matter how much benefit you believe you will receive from the software or hardware. It is essential to identify these untenable strategies. Also, having this mindset makes you more likely to work effectively with IT professionals, who will respect that you are thinking through how much a strategy will affect them and their established systems.

So, you must be aware of security and sustainability when researching and promoting specific tools. However, I also encourage new behavioral health consultants to be persistent in pushing their administrators and IT professionals to create more flexibility, especially when doing so has significant benefits. I've seen clinics where purchases are made reflexively based on the personal preferences of the IT professionals without consulting the teams for their preferences. In these instances, becoming respectfully involved and challenging the status quo is helpful; this does not require being confrontational, but it does require being persistent and highly relational. Even when disagreeing, I've always tried to befriend and understand my IT brethren. And I don't pretend to know as much about the intricacies of computing as they do. But I also don't abdicate my responsibility to participate in the decision-making around technology.

A Final Note About Generative AI

One tech trend to keep an eye on in the coming years is generative artificial intelligence. This technology has significant promise for improving various aspects of primary care medicine. A short list includes:

- Listening to consults in exam rooms and auto-generating SOAP notes
- Automating responses to patient patient portal inquiries (or at least suggestions for providers)
- Assisting with diagnostic clarification and best practice interventions

And this is just a short list of what is likely to become a major shift in the practice of medicine. Use the same principles we have discussed above when you participate in conversations with your leadership about implementation decisions. This requires you to get in early on these conversations, even if you feel uncomfortable with the technology itself. A good first step is to begin to use the technology yourself (eg. ChatGPT) for other purposes.

About the Author

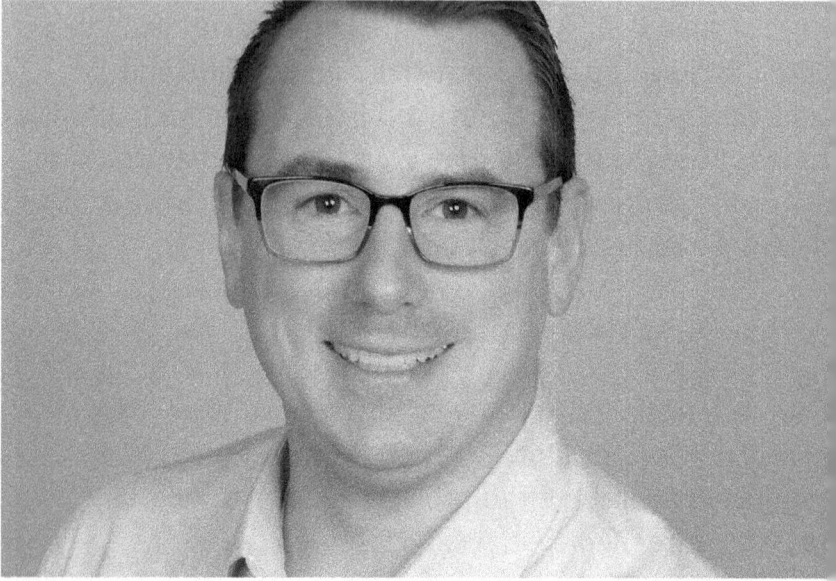

Alexander Smith, PsyD is the Behavioral Health Lead and Liaison at Access Community Health Centers. He has 8+ years of working within an integrated healthcare setting. He relocated to Madison, WI after obtaining his doctoral degree in clinical psychology at Adler University in Chicago, IL. He co-authored "Primary Care Behavioral Health (PCBH) Model and Suicide" in Suicide Prevention and is a member of his local Zero Suicide Collaborative. He is passionate about working with vulnerable and underserved populations.

Chapter 27: Building A Training Program

By Meghan Fondow, PhD

The Behavioral Health Consultant training program at Access Community Health Centers (Access) existed almost from the beginning of the program. Our program founder, Dr. Serrano, committed to the idea of a training program from the outset and was able to communicate the importance of training future behavioral health providers in the PCBH model to the administration of Access by selling the notion that cultivating prospective hires could happen best through the training program. It is essential to have support for the training from everyone involved, from administration to medical providers to support staff. Establishing a training program should not be a side project of a clinic but rather a central part of a workforce development strategy.

When I began working at Access in 2007, the behavioral health consultant team consisted of one BHC (psychologist), an MFT student, a fellow from the hospital, and myself as the first Access post-doctoral fellow. At that time, the team worked at two clinic locations; this presented a rich and robust training experience, as I could do a significant amount of direct patient care and administrative tasks. It also provided a rapid, if steep, learning curve and helped shape how I formulated future training experiences for other students. I found medical providers and all the other staff at Access to be quite welcoming, which was refreshing because, as a student, I had had plenty of experiences of feeling that I was tolerated but not perceived as helpful.

Our basic training model has remained the same since my training year, with fine-tuning and adjustments as the team grew and expanded. I read the "purple book," which is our affectionate name for "Behavioral Consultation and Primary Care" by Robinson and Reiter (2007), now the "blue book" when the second edition came out in 2016. This text provided an invaluable background to the PCBH model and population-based care. I discussed the model in detail with Dr. Serrano, the BHC who started our program, reviewing core components and comparing it with specialty mental health, as this was the framework with which I was most familiar.

Training began with shadowing experiences of a medical provider and Dr. Serrano. Shadowing experiences allow students to observe the interactions between behavioral health consultant staff and the medical providers in the clinic, as well as the direct patient contacts. During my training year, Dr. Serrano would explain his thought processes in managing a consult as I followed him around the clinic. He emphasized the importance of having a clear consult question, as we are working as consultants to the providers and are there to address the concerns they bring to us. Watching Dr. Serrano work directly with patients was one factor that helped accelerate my learning, as it helped me develop my sense of timing regarding working within the behavioral health consultant model and the reality of a 15-30 minute patient contact. We would then discuss the case after the patient visit, and I would observe Dr. Serrano provide feedback and recommendations to the referring provider.

After observing for a time, Dr. Serrano had me begin to write SOAP notes for the patient visits I observed. Initially, he dictated the notes to me, then later allowed me to try it on my own; this was an instructive training step and less intimidating than simply starting to see patients independently. Helping to write a note when both of us had been present with the patient allowed me to deepen my case conceptualization skills and better understand the behavioral health consultant model in practice quickly. We could discuss differences in our perceptions as well as similarities.

The behavioral health consultant training program worked initially within a preceptorship model of supervision, meaning that once I was done seeing a patient, I would report to Dr. Serrano, who would also check in with the patient to review my visit and the plan of care. Being able to receive on-the-spot supervision was one factor that provided a rapid learning curve for me because I could discuss my thoughts, concerns, doubts, etc., at the moment and receive feedback immediately. While initially intimidating, it quickly became apparent how useful this would be in developing my skillset within the behavioral health consultant model. It is also an efficient supervision model, as it allows for direct feedback on every patient rather than just patients selected for discussion in a traditional one-hour supervision session.

As I mentioned, direct patient care was only one part of my training year. I assisted with follow-up phone calls, crisis management calls, curbside consults, and staff development training. By the end of the training year, I was more than ready to begin working as an independent psychologist and BHC. I started taking over the scheduling for our team at the end of my training year once we hired another staff BHC. I was ready to take on extra administrative responsibilities due to the excellent clinical training I had received all year.

Core Components of The Training Model

Currently, the beginning of the training year includes a training sequence similar to the one I started with. We formalized an orientation process and internal training manual for students, including an orientation checklist, staff information, patient care logistics, and training program logistics. Students work through introductory readings regarding the behavioral health consultant model of care and videos from various sources, including CFHA Learns and Drs Beachy and Bauman's website (PCBH Corner | Beachy Bauman PLLC). We have didactics on a variety of topics, including BHC workflows, crisis management, theoretical orientations such as CBT, ACT, MI, and DBT within primary care, functional analysis, contextual interviews, working with different presenting concerns such as severe and persistent mental illness, substance use, chronic pain, sleep, and working with pediatrics. Various team members lead the didactics and provide ongoing learning opportunities for students and any staff who wish to join. The training program is very much a team effort, with all staff participating; all staff serve as on-site supervisors for students as well. My role as Clinical Training Director includes interviewing students (from post-docs to practicum students) and selecting students who appear interested in working in primary care and are a good fit for our program.

Introduction Of Services

Once students are comfortable with the basics of logistics, we have them work on their ability to introduce our service to patients. The ability to provide a clear introduction is linked to the student's understanding of the PCBH model. Suppose students begin seeing patients before they clearly understand the behavioral health consultant model; this will be communicated explicitly or implicitly to the patient as the student fumbles through an introduction. Therefore, we have found that introducing services is crucial to patient buy-in to the model and helps avoid false expectations regarding care. Assisting the students in learning an appropriate introductory script is essential.

As mentioned in previous chapters, this introduction should be simple and brief, communicating essential expectations efficiently. We have students practice this introduction with several BHC staff and provide feedback about missing elements. Core pieces to include in an introduction are:

- All treatment providers work collaboratively and share information.
- The estimated time frame of the visit with the BHC. (typically 20 minutes)
- The behavioral health consultant records information directly into the patient's electronic medical record (EMR) to facilitate communication with the team, and this is protected just like any medical note would be.
- Patients can request a consultation with a behavioral health consultant during future visits with a medical provider.
- Patients can schedule separate appointments with a behavioral health consultant if they wish. Each visit will include a determination of whether future visits are needed.
- We include information on confidentiality and reporting requirements when working with pediatrics and share that the BHC team bills for services.
- Students also need to communicate that they are in training and will have their supervisor check in at the end of the visit.

Patients are remarkably accepting of the supervision model, and anyone who has worked within a teaching hospital or clinic can attest that this is a common practice.

Direct Patient Contact: Starting With Shadowing

We begin by having students shadow their supervisors or other current students. Shadowing provides an opportunity to see the model directly in practice, bringing the concepts and logistics they are learning to life and providing immediate context. As a team, we try to be transparent in our work as students shadow us, often taking time to explain not only how to do something but why. When debriefing with a student following a patient visit, we share our thoughts about the visit process and explain the thinking behind clinical decision-making and assessments. How long each student spends in the shadowing phase depends on their previous experience level and comfort with the model. More advanced students typically begin providing direct care sooner, but this is tailored to each student, meeting students where they are with a developmental lens—a typical minimum may be two weeks for a well-prepared student.

Note Writing While Shadowing

Students assist in writing APSO notes for patients they observe as another training step; this allows the student to begin to learn how to condense information into a reasonable note, how to write for the intended audience, and how to start to develop skills at writing a precise assessment. Writing a note for a session conducted by their supervisor is helpful, as the student is focused on the content of the visit since they did not run it; this allows students to pay more attention to process issues early on in the training year.

Beginning To See Patients Independently

It is helpful to be conscious of the type of consult or complexity of the consult when beginning to allow students to see patients independently. While the expectation is that at some point, students will handle all consults, at the beginning, when they are still becoming accustomed to the model, it can be helpful to have them see the more basic or straightforward consults first; this can also help to increase the student's confidence in their abilities. Follow-up consults can often be easier, but not always. Before seeing the patient, students are encouraged to review the patient's chart and develop a plan to discuss with their supervisor.

Either way, it is helpful to work with the student to create a plan for the visit and how to address the consult question; this is called pre-staffing or pre-visit planning. In practice for our team, this often includes discussing content issues (i.e., reviewing symptoms of depression) and options for intervention (i.e., consider talking about behavioral activation or medication depending on patient preferences and motivation). Students at the beginning of the training year often say, "I don't know what to do with this patient," and supervisors can provide teaching and offer suggestions.

Some students become intimidated by the breadth of issues patients present with or create plans to cover too many areas during one visit; this often comes up as confidence grows and the student has more ideas on interventions that could be useful for a patient. Pre-visit planning can be a valuable way to decrease anxiety in the student and increase confidence. The goal for all students is that by the end of the training year, they will be able to manage a clinic independently, manage the flow of patients, curbside consults, attend to phone calls, and complete charting on time.

Content And Process Of The Visit: Contextual Interview, Functional Analysis, And Evidence-based Practices

Another aspect of training is assisting students in conducting a contextual interview (also called a functional assessment.) The diagnosis of a patient is, of course, helpful in guiding care and communicating with the treatment team. Still, understanding the context of a patient's life and current functioning is much more critical in developing the actual step-wise care plan; this can be difficult for some students to grasp, and they may continue to spend the majority of a visit probing for diagnostic criteria rather than understanding how the patient functions on a day-to-day basis. Students may also underestimate the importance of a solid contextual interview and how this information is helpful for the care team in moving care forward.

Gathering information on a patient's life context will help inform interventions by meeting patients where they are to be responsive to what is happening within their lives. Reviewing the elements of an efficient contextual interview is crucial, as there are times when students perform an excellent contextual interview but are not explicitly aware of it. I have found that many students have trouble verbalizing why they are doing what they do in the room with patients and that they have an implicit understanding of the need to explore current functioning. Talking about context directly can help students be more explicit and direct with their case conceptualization skills, which can help guide thoughts about interventions.

Critical components of a functional analysis include:

420

- Identifying the problem or target behavior.
- Describing the onset, duration, frequency, and intensity.
- Understanding what the patient has already tried to do to manage it.
- What has worked and what has not worked? What are the triggers, where does it happen, who are they with when it does, and what happens after the behavior?
- We also encourage students to develop skills in assessing the basic context of the patient's life. One fundamental question to help with this can be to ask patients to describe a typical day from when they wake up to when they fall asleep; this can provide a wealth of information in a brief format.

Our team uses clinical skills from evidence-based practices, including CBT, ACT, and MI. We train our students in the basics of these models of care, and students have exposure to brief interventions aimed at increasing the functional abilities of patients. We also train students on the concept of step-wise plans of care, as most of the patients we see may have multiple issues with multiple avenues for intervention. Students learn to work collaboratively with patients and the medical team to develop plans of care that provide something substantial in the current visit (i.e., psychoeducation, plan for behavioral activation, relaxation skill training, etc.) and lay the groundwork for future visits.

Reverse Shadowing/Direct Observation

Once students see patients independently, supervisors will engage in reverse shadowing, stepping into the room, or into a telemed visit to observe the student working with the patient directly. We do direct observations for two reasons:

to allow for enhanced feedback to students and for billing purposes in the state of WI. I have seen students' growth curves improve significantly using direct observations. We can see and hear directly what is happening with the visit. We can then offer more specific feedback with encouragements and reinforcements for what is going well and suggestions for areas of improvement. Our team has utilized reverse shadowing as an opportunity for a co-visit if a student is not entirely comfortable with a particular clinical concern or population. Many students come to BHC work in primary care with gaps in their knowledge, given most graduate schools are not training students as generalists. For example, many students may come to us with limited experience with pediatrics. Conducting visits with BHC staff and a student allows for enhanced training within the moment of learning.

Debriefing With The Supervisor

Once the student completes a consult, they debrief with their supervisor. We work with the students to report efficiently and succinctly, which can be difficult for some students who want to process the visit rather than offer their assessment, which is the primary goal. We ask students to begin with the assessment and plan for the patient in line with how they would write their chart notes; this helps students to come up with that basic conceptualization more quickly and to develop their clinical skills rather than just reporting verbatim what happened in the room with the patient. Of course, there are times when the student has trouble with the assessment, which can occur for many reasons. We encourage students to be open about this, to indicate what they do and do not know, and where their questions are. As we are all aware, there are times when patients present with issues that do not fit neatly into a diagnostic category or plan of care. A formula you can provide trainees to present a case to a supervisor could be something like this:

> PT is an XX-year-old Race, Gender ID, presenting with XX (symptoms, issues) who would benefit from/ is struggling with (conceptualization). Our plan was: XX. My question/ concern is XX.

Supervision

We utilize a developmental approach to supervision, following students' needs for the skills and knowledge they need to develop. Supervision is available on-site every day. Additionally, I have been meeting with full-time post-doctoral fellows in the clinic for 1 hour of supervision per week. This additional supervision started during the COVID-19 pandemic when the clinic had so many operational changes in order to provide additional support and opportunity for growth and development. This extra hour of supervision has provided a time to talk about bigger picture things, such as trends a student has noticed in growth or a skill they have realized they are lacking.

During supervision, we listen to students' reports of their visits and ask questions to clarify and direct conceptualizations and care plans. We discuss content and process (e.g., time management) issues related to the visit. One crucial goal with supervision, different than specialty supervision, is to provide coaching on consultation skills in working with the medical providers and other healthcare team members.

We coach students on writing SOAP notes in the APSO format, which involves learning the basics: what information goes where, progress vs. process notes, and their target audience. We often have to work with students on writing more efficient and concise notes rather than a visit transcript. The most challenging part of the note for most students is the assessment portion, which makes sense as this is where their clinical judgment and conceptualization are needed. These are the skills that usually take the longest for students to develop. For more on documentation skills, see our chapter on charting.

Encouraging students to use portions of their notes together can be helpful. For example, subjective + objective = assessment; therefore, plan (S+O=A, therefore P) is a useful shorthand. It helps to describe the merging of the actual content of the visit and the process or subjective experience of being in the room with the patient to form a complete clinical picture. We work with students on their ability to report their assessments to us first because it is the most challenging for most students. It is a critical skill in the PCBH model. The assessment is what the medical providers are asking for, as this is where you are answering the referral question and fulfilling your role as a consultant.

Evaluation

As our training program has evolved, our evaluation practices have become more formal. Initially, supervisors just completed evaluation materials for students as required by their programs. It became clear, however, that these tools needed to be more specific for our setting and specialized model of care. We again turned to the "purple book" and began using the PCBH-specific evaluation tool described there (Robinson & Reiter, 2007). This tool allows for the evaluation of the various core components of the model, from understanding population-based care to working within a team, brief and efficient visits, and charting. More general components are included, including responsiveness, timeliness, and productivity.

I meet monthly with the other staff BHCs for supervision of supervision meetings. During this meeting, staff can share their impressions of students, what is going well, and areas of needed growth. We can talk as a team about what to focus on next for development, coordinate together, and make working with multiple supervisors smoother.

Selecting Students

Our team decided early on that we would accept students from various training backgrounds within the mental health field, including clinical and counseling psychology, social work, marriage and family therapy, rehabilitation psychology, and Ph.D. and PsyD programs. We have found that overall, cross-training and cross-pollination work well. In addition, we have found that other factors more important than training background dictate students' success or lack thereof. Since the last version of this book, our team has evolved to take on a blend of practicum-level students (still in their graduate programs), interns (last year of graduate programs), and post-doctoral/post-graduate students.

The COVID-19 pandemic created challenges in so many ways, and one impact was on the amount of space we had for students. With the need for social distancing, we had to restrict our training program to post-doctoral fellows. As the pandemic continued, we have looked towards re-growth, including planning ways to re-develop relationships with our local social work program. We created a social work post-graduate fellowship to encourage the outstanding social work students we've worked with to continue their training in integrated care and PCBH. Our program serves as a rotation site for a local psychology internship, creating another pathway for student recruitment that has been valuable as state licensing laws change.

Effective selection of students is an essential part of recruiting people who will thrive in the culture of primary care. Students need to be:

- compassionate, respectful, non-judgmental, and empathetic, or in other words, to have strong humanistic characteristics,
- enthusiastic and share our sense of mission to provide population-based care, particularly to the underserved,
- flexible and exhibit the ability to shift from one task to another,
- able to work within a team, both the behavioral health consultant team and the larger medical team, so assessing motivation is key,

- able to establish rapport quickly, as the first five minutes of the consult can demonstrate. If the initial connection is poor, it will impact the rest of the consult and possibly future consults if the patient is even willing to meet with a behavioral health consultant again;
- flexible, adaptable, and motivated to be in the training role (they get lots of feedback);
- approachable and open to consults to build rapport with providers and encourage future consults.

Over the years, we have developed a more formal interviewing process for students, which involves reviewing their application materials, mainly their cover letters. We ask students to come in for an interview and observe the clinic for an hour or two; this may involve directly shadowing a patient consult or simply seeing the interactions with providers and other staff. There is no alternative to seeing primary care in action to understand what you are getting into as a student!

During the COVID-19 pandemic, we shifted to virtual interviews for post-doctoral fellows. We found that this can work well, though the student does miss out on experiencing the "feel" of our setting and the welcome of other staff and medical providers that happens when applicants are on site. The ability to offer virtual interviews will continue to be an essential tool in our recruitment process, creating more equity in the application process for those who do not have the time or funds to travel across the country for interviews.

For those who come on-site, this observation opportunity has helped weed out students who are not a good fit. I had one student ask where their office would be during the interview, and she was less than receptive to learning that there is no "office" - we share exam rooms and workspaces with the team! At the outset, exploring whether a student is ready for the fast-paced, ever-changing milieu of primary care before agreeing to a training experience is best.

All cautionary tales aside, we have found that students from various training backgrounds, as mentioned above, can be successful and enrich both our program and their training. Students get to see many patients not readily available in other settings in terms of presenting problems, intensity, and complexity of medical and psychosocial issues. After the initial training period, students are exposed to all types of patients without any sheltering. The expectation is that they will work with even the most complex patients, with support from their supervisor.

Medical Provider Concerns Regarding Students

As our training program grew, we did encounter issues with medical providers who were, in theory, receptive to the idea of students. However, there began to be times when medical providers would ask to have staff see a patient because of the complexity, intensity, or because it just seemed easier to them. The BHC staff chose to take a few minutes to discuss medical provider concerns at the moment, sorting out assumptions from the medical provider and offering reassurance that the student is not operating in isolation but with their supervisor. We also reassured medical providers that it is part of our job as supervisors to determine what our students can handle and how to guide them appropriately; this is not a role the provider needs to take on. Now, our medical providers are firmly on board with our training program, over 15 years since the training program started. We often hear questions about who the next round of students will include. We are fortunate at Access to work with such supportive and welcoming medical providers overall, as they have supported the behavioral health consultant team and the idea of training future professionals.

Development of Professional Relationships Between Medical Providers and Students

The strong relationship that the behavioral health consultant staff has developed with medical providers is one reason our training program has been successful. Our medical providers have been willing to take that leap of faith that we are selecting appropriate students who can handle the work and contribute meaningfully. We discuss with students how they can initially "borrow" our relationships with providers, essentially riding on our coattails regarding gaining medical providers' confidence. However, we warn students they cannot always behave as we do. While staff can get away with multi-tasking as a medical provider discusses a patient with us, students may not. They need to show medical providers they are listening to consults and that they are, in fact, receptive to these consults in the first place. Students need to attend to relationship building with providers directly and with intention.

We coach students on interacting with medical providers regarding what they say and their non-verbal communication. Suppose a student never looks up from their computer when a medical provider gives a warm handoff. In that case, the medical provider may feel the student is not listening, even if the student is looking up the patient's chart while the medical provider is talking. Additionally, we encourage students to be assertive in communication, as this will help medical providers address referral questions directly to the students rather than to the supervisor present.

The Tendency of Students To Refer Out

A trend that has become more obvious as we have had more students over the years is for students to want to refer patients out to the community for specialty mental health care within the traditional model. While there are certainly times when this is entirely appropriate, there are many more times when the referral is unnecessary, as the issue could effectively be handled within the primary care setting. In addition, the barriers to specialty care still exist for patients. We know most patients will not make it to specialty care for various reasons. Therefore, we have begun to spend more time on this issue with our students.

The issue is again linked to the student's understanding of the PCBH model of care, combined with a knee-jerk reaction to refer out the more complex patients. I have found that students often underestimate the impact of behavioral health consultant services on patients and often believe that patients with more complex issues (i.e., trauma, AODA, severe and persistent mental illness) need more intensive specialty services. Students may also refer patients to the models of care they are already familiar with from previous training settings. The reality, however, is that patients often either do not want the outpatient specialty mental or substance use services due to the usual barriers, or they have no access to these services.

Reminding students that the goal for each visit is to provide the patient with something of value can be helpful. That is the purpose of the behavioral health consultant team: to complement and enhance the care they already receive from their primary care clinician. Students seem to run into this issue even after working in the model for several months as if they lose sight of the value they provide. At this point, it can be helpful to review with students all the intervention strategies they have in their "toolbox" and to remind them of how powerful these strategies can be when delivered when the patient asks for them. Reviewing the utility of humanistic skills, validation skills, and contextual interviews is good as the student's skills grow. I don't think I can count the number of times patients have shared how impactful it was for them to be treated with respect, listened to, seen, and heard as a fellow humans. Often, students take these fundamental skills for granted and stop seeing the value they add to the patient and the whole medical care team.

Billing

Rules for billing students vary from state to state and site to site (i.e., FQHC vs. community mental health center vs. private practice and more). Sometimes, it is possible to bill for student-provided care if the supervising (licensed) behavioral health consultant has face-to-face contact with the patient or is on-site (Qualified Treatment Trainee or

QTT). In some settings, the patient contact will need to be substantial, such as the minimum amount of time required to bill a visit: 16 minutes for a 90832 coded visit, and include double documentation from the supervisor. In the end, your goal should be the highest quality patient care. So, we spend whatever time is necessary to ensure that the patient has received what they needed that day and that meets billing requirements. Our current workflow is to step in on the patient consult about 10 minutes into the consult and shadow/ participate as needed, which usually gives us the time required to bill. The student then documents a note, and the supervisor must also write a note according to Wisconsin regulations. Creating relationships with your local coding and compliance people is extremely important.

Given that our work in integrated care is infrequently articulated in coding rules, the appropriate course of action for billing student-led care can be unclear. Suppose there are no provisions for billing for unlicensed trainees in your region. In that case, you will either have to get creative about stepping in on patients to meet billing criteria as the provider of record, or you will have to sell a strategy to your administration that involves not billing for these visits.

Other Training Options

Our team also provides training opportunities for medical residents from three specializations: family medicine, pediatrics, and psychiatry. We offer rotations for the first two groups where the resident can shadow behavioral health consultants directly for one or two clinics; this includes an opportunity to discuss the behavioral health consultant model, the idea of population-based care, and how we work as a part of the larger medical team. Residents can observe warm handoffs and then shadow during patient visits to see what we do in the room with a patient. In between patients, residents will often ask about ways to cope with patient issues they commonly see, such as behavioral issues with children, parenting issues, smoking cessation, or anxiety.

One of our medical clinic sites is affiliated with the University of Wisconsin Madison Department of Family Medicine and Community Health. It serves as a training site for three years of residency for family medicine residents. Our Behavioral Health team staffs this site, and we often work with residents as they see their patients for warm handoffs or curbside consults. These serve as real-time training opportunities for residents to deepen their knowledge and skills in working with behavioral health concerns. Each time I hear from a resident that they only want to work in a future clinic where integrated care is present, I feel an enormous sense of accomplishment. We have recruited many residents as medical providers for our other two medical clinic sites over the years, a mutually beneficial setup.

The second group of residents are the psychiatry residents from the UW Department of Psychiatry, who rotate through Access for a three-month rotation in community psychiatry with our consulting psychiatrist; Dr. Kelly Clements, our consulting psychiatry program manager, manages this. The psychiatry residents who go through this rotation learn how to work in a consulting role, as described in the consulting psychiatry chapter.

Conclusion

If you are considering offering training in your integrated care program, I highly recommend proceeding even with the work involved in setup and maintenance. Working with students is rewarding on many levels and offers a diversity of work tasks each day. Training to create future integrated care behavioral health providers fulfills the "Educator" role in the GATHER acronym. Training more behavioral health providers also means that access to PCBH services will grow, making integrated care more universally available and benefitting the field overall. And in areas of the country where hiring mental health professionals is challenging, there is no better way to have a pipeline of talent for future positions.

Chapter 28: The Trainee In PCBH

By María I. Lázaro-Escudero y Nydia M. Cappas

María Isabel, Day One

A roller coaster of emotions flowed through me as I approached the entrance of the clinic: excitement, gratefulness, fear, and nervousness. This first day marked the beginning of a new professional and life phase. I was now officially a psychology intern, meaning I was expected to be more independent, self-sufficient, and assertive in all dimensions of my clinical work. As a student in training, transitioning from an "amateur" level of practice to becoming an intern in a primary care setting, I had many expectations. I expected this clinical experience would be different from others. I imagined fast-paced workdays, a more significant workload, constant interdisciplinary teamwork, a pro-learning environment, personal/professional growth, and, most importantly, guidance and feedback. As with all great expectations, there also comes fear. Fears that I would be too slow to adapt to the workspace, unable to meet demands, reach burnout, or manage time effectively. Though I tried not to let these fears keep me from enjoying the excitement and pride of achieving this professional milestone, they were unavoidable. These fears helped me acknowledge that I had to prepare myself for the journey I was about to begin.

My first order of business was to meet everyone. I met many of the clinic's healthcare providers, including a nutritionist, a clinical social worker, a speech pathologist, a case manager, medical secretaries, a health educator, primary care physicians (including family medicine and pediatrics), a gynecologist, a substance abuse counselor, and a psychiatrist. These were only some of the health providers at the primary care center. It seemed surreal that my welcome was so warm. I can say that my first-day anxiety was reduced exponentially by how the team greeted me. Everyone I met treated me kindly. That was fundamental in helping me overcome my initial fears and embrace the excitement of the journey I was about to begin.

As I became comfortable in my new workspace, my supervisor entered the office, and we welcomed our first patient. I did not expect to see patients so quickly, but I knew that was my job. And so, with the usual first-day butterflies in my stomach, I completed my first behavioral health screening and conducted the initial interview. It all went smoothly during the first consults (except I felt like a mess while navigating the electronic record). Afterward, I discussed the cases with my supervisor and was greatly relieved to receive good feedback. I finished preparing my workspace for the next day and took a deep breath. It was a relief to have completed and survived my first day of the internship. I still remember how happy and excited I felt at the end of the day though I was tired and overwhelmed.

My name is María Isabel Lázaro-Escudero. I am a Ph.D. Clinical Psychology graduate candidate (6th year) of the School of Behavioral and Brain Sciences at Ponce Health Sciences University. I was born and raised in Puerto Rico, where I completed all my professional training, including a Bachelor of Science in Cellular Molecular Biology. My combined biology and clinical psychology training has given me a holistic approach to health; this led me to pursue my current internship in health psychology, which focuses on the biological, psychological, and social factors that influence health and illness. To gain practical experience in this field, I completed a clinical practicum at a teaching hospital. I performed brief interventions on patients in critical care units and provided psychological consultations. I also completed a year-long clinical rotation at a private oncology practice, focusing on providing psychological care to oncological patients. Through biweekly case discussions with an oncologist, I saw firsthand the benefits of integrating mental health services in medical settings.

Alongside these clinical experiences, I was also dealing with the social circumstances the island faced. As a student, I met many challenges stemming from natural disasters such as hurricanes Irma and Maria, as well as the 2020 earthquakes, the COVID-19 shutdown, government corruption, the collapse of public education, the exodus of doctors, and significant gaps in access to healthcare, to name just a few. These experiences exposed me to the realities Puerto Ricans face (patients and health providers). Practicing in the context of these experiences reinforced and fueled my passion and belief in affordable and accessible integrated health care as a birthright. There is no logical reason for separating mental health from physical care. I was able to witness, through my clinical practicum experiences, how physical and mental phenomena are intrinsically one, and I developed a passion for advocating for integrated behavioral health. These challenges motivated me to apply for an internship in Primary Care Psychology. I wanted to immerse myself in this practice and see how this philosophy was being implemented in Puerto Rico. I was accepted at my school's Psychology Internship Consortium, specifically the Primary Care Psychology Program (PCPP). The director of PCPP, Dr. Nydia Cappas, will describe some details about the program, the clinic, and the feedback received in the sections below.

The Primary Care Psychology Program

María Isabel's accounts are part of her internship experience with the Primary Care Psychology Program (PCPP), a service and training program housed at Ponce Health Sciences University in Puerto Rico. Originally established to train clinical psychology doctoral students in providing care to people living with HIV/AIDS in the municipality of Ponce, the program has since expanded to provide services and training at 27 clinics throughout the island. PCPP has trained more than 150 practicum and internship students in delivering effective psychological care within integrated health teams, including primary care medicine, nursing, public health, case management, substance use specialists, and other health professionals.

PCPP provides more than 6,000 consults annually across primary care and immunology clinics. Our internship program is part of the Ponce Internship Consortium and is accredited by the American Psychological Association. With support from HRSA and State grants, we integrate our interns and professionals into health teams using the PCBH model of services. María Isabel is one of 11 students completing their internship year with PCPP in 2022-2023.

To provide some context for María Isabel's internship experience, it is essential to understand our program's approach; we call it RTDM (recruit, train, deploy, and monitor). The recruit portion refers to the PCPP process of recruiting clinical psychology interns and primary care sites. The sites recruited are part of a decade of collaborations (formal and informal) among primary care settings and the PCPP. Recruitment of interns follows the APPIC guidelines.

The training portion is perhaps one of the most critical aspects. Over the years, PCPP has developed a training that includes a boot camp offered to interns before they enter a clinical site, ongoing training on issues related to integrated behavioral health every other week, and weekly group supervision with an interdisciplinary team. The team comprises a family physician, a nurse practitioner, an epidemiologist, a substance use specialist, and clinical psychologists. Once the interns have gone through the boot camp, the program deploys the student to the assigned clinic. During "deployment," interns have the experiential portion of their training for one year at one of the eight collaborating primary care clinics. Except for Fridays, interns attend their assigned clinic every weekday. On

Fridays, we have educational training and group supervision involving multiple disciplines.

Once the intern starts their "deployment," the program uses a software system to monitor their progress. Because PCPP is not a clinic, nor do we own any clinics where our interns train, it is essential to monitor their progress effectively. We collect data daily that allow us to approach a student early if any data indicates they are not successfully adapting to the clinic's service model. Finally, the program continuously assesses its outcomes and modifies anything as necessary, from training to systems; this is a natural extension of the monitoring process that allows us to be more efficient.

The Clinic

The primary care clinic María Isabel is assigned is <u>Concilio de Salud Integral de Loiza (CSILO)</u>. CSILO is a Federally Qualified Health Center (FQHC) located in the island's eastern region. The center serves more than 12,000 patients each year, and almost all (98%) of the patients served have incomes at or below 200% poverty level, according to HRSA's Uniform Data System. CSILO is the only clinic serving more than three adjacent municipalities. Their services include general primary medical care, ob-gyn, oral health care, family planning, HIV testing and counseling, immunizations, health education, X-ray and sonography, pharmacy services, and home and nursing home visits.

The center is a certified Primary Care Medical Home and hosts a Residency in Family Medicine. They provide integrated care services, including services for substance use disorders. CSILO collaborated with PCPP in 2020, hosting one of our interns each year. Now that the reader has a panoramic description of the program and the internship site let us continue with María Isabel's narrative on her experience.

María Isabel's Story

There is more to the internship experience than the feelings I shared about the first day. Throughout the twelve-month training program, I learned and adapted a great deal. Let me share some of these experiences with you.

I started at the clinic in mid-July, but I had already received two weeks of skills and administrative pre-training or "boot camp" offered by the Primary Care Psychology Program (PCPP). These trainings were vital since they allowed me to polish practical skills tailored to the clinical setting I would face. During these pre-trainings, I met with colleagues (other interns) that were going to be in similar clinical scenarios as me; this helped to develop a sense of community and support network, as we were able to share fears and worries before starting the internship; this also conveyed a sense of unity that felt like we were all in this together.

We also met with the PCPP supervisors (different from the assigned supervisor at the clinic). Supervisors from the PCPP's multidisciplinary team meet with us each week for group supervision. This weekly supervision became our safety net, a space to extend our case discussions through group supervision and be vulnerable and honest about our learning process. The pre-training received, and the interpersonal connections that resulted from it fueled me with motivation and enthusiasm for the beginning of my internship.

My first months at the clinic were all about adaptation. When I started, I remember feeling overwhelmed after reviewing all my responsibilities, and I never had so much work expected from me all at once! My schedule was as follows: I attended the clinic from Monday to Thursday (from 8 AM-4 PM), and on Fridays, I attended group supervision with PCPP's interdisciplinary team from 8 AM to 10 AM and attended advanced training from 10 AM to 12:00. Friday afternoons were reserved for administrative work, dissertation work, or self-care activities. I supervised family medicine residents performing behavioral health interventions on the first Friday of every month.

In clinical work, I performed screenings, intake interviews, targeted interventions, administered psychological tests, completed written reports, and had case discussions with primary care physicians and other relevant health providers. These discussions are concise, focused, and informal. Discussing every new case with the respective primary care physician was mandatory to ensure integrated health management and intervention. In addition, I was part of each Wednesday's Diabetes Support Group, whose purpose was to increase awareness of the condition through education and provide resources, tools, and tips to improve the quality of life of people with diabetes. My role was to give 30-minute workshops to increase participants' awareness of mental health and provide simple strategies to improve their well-being. I also had to complete patient documentation in the EHR. On the 10th day of each month, I had to hand my supervisor the signed treatment plans formulated for each new case admitted to mental health services and a registry list containing all the patients seen the previous month. So, of course, the first months were all about figuring out how to keep up with all my responsibilities. During this time, I mainly focused on mastering the electronic health record, improving my clinical note-writing skills, engaging hospitably with the clinic's staff, and making myself available. One mistake I think I made during those first few months was that I said yes to everything, and in the long run, it had its disadvantages: burnout. I will come back to this later.

At this time, I had a hard time conducting case discussions with the medical team. I wasn't completing the monthly case discussions required. Some doctors were not available for case discussions every day, and my clinic schedule changed throughout the day at other times. I ended up missing the opportunity to discuss the cases with other professionals.

After three months at the clinic, I felt more comfortable engaging with the staff and patients. My day-to-day tasks felt more balanced, and I felt like I belonged in this workspace, which was exciting. However, I also realized I needed to improve my clinical note-writing skills to be even more concise, as it took too much time. After consulting with my supervisor, we carefully reviewed the patient data that should be included in my progress notes. This supervision exercise helped me improve my efficiency and time management skills, which helped everything flow more smoothly.

During the second quarter of my internship, I started to face the reality of the population I served. The municipality of Loiza is recognized for its cultural value and natural beauty, exquisite food, and loving people, but all the same, it is a marginalized and impoverished town. By this time, I was beginning to see a trend, a norm that alarmed me and faced me with a harsh reality. Most of my patients were victims of criminal violence, had a history of personal or family sexual abuse, presented some health disparity, or faced structural violence. This realization made me adapt the approach toward my clinical interventions. Behavioral health interventions in medical settings tend to be targeted, solution-focused interventions. However, brief interventions were not always possible.

Our population faces severe and complex issues and symptomatology, and specialized mental health is not easily accessible. Where would I refer these patients to receive specialized mental health services if they did not have the financial power or transportation to get there? And so, I adapted my treatment approach accordingly. After all, implementing integrated primary care does not have to mean imposing a rigid structure on different clinical settings with unique needs.

Remember the difficulty discussing cases with other providers? Towards the middle of my second quarter, I began creating a monthly registry of all the patients that needed to be reviewed with a primary care physician or any other clinic member. I wrote down the dates that the physician would be at the clinic, which I checked on the calendar of the electronic record. I then made sure to make one or two case discussions daily (depending on the load) until the end of the period. This strategy helped me increase my interactions with the team and meet the internship requirements; this was a welcome change from the experience at the beginning, where I felt restrained. In retrospect, this restraint or difficulty mainly stemmed from fear of reaching out to another health professional in another health field whom I did not know personally. But like any other interpersonal relationship, through frequent interactions, the relationship evolves, transforms, and becomes more familiar.

By this time, my relationships with the staff also became closer. The case discussions became more fruitful, effective, and straightforward. I felt more comfortable interrupting the physician during work time; I sensed the physician felt that way too. During case discussions, I eventually tended to ask physicians if there were any barriers the patient experienced toward treatment adherence (even if there was no evident health issue). This way, I could incorporate the physician's concerns into the treatment plan creating instant common ground. With the patient, this question allowed me to explore the root causes of those barriers. I found that most patients could benefit from connecting the treatment benefits with their values and needs and that psychoeducation and value-centered approaches were the most effective in these cases. This approach also let physicians know I acknowledged and respected their work and that integration was practical and beneficial for advancing the patient's health.

Another helpful strategy was to review each patient's most recent medical progress notes to identify any previous physician referrals and their follow-up; this helped me corroborate any contradictory or missing information relevant to the patient's treatment. If something were identified during the case discussions (e.g., missed follow-up to referral, failure to bring lab results, poor adherence to treatment, missing relevant medical/psychiatric history or symptoms, etc.), I would incorporate 5 minutes to follow up on these issues with the patient. Experience and training have shown me that physicians have so much workload that even if something is documented in a progress or health management note, they commonly miss it (and I don't blame them). That is why case discussions are even more valuable when multiple providers treat one patient. The behavioral health provider fills in the gaps and builds a bridge within the medical team so we can all be on the same page.

My clinical skills had significantly improved by the end of my second quarter. I started feeling more assertive in decision-making and thought I could formulate and deliver strategies for patients immediately. My skills in identifying and defining the patient needs improved. I also developed a much more clearly defined identity as a therapist. I was confident that I had a person-centered approach and was aware that my unconditional positive regard in therapy was central to generating better patient outcomes; this also applied to my experience in the diabetes support group. In the beginning, I gave very structured workshops. However, with time I realized it was much more effective to mediate the support group through direct discussions around the relevant barriers participants faced in managing the condition and balancing their mental health during their journey with the diagnosis. Participants were more open to being vulnerable about their experiences and felt seen when other participants shared their struggles. Through this change in approach, I facilitated a supportive and safe space that responded to the participants' felt needs at each session.

Unfortunately, right around this time, my health started deteriorating, and I failed to listen to my needs. I attended the clinic on days when I shouldn't have and depleted my body and mind of vital energy; this, together with all the extra load I took on at the beginning of the internship, resulted in a diminished capacity to balance work and self-care. The work piled up, and I had too many due dates and too little time. Through this challenging phase, I learned one of the most important lessons during my internship: self-care is non-negotiable. Supervisors should keep an eye on this since it is easy for a trainee in a primary care setting to work at a very high pace and lose track of the appropriate balance of self-care. Thanks to the support and validation received during the PCCP group supervision, I recognized that I was burning out, and this was the first valuable step towards assessing and meeting my needs.

Despite the heavy days in which burnout took hold, the light was at the end of the tunnel. My Christmas vacation had arrived. I promised myself I wouldn't do any work during this period, and I kept my word. How can I even begin to express how important this time was for me and the months following until the end of my internship? I came back from my vacation revitalized. I was astonished at how clear-minded and energized I had become. I started taking care of myself consciously by paying attention to my daily needs and meeting them through consistent weekly planning. I also changed my diet by adding more greens and fruits and working out more.

Most importantly, I started setting boundaries and felt comfortable saying no to additional work I knew I could not complete promptly. I finally began to practice what I preached; this directly impacted my clinical interventions and how I managed my workload. When I compared myself to the version of me before my vacations, I felt like a completely different person.

Thanks to these basic adjustments, the third quarter of my internship felt like I had reached my potential for this level of training. I felt in control and balanced because I knew I would care for myself unconditionally. The mental strength this provides helps endure the hectic scenario of primary care. With this state of mind, I served my patients more mindfully and delivered the type of care they truly deserved. Supervisors should look forward to their trainees' vacations and resting periods because it impacts their mental health and the quality of work they can deliver.

As I write this chapter, I am approaching the last quarter of my internship and beginning to understand what this experience means to me as I enter the professional world. Working in an integrated primary care setting and serving the community of Loiza forever changed me. It has sharpened my clinical skills, challenged me to adapt in ways I didn't know I could, revealed the true embodiment of self-care, and, most importantly, transformed and redefined my love for my country. This love reassured my commitment to be an agent of change through my work. I believe integrated behavioral health is a promising field that offers realistic and viable solutions to address the relevant mental health issues this era faces.

Nydia: Giving Feedback

When we finished this chapter, Maria Isabel was about to complete her internship year. Her account does much more to convey what an awesome intern she has been than any statistics can. However, for the sake of objectivity, I will share some feedback and numbers that can help paint the picture of her training at the site. María Isabel is well on her way to finishing the required intervention hours. Her report shows that she discussed at least 51% of her interventions with other health team members. Her supervisor evaluations are excellent, with most skills ranked at the proficiency or mastery level (2 highest levels). Her direct supervisor expressed in a meeting: "María Isabel has been able to work with the flow we need. She is very thoughtful and analytic and always includes a broad look at the social determinants of the health of our patients...."

Like María Isabel, many other interns have completed our internship program. Since the beginning of the program, 86 students have completed their internship at PCPP. All those interested in following a postdoc have found placements, and our last review of graduates (2020) showed that 58% are working in integrated care as clinicians, leaders, or teachers. Collectively supervisor evaluations rate students with the highest ratings in the competencies of Science, Application, and Professionalism related to integrated primary care. As the program prepares for its next cohort of interns, accounts like Maria Isabel's energize, humble, and equip me to apply the lessons learned to teach a better and balanced healthcare workforce. She deserves the last word.

María: Final Thoughts

As I write this conclusion, I am weeks away from the end of my internship. I hope my perspective is helpful to anyone thinking about training or working with trainees in behavioral health. Through my internship, I have come to appreciate the value of a well-planned integrated behavioral health program that prioritizes the biopsychosocial needs of the population it serves. I have learned that it is essential to fill gaps in care, support the well-being of all professionals (including interns), and remain focused on improving the lives of those we serve.

There is one unexpected outcome I have left to share about this journey. During my internship year, I developed a particular interest in public policy. I became acutely aware of the importance of addressing the social determinants of health through relevant political actions. My experience with my patients highlighted the need to reinforce laws that protect fundamental human rights; this, I consider central to advancing and bettering the health and eradicating social and health inequities that feed off of the current political (and health) paradigm. I will hold myself accountable because who will if we don't act against the social injustices we see in our therapeutic spaces?

As we come to the end of this chapter, I am reminded that while the experiences shared here are personal, they are not unique. I hope that through my narrations, I have captured the feelings and experiences of many other interns embarking on their journey into the world of primary care. The training in behavioral health goes beyond just acquiring skills and competencies; it is a transformative journey filled with highs and lows. The clinics, behavioral health teams, supervisors, colleagues, and all providers play a crucial role in supporting the growth and development of interns in these environments. Along the way, we discover our skills, strengths, needs, and styles. And most importantly, we can utilize these experiences and learning processes to improve the health of our communities.

About the Authors

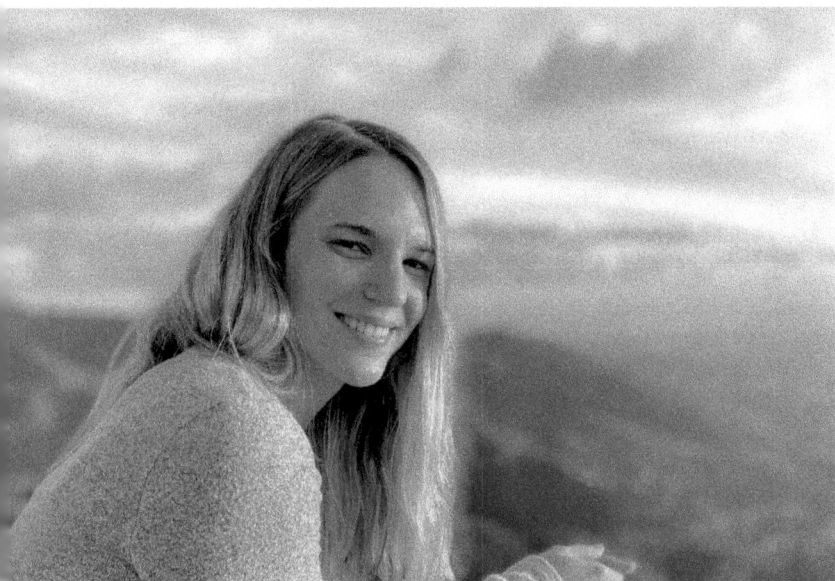

María I. Lázaro-Escudero, B.S., is a Ph.D. candidate in Ponce Health Sciences University's Clinical Psychology Program. Throughout her doctoral training, she has gained experience in health psychology, with a specific focus on psychoneuroimmunology. Her research aims to explore the biobehavioral mechanisms through which stress and social adversities synergistically impact diseases, particularly cancer, within the Hispanic/Latino population. As a therapist, she advocates for integrated care and envisions herself implementing this holistic approach. Beyond her clinical work, she aspires to translate research findings into public policy to help mitigate health disparities and address social injustices. Outside the academic realm, you can find her engaging in deep existential conversations and spending time with loved ones. She also finds joy in hiking in nature, journaling, practicing mindfulness, exercising, and ensuring there is always ice cream in her freezer!

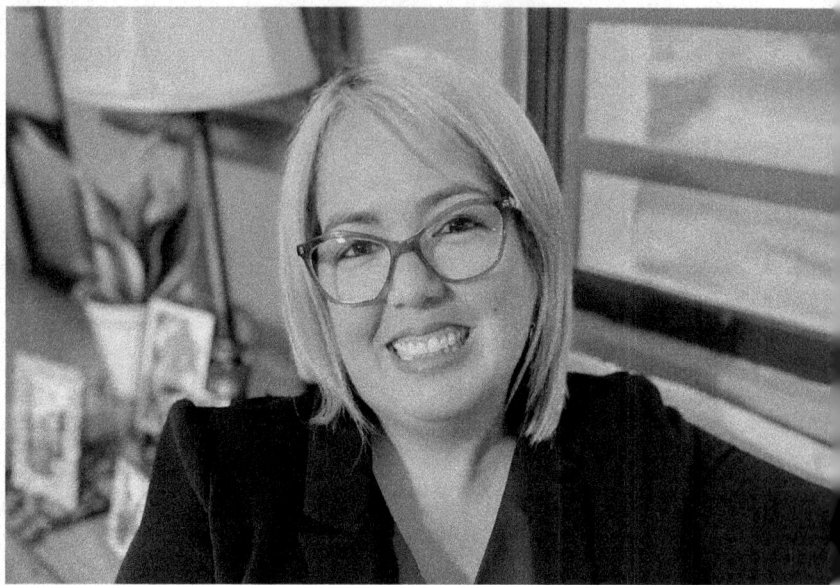

Dr. Nydia Cappas is a clinical psychologist, administrator, and academic committed to the integration of Psychology into Primary Health Care. She is a graduate of the University of Massachusetts and the Ponce School of Medicine, with postdoctoral studies at Yale University and an MBA from Temple University. She has been leading the Primary Care Psychology Program (PCPP) at Ponce Health Sciences University since 2007, contributing to the training of psychologists and health professionals in numerous clinics across Puerto Rico. Her work fostering service integration in Puerto Rico has earned her awards such as the Psychologist of the Year from the Puerto Rico Psychology Association (APPR) and the Wingspread Award from the Collaborative Family Healthcare Association (CFHA). Her most recent project, Psicología Todo Terreno

(All-Terrain Psychology), seeks to expand the way we integrate psychology into our lives and work environments through education and consultancy. Her podcast, which has the same name, reviews examples of integration through reflections and interviews with guests from different personal and professional backgrounds.

Chapter 29: Self-Care

By Neftali Serrano, PsyD with Elizabeth Zeidler Schreiter

T he life of a behavioral health consultant has many of the same risks as primary care providers. If national surveys of workplace stress are any indication, that is not a good thing. Here we review some of the critical threats unique to the work of behavioral health consultants and their directors. Since I moved on from my role as Chief Behavioral Health Officer at Access, I also provide running commentary in the narrative, updating my perspective almost a decade after the original narrative was written; this should give the reader a longitudinal view on the topic of self-care in PCBH. Note that the narrative is written as if I was still the director, and the commentary is indented and in italics for clarity.

Multitasking

One of the essential traits of the behavioral health consultant is the ability to handle multiple pieces of information and tasks simultaneously while prioritizing effectively. This aspect is magnified for those who assume leadership for behavioral health consultant teams, who have to add various administrative and program development tasks and relationships to the clinical work. This aspect is not unlike a computer's central processing unit (CPU), which must handle various inputs from the software and hardware of a machine simultaneously. And just as a CPU can overheat and either become damaged or slow down, human beings engaged in multitasking over an extended period can suffer consequences. Here the analogy with a CPU can be helpful since computer makers build in functions to help avert disaster. For example, a computer will have a fan or other cooling mechanism to help mitigate the heat generated from a CPU engaged in multitasking over an extended period.

Furthermore, the software that controls the central processing unit will limit its workload to a specific rate to prevent it from overworking and causing damage. Finally, computer makers work overtime to improve the efficiency of the central processing unit, for example, by adding cores (additional processing units) and improving transfer rates between the processing unit and other components in the computer. For behavioral health consultants, it is essential to recognize that multitasking is a serious threat and must be addressed proactively; this is similar to how computer manufacturers anticipate the potential harm of multitasking even before the user interacts with the computer. And just like computer makers, the good behavioral health consultant will have built-in functions that operate like a fan that help mitigate some of the sequelae of multitasking and hard stops that help set limits on the demands.

One example of this was a decision we made early on as a team that if a behavioral health consultant had an excessively heavy day or series of days, the rest of the team would pitch in to help that behavioral health consultant gets caught up with notes. For example, a behavioral consultant may have seen upwards of 15 people on a particular day. Because they're working with another staff member or student the following day, they can ask the staff member to cover their clinic the next morning for a few hours while they get caught up. Over the years, there have been very few times when we have had to implement this policy. However, the very presence of the policy has helped mitigate stress since people know that others care and are willing to help them even when they're swamped. In fact, as a general rule, our experiences have been that some of the most potent mitigators of stress, in general, are related to interventions that leverage our community as a team.

The culture remains the same even almost a decade removed from my time as the Chief Behavioral Health Officer at Access. The PCBH team mitigates stress by supporting one another proactively.

Vicarious Trauma & Moral Fatigue

The caregiver burden is a substantial strain on the behavioral health consultant. An aspect of this burden is the sheer volume a behavioral consultant will see and the pace at which the behavioral health consultant works. Hearing story after story of trauma and suffering has been well-documented to impact professional and nonprofessional caregivers significantly. Here too, it is helpful to have some signs and markers built in to help identify when caregiver burden is becoming problematic.

For example, it is common for caregivers to begin to adopt a negative attitude or perspective after they have been exposed to enough vicarious trauma. These signposts serve as signals that some form of self-care must be initiated to counteract the impact of the trauma. Cynicism decreased empathy capacity, and irritability are other common signs of caregiver fatigue. Working in primary care has some built-in mitigators that help with the issue of the content and pace of the consults, but these must be leveraged well by the behavioral health consultant team. Again, we have found that our team cohesion is the most significant factor in dealing with this threat. For example, when one of our behavioral health consultants feels particularly affected by their work, they know they can quickly videoconference another behavioral health consultant and debrief. This simple intervention is powerful and immediate and builds upon itself as, over time, team cohesion and communication reinforce themselves.

Another aspect of vicarious trauma is feeling over-responsible for one's patients. I found this true, especially for newer behavioral health consultants who may work harder than their patients to achieve health outcomes and feel personally responsible when patients do poorly. Managing the emotional investment one gives patients should be an intentional aspect and a growing skill for a behavioral health consultant. This calibration differs significantly from a population-based model to a specialty care model. However, even seasoned therapists will develop good boundaries and skills in this area to avoid burnout and decreased clinical efficacy.

Simply put, the behavioral health consultant has to understand that they are spreading themselves across a large number of patients, some of whom will require somewhat more of them than others but in the end, they are responsible for all of them. They thus must consciously consider how much they have to give emotionally and otherwise. This calibration gets much easier with time and experience. As a new behavioral health consultant, I struggled with feelings of guilt and inadequacy, mostly because I didn't know how to judge how much I should give to a particular case or situation - and that self-doubt quickly gets morphed into feelings that impact our self-efficacy and sometimes our self-worth.

While working at Lawndale, I gave primary care providers a burnout inventory called the Maslach Burnout Inventory and offered feedback based on the results. This inventory is considered the standard in the field. The clinicians filled out the inventory and then met to discuss aggregate findings and directions for interpreting their confidential individual results. What was most surprising from that intervention was that compared to norms, the rates of burnout were not as excessive as they had anticipated, and the distribution of burnout scores of the group took the shape of a standard bell curve. This feedback provided helpful information to them as a group (i.e., we are similar to other workers). Also, it helped individuals who were struggling to label their struggles and, in some cases, take personal action.

We have since experienced a pandemic, an upsurge of mental health needs in the community, and significant strain on the health system and its providers. Moral injury and compassion fatigue are real threats to the workforce. What has been encouraging is that BHCs were part of the buffer for many clinics during this period. BHC teams were called upon by their organizations to support other staff members and each other, and many stepped up to the plate, including the Access team. My perspective on this has not changed: the teams that mitigate burnout well have a culture of shared responsibility and mission and actively deal with vicarious trauma as immediately as possible. The Access team does not use videoconferencing as much now, but they do use an instant messaging platform to share the burden of care as they go.

Performance Anxiety

Pressure to perform is often a constant in many primary care organizations. Veterans of primary care have been through many cycles of threats by clinic administrators of impending doom if productivity is not improved. In fact, generally speaking, the more dysfunctional the organization, the more productivity threats there are (as measured solely by the number of patient encounters); this reality, coupled with what I find to be a common trait in mental health professionals - the desire to please authority figures - often leads to a significant amount of consternation whenever productivity is called into question; this is particularly true in the first few years of program development when productivity tends to be uneven.

My advice to behavioral health consultants and directors alike has been to focus on doing the absolute best job while trying hard to ignore the background noise of an organization's anxieties. The truth is that telling someone to do more work or to work harder is rarely an effective strategy for improving productivity; this is why for behavioral health consultants, I focus on the commitment to the mission of the work and the removal of barriers to efficiencies to maximize productivity. But in the end, it is hard to ignore that in the context of other stressors, demands for productivity can feel onerous and uncaring. In many cases, it affects the work environment, such that personnel begins to talk about this anxiety in unhealthy ways that only heighten the fear of losing employment or other penalties.

One other facet related to performance anxiety can occur as a byproduct of a good thing, namely, the mission focus. I've met many dedicated individuals who are passionate about their work, and this passion itself creates performance anxiety. Maintaining a "big picture" perspective is vital when dealing with feelings of inadequacy or feeling as if you are underperforming or not effectively meeting the PCBH mission. After reading a book like this one, it is easy to feel inadequate after seeing just a few patients in a day when launching your program. It is essential to understand that you cannot be judged by your work's day-in and day-out productivity, especially in the first few years. The wise behavioral health consultant director will keep an eye on the big picture of transforming the primary care practice over time, which means winning hearts and minds such that behavioral health becomes a natural part of primary care practice. This takes time.

Access's leadership gave me the room as a director to instill this philosophy, which paid off. During my tenure, the best we ever did financially was break even. Since then, the PCBH program has brought in more money between grants and fee-for-service work than it has cost the clinic, and staff turnover has been reasonably low. In other words, it does pay to have a long-term perspective that does not focus obsessively on productivity as defined by patient encounters alone. Access BHCs work hard because they feel enabled and motivated to work hard, not because they have productivity standards looming over their heads.

Feeling Stretched

Although this threat category could go along with multitasking, it deserves special attention. In the context of behavioral health consultation, feeling stretched relates to beginning to take on multiple responsibilities within an organization; this often happens as a positive development, namely that the organization recognizes the unique skills of mental health professionals that apply across aspects of organizational functioning.

For example, in my case, after several years of developing the behavioral health program, the organization began to recognize some of my skills in leading teams, managing process improvement, ability to handle data, and general insight into organizational dynamics; this led to my assignment as a member of the senior leadership team. In other organizations, I have often seen behavioral health directors in charge of or participating in efforts by clinics to achieve primary care medical home certification, training providers in motivational interviewing, and helping poorly functioning teams. These are all good things, but they are time-consuming activities that can detract from the development of the behavioral health program and stretch the individual. For this reason, managing a manager's range of responsibilities is vital. In other words, only some good opportunities are ones that a director should take.

This is both a pro and a con of a career in PCBH. There is much room for career growth for mental health professionals in healthy organizations. Navigating the various responsibilities that come your way requires wisdom. One of the reasons why I left Access was because I needed time and space from these responsibilities to recalibrate my professional life. In retrospect, I would have sought career mentorship to think through how I could develop as a leader and manage the growth of my role. I engaged an executive coach during my tenure as CEO of CFHA and found it worth every penny. Sometimes we need an external voice to help us make choices that match our skills and values.

Isolation

Perhaps the most pervasive and threatening stressor not only for behavioral health consultants but for human beings, in general, is the threat posed by isolation. The first few years of program development at the two clinics I worked at were frankly painful. They were painful mainly from the perspective of the amount of work that had to be done initially and the relative isolation I felt when building the programs.

In the case of my time at Lawndale Christian Health Center, the isolation was heightened by the lack of general development in the field. In other words, there were very few people that I could talk to across the country who could understand what I was working on and why. Fortunately, that is not the case today. In the case of my time at Access Community Health Centers, the isolation was a product of simply starting a new program with me, myself, and I. Indeed, there was excellent support from administration and providers alike, who helped to diminish my sense of isolation. Still, the absence of a team of professionals working directly with me on the program development task made it difficult.

I distinctly remember one moment early on when I was so overwhelmed with the intensity of patient care and the range of things I had to do that I left the clinic building, sat in my car in the parking lot, and cried for lack of a better alternative. I called my father and had a brief conversation that helped me some. Fortunately, that same depth of feeling overwhelmed has not returned since then, primarily because I'm no longer working alone. As human beings, we are made for community, and the absence of community damages our well-being; this is why I consider my most significant accomplishment at Access Community Health Centers to be the development of a community of behavioral health consultants who care for one another, have a common understanding of the work and mission, strive continually for excellence, and understand that achieving excellence is a communal task.

Many behavioral health consultants in small clinics and remote communities do not have the luxury of having this kind of team around them. It should be a core task of behavioral health consultants and their clinics to mitigate this isolation because there is no more significant threat to staff retention and well-being than this singular factor. Behavioral health consultants who have effectively counteracted their isolation tend to develop mutual consultation arrangements (for example, calling or videoconferencing colleagues in other clinics), participate in online forums and organizations such as CFHA, and generally work hard to develop good relationships with coworkers. It has also often been the case that organizations have contracted with consultants for technical expertise and to support the lone BHC. CFHA offers this kind of support through its technical assistance program.

As CEO of CFHA, I have emphasized providing avenues for isolated BHCs to gain support from the director's peer groups, consultants, and mentoring programs. Please don't try to do this on your own.

Life

It may seem odd to list life as a threat, but, generically speaking, it is. Positive and negative life events are - and should be - an expected threat to program functioning. Some of the most challenging times for myself and my staff have come when balancing the demands of new additions to our families amid the intensity of our work. As a team, we have learned to recalibrate when we have staff members who have young children; this is not a negative threat in the sense that it is a bad thing, but it is something that needs to be taken into consideration since, as human beings, we do not have infinite personal resources. There are stages of life, such as when caring for young children, during which a behavioral consultant has less to give. It is my philosophy that a workplace should accept this, encourage it, and, within reason, support it.

Other life events can also threaten our well-being, even if they do not directly impact our persons. For example, several of our staff have had spouses in transition times such as unemployment or over-employment (as in my wife's case during medical residency). The point is that life events are part of who we are when we come to work. However, it is essential to maintain professional boundaries and general professionalism; an excellent behavioral health director will attend to these factors within limits and make reasonable adjustments.

I now have teenage children and can attest to the reality that each stage of life presents unique challenges. As CBHO at Access, I paid attention to where my staff were in their personal lives, which paid off in staff longevity with the organization. Very few staff left as a result of disaffection with the organization. The staff that did leave typically left due to family transitions or a desire to switch career emphasis. If you support your moms during their pregnancies, they will reward you with high-quality work and leadership over the long term. If you support your dads to be engaged in their little kids' lives with flex around scheduling, they will remain engaged and productive. The key is having a long-term vision for investing in your staff.

What To Do

The following section will focus on self-care skills and ways to mitigate the work strain. However, it is worth noting that one of the first steps to successful self-care is identifying the particular threats you are facing and then building in proactive elements, whether it is into the work itself, the BHC team functioning, or the self-care repertoire. The effective behavioral health director will be mindful and aware of threats. Likewise, a successful behavioral health consultant will regularly check in with themselves and recalibrate as needed. While each workplace will have unique needs, one common thread can serve as an antidote to virtually all threats, namely community. A well-functioning behavioral health consultant team or a well-connected behavioral health consultant can cope with the work demands and deal with the ups and downs of life in primary care over time. A fragmented team and an isolated behavioral health consultant will constantly be under threat. So if there is one area to work on, this is it: developing a sense of community and feeling connected to others around you.

Any discussion of self-care skills must begin with the caveat that individuals respond differently to different strategies. Good behavioral health consultants know this since teaching self-care skills is one of the more common clinical activities. However, applying self-care skills to one's life differs significantly from teaching them to others. So in one sense, much of what will be discussed here in this chapter should seem redundant to a behavioral health consultant;

however, it will serve as a good reminder of the importance of continually working on this area.

Time Off

One of the more effective strategies for mitigating stress for behavioral health consultants is strategically taking time off. In our case, this requires some planning since our schedules are determined one quarter in advance; this has been helpful because it has forced me to think ahead of time about my needs in the future. So at the end of each quarter, when we begin planning the schedule for the next quarter, I am forced to sit down and think about when I might need respite. In doing so, I consider various factors, such as how many weeks in a row I may work without a day off and any seasonal variations in work responsibilities, such as interview season for interns, budget creation season, and the orientation of new trainees. I have learned over years of experience that different times of the year require different calibrations of my efforts and resources. Again this is unique to me, but it may be instructive in your thinking.

For example, there are two lull periods in the year, summertime between late May and August and late November through December. These are times when many people take vacations, and as such, I typically do not plan any large projects that require collaboration. As a result, I also tend to take fewer days off during these periods, especially since there are already holidays during the November-December period. I also feel less need for days off in the summertime since other aspects buffer stress for me, including the sunshine and many outdoor activities.

I've also learned that there are particularly stressful periods that are reasonably consistent year-to-year, namely the months of September through November and the months of January through March. These tend to coincide with times during which organizationally there is a lot going on and times when, for whatever reason, there is more of a clinical load. I suspect that, generally speaking, the change of seasons and the beginning of a new school year tend to ratchet things up for everyone in the community in September. I also suspect that getting into the heart of the winter months tends to impact patients' mental health and social issues. So during these times, I am conscientious about taking strategic days off, usually Mondays and at least at a rate of one day a month.

The bottom line is that the intensity of behavioral health consultant work is such that removing yourself from the environment is crucial to gain a new perspective and energy and climbing out of the ruts that develop when engaged in any repetitive task. What people do with their days off will vary as much as how often they take time off. I enjoy lounging around my house, running basic errands, having quiet time, etc. A good day off for me is a day when I don't think about work. In rare cases, I will schedule special activities on a day off, such as a massage or a trip to a local spa.

Others may choose different strategies for taking days off, including more extended vacations. I need regular days off at reasonably regular intervals instead of extended periods. But again, this is a function of individual differences. Despite changing roles, my strategies have mainly remained consistent. I plan a day off every six weeks to complement formal vacations. I have added a couple of strategies that bear mentioning. One is that I regularly meet with close friends to debrief life, especially friends who understand the burden of leadership; this helps clear my mind and reduce leadership fatigue.

Another is a sabbatical; this second edition was written mainly during that sabbatical and was revolutionary for me. In contrast to a vacation, a sabbatical is a time for professional and personal self-reflection. I shifted my energy during my six-week leave from work to work on myself; this is well worth the time and money for any professional, especially those in leadership and caregiving roles.

Scheduled Wellness

I've learned that a critical aspect of self-care is scheduling activities and experiences that prioritize our overall health and well-being. I call this practice scheduled wellness. This takes the form of several commitments I have made to myself and built into my schedule. Some of these routines are monthly, and others are seasonal. For example, every month, I will schedule a massage through a membership with a massage company and get a haircut. Seasonally I will play indoor soccer weekly and play baseball. These planned activities are crucial for self-care because they take the thinking out of it; this is especially important because making decisions during times of high stress often results in poor decision-making. Somehow it always seems harder to spend money on yourself when you're most stressed. This regularity also helps us internally anticipate respite times versus needing to plan rest when we are already exhausted.

This is crucial and has not changed for me in the ensuing years. Anticipating maintenance, be it physical, mental, emotional, or spiritual, is essential for all healthcare providers. These routines will change over time; for example, I no longer get monthly massages and play soccer, not baseball. However, the routine of planning self-care has stayed the same.

Physical Health Maintenance

Maintaining your physical health should seem obvious to the behavioral health consultant, but it bears mention because of its importance. Helping the mind through the body is an age-old strategy. Exercise is one of the antidotes to mental strain, but it is also very difficult to maintain consistently, as our patients can attest to. Here too, finding seasonal rhythms that work well with your schedule and that are preplanned our most effective. For me, the seasonal variations are significant. Most of my exercise comes naturally during the summer through family events, baseball, and swimming.

During the fall and winter months, I get some exercise through indoor soccer, but I have to supplement with one to two trips to the gym each week (which doesn't always happen). In my case, I take a very "BHC" approach to exercise and set very small goals and engage them in small increments. I do not tolerate long periods of exercise other than athletic activity, so a quick 30-minute trip to the gym is good enough for me.

Other than formal exercise, one of the other activities that I found to be helpful is utilizing a standing desk. Every so often, I will bring a portable keyboard stand that allows me to stand at my workspace at work, and this helps me to feel healthy for the half day or so that I use it. I will also practice walking through the clinic periodically during shifts to increase my visibility and help my mind defocus.

It should go without saying that diet is also an essential component of self-care. Our most stressful family times coincide with times when we do not go shopping regularly enough (probably because we are too busy); this will result in poor lunches, eating out more, and generally snacking unhealthily. To help combat this, we will periodically shop online for groceries and have them delivered. Although there is a small extra expense, it helps ensure we have the right foods at the right time. I have observed many of my colleagues also work hard to bring healthy snacks to work, which also takes some planning.

The importance of exercise and diet has only grown for me in the ensuing years.

Finding Your Moments Of Zen

Grounding oneself is a crucial strategy for a behavioral health consultant since the burden of patient stories and other demands can quickly make you feel rudderless. Here again, individuals will vary dramatically as to what helps them. I found several essential components I must build into my life regularly to avoid this feeling of being lost. The first and most vital for me are spiritual disciplines. These include things as simple as finding a few minutes each day for prayer, meditation, reading, or just simple, quiet moments. During these moments, I'm able to extract myself from all the "stuff" of life and work and focus on things bigger than me, which in turn helps me to have a new perspective on my work and also helps to sensitize me to particular needs that I may have and that I perhaps may have been ignoring.

Another grounding place for me is water. I've long known that I have a special relationship with water for reasons that I do not know. I love being in a swimming pool or a beach more than anything else. During the summertime, I go to the swimming pool virtually every day, and in those moments when I'm under the water, I'm able to block out all my senses and somehow recalibrate such that when I come out of the water, I feel like I've started a new day. Similarly, the experience of the power of waves at Jones Beach in New York, near where my parents live, and witnessing the beauty of the water, sun, and sand has life-giving power for me. Unfortunately, being that I live in Wisconsin, I haven't found this true of the snow.

Finding these grounding moments and strategies is essential for the behavioral health consultant, who must be rock solid in the face of the trauma and adversity that patients present to them regularly and the demands required of working so closely with other team members. Again, a critical undergirding principle is scheduling or accessing these moments readily and consistently.

One of the top reasons for my departure from Access was the difficulty I experienced during winter months in the northern US. My move to North Carolina reinforced how helpful Access to water (the beach) and sun are to my well-being. Even so, the routines I mention above have primarily remained part of my self-care, particularly the moments of quiet and centeredness that I require to operate well at work.

Relationships

A central theme of this book is the importance of community. Here too, community plays a significant role. Working on and maintaining relationships at work and in your own life is crucial to mitigating work stress. There are times, for example, when I purposely stop what I'm doing at home and start playing with my children in recognition that my mind has developed a rut where it is constantly thinking about work. Thus I will counteract that by focusing my energy on my children. My wife and I are busy professionals who continuously need to check in with each other about our work-life balance (or lack thereof). I have found myself less effective, more distracted, and more dissatisfied when my core relationships with my wife and children are not working well. I need those to be good for my work to be effective. So this requires maintenance and regular attention.

The main challenge in this area is that relationships are moving targets. Things that work for us in certain seasons don't work so well in other seasons of our life. For example, my wife and I have gone through seasons when we will schedule monthly dates; this has worked well for certain periods and then will not work well during others. Your children will enjoy different activities at various stages of their lives, and your connection to them will change over time.

The bottom line is that no singular strategy can perpetually help with this issue. What does help is having a consistent approach where you check in with your key relationships regularly to problem solve and (here is that word again) plan for what that relationship needs to sustain itself. More recently, for example, my wife and I decided that travel is important for us to reconnect. We decided that we needed to use our money in this way to help us form new shared experiences and have time with our children and time for ourselves; this makes sense during this season of our life as our children are no longer infants and toddlers, for example.

Non-work relationships are crucial for the effective BHC and BHC director, requiring regular maintenance and attention. While I did not inappropriately insert myself into my staff's relationships, I did make it a point to communicate the cultural value of our team and that these relationships are essential parts of ourselves that we bring to work with us. Occasionally, this led to staff sharing needs outside of work with one another. When possible, our team would support one another as a result, and many staff became friendly with each other's families.

Building Community at Work

Finally, it should come as no surprise to a reader of this text that the most critical self-care strategy we recommend involves how you put together and maintain your team. In the pages of this book, you have read about many methods for organizing the behavioral health consultant's work and managing communication between team members. An undergirding principle of all this is the centrality of having a healthy community, which includes not just the behavioral health consultants but all of the medical staff and organization, to promote health in patients. In other words, it is essential to have health in your community to give health to those in your community.

For example, it means checking in with each other regularly. I check in with staff individually three to four times a year formally and many more times informally. We have regular videoconferencing meetings every three to four weeks. We have an annual seminar series where we take four half days a week and spend time together in training, then end that week with dinner. Many of our staff do things together outside of work, such as participate in book clubs or go out for drinks. We create opportunities to get to know each other's families and thus can share these parts of our lives as well. In sum, it is clear that we have made it culturally essential for us to care for one another. There is no more critical, sustaining aspect of what we do that helps us mitigate the stress and the strain of our work and promote a sense of well-being and purpose than our community.

Hopefully, the many strategies for building community and communication have been clearly outlined in this book, not to be carbon copied, but rather to stimulate ideas and the vision for what an excellent behavioral health consultant team is and, even more so, what a great organization can look like. A primary key is understanding that self-care is not something you do as a last resort or reactively in the face of stress and strain. Self-care is part of your job. We believe this so profoundly that we built it into the behavioral health consultant job description. We suggest you do so as well.

So, why would I leave such an incredible organization and PCBH team? Trust me, I have asked myself this question on occasion. I did not go because I was burned out. I left for two reasons: 1. I sensed a need to create space for some of the rising talent on the team to take the helm, & 2. I needed to recalibrate my career while moving geographically to a warmer, sunnier climate (If I could have moved Madison, WI, to a different latitude, I would have.) I would encourage you to pay attention to the longevity of the wisdom in this section. In other words, these principles and approaches bore good fruit over 15 years. That long-term approach to staff wellness, personal wellness, and team cultural development led to sustainable and profitable results. Your solutions will differ, but the pathway is likely similar.

The New Chief Behavioral Health Officer Gets The Last Word

By Elizabeth Zeidler Schreiter

With my role as the Chief Behavioral Health Officer balancing leadership demands, managing a growing team, and clinical care, the work demands can exceed my internal resources. I have become much more mindful of over-extending myself and carefully examining what factors may contribute to this feeling. I have had to find ways to recalibrate and re-prioritize my self-care.

As Neftali mentioned, boundary setting has been a critical leadership skill required to sustain and do this work well.

For me, external boundary setting came much more effortless than internal. I have always been a high achiever and am highly passionate about my work and the patients I serve. I can "overfunction" sometimes, putting my self-care on the back burner; I have found this is a recipe for burnout. Awareness of my resources and learning to allocate them most effectively has been the most significant area of my personal and professional growth. I feel fortunate to work in an environment that fosters such growth. It has been essential for me to have the freedom to communicate openly about the amount of work I can effectively take on from day to day. Sometimes, this may require me to pull back on new initiatives or collaborations. I remind myself that this work is a marathon, not a sprint, and to permit myself to be present on the journey at the moment to promote sustainability.

This boundary setting and intentional awareness of the demands to do this work effectively has assisted on an organizational level when we discuss new initiatives, projects, strategic plans, etc., in ensuring we keep employee/staff wellness and work-life harmony at the forefront when pursuing initiatives. We meet weekly for 30 minutes as a team to discuss clinical and operational challenges and wins. I also "round" monthly with each staff member to check in on self-care sustainability, express gratitude/appreciation for their work, and support professional development.

Functioning as a behavioral health consultant is highly fulfilling but also hard work. It can be both physically and emotionally taxing. The significant emotional labor associated with this work makes self-care paramount to sustainability in this setting. All full-time BHC staff are given one day per week of administration time, which provides vital opportunities to engage in other areas of leadership, catch up on note writing, flex time for intentional self-care, and pursue other passion projects related to clinical excellence; this also provides team members with diversity in the workweek, which has been another protective factor from burnout. As the Chief Behavioral Health Officer, I have 0.2 clinical FTE and 0.8 administrative FTE. I can direct all my energy and efforts to patient care and availability to our primary care clinicians in the clinic without feeling pulled to complete other administrative tasks.

Self-care is an area I continue to develop and prioritize to bring my best self to work every day. For me, self-care has involved setting limits and boundaries regarding the work I take on and in my day-to-day practice habits. Previously, there were numerous days in which I would work through lunch. However, if I did not take the time for lunch, I felt scattered, slightly irritable, and hungry later in the afternoon. While basic, simply leaving the clinic to eat lunch (even for only 15 minutes) and taking a brief walk leaves me feeling refreshed, recharged, and ready to tackle whatever the afternoon offers.

In addition, the BHC team has been instrumental in supporting clinic-wide wellness activities related to the 4 R's (Ready, Refresh, Recover, Recharge); thus, it is an added incentive to "practice what I preach." My self-care took on a new level of importance since becoming a mother. My typical self-care behaviors were either no longer effective or were too challenging to fit into my new routine as a full-time provider, leader, mother, wife, daughter, friend, etc. I intentionally complete all notes before leaving for the day to minimize how often I take work home with me (I typically document in the EHR while I am in the room with a patient). When that is impossible, I limit the time I chart from home (our electronic health record allows remote access) to protect family time. Family is one of my core values; thus, this will enable me to engage in values-based behaviors and bring peace and balance when I can live according to my values.

During the day, I consult with my behavioral health consultant colleagues regarding particularly challenging patient situations. Regular exercise, time with family and friends, a healthy diet, and good sleep habits also help to keep me grounded.

For those just getting started as a behavioral health consultant, please be mindful of forming a good team with individuals who can bring different attributes and talents. Given the nature of primary care, there is always more to be learned by surrounding yourself with colleagues with differing skill sets. Keeping your team diversified will promote continued growth and professional development.

Do not pressure yourself to learn everything simultaneously; this is a familiar feeling. Learn to notice this pressure and continue to take one day at a time. Starting as a behavioral health consultant involves navigating so many changes co-occurring: a new environment, new relationships, and your new role/ identity as a behavioral health consultant. Allow yourself time to get acclimated to your surroundings, and don't be afraid to ask questions of your new PCP colleagues. These inquiries can assist with building relationships, expanding your medical knowledge, or simply gaining a better understanding of how the provider you are working with thinks. Don't be afraid to speak up if you hear a provider discussing a challenging patient situation; this may be an opportunity to offer your expertise and further facilitate reciprocal learning, which is essential in primary care.

Chapter 30: Ethics, FAQ

By Neftali Serrano, PsyD

thical issues are part of working in healthcare. The issues that arise in integrated care are mostly the same ethical concerns that permeate all of healthcare, but some nuances are worth discussing. Here, we will not cover all of the ethical issues in healthcare as those are well covered elsewhere but instead focus on those pertinent to PCBH implementation specifically.

1. *Patient Privacy and Confidentiality: How can the clinic ensure the confidentiality of patient information, especially when sharing it with behavioral health providers?*

Privacy and confidentiality are cornerstones of healthcare, but they should not impede quality, integrated care. Training ensures that your care teams respect patient rights, not arbitrary limits on information access. All patient information is equally protected under HIPAA (federal law governing patient records); therefore, arbitrary limits on information access, such as break-the-glass features for record access, only create the illusion of protecting some information more than others. Our recommendation is to focus on robust and routine training on how information is shared verbally (e.g., curbside consults not occurring in vulnerable areas), on software platforms (e.g., EHR, texts, etc.), and with external agencies (e.g., internal processes for record releases and verbal communication). As usual, we recommend using the golden rule in most cases: "Do as primary care does."

What measures should be in place to protect patient records and information in an integrated care setting?

As per the above, we recommend a strategy that mirrors what primary care is already doing to protect information in the EHR. If specific staff do not have access to PCP documentation, they shouldn't have access to BHC documentation either. If notes are automatically sent to patients upon completion through a patient portal for the PCP, then the same should occur with BHC notes (most systems provide an opt-out option). The key, again, is training, particularly for appropriate documentation for primary care. Your teams should be trained on what content is suitable for the EHR and should be written with the patient, PCP, and other care team members in mind when writing (and the insurance company). Beyond this, what will ultimately protect your PCBH service are the same policies and procedures that protect the rest of the primary care team.

2. *Informed Consent: How will patients be informed about integrating behavioral health services into their primary care, and how will their consent be obtained?*

The same way that consent for all of the services at your clinic. Once again, we do as primary care does. All patients seen by the PCBH service should be enrolled as clinic patients with an assigned PCP. This process usually involves paperwork describing the services and team members the patient will work with and various disclaimers related to financial obligations and patient rights. A new PCBH service should review this paperwork and suggest additions to ensure that the PCBH service is represented as part of the primary care team services the patient will experience. Typically, it can be helpful to add a statement noting that additional services provided on a visit may incur additional charges based on the patient's insurance, such as a copay. Look at state regulations for the license types working on your PCBH service and refer to applicable ethics codes (e.g., the American Psychological Association ethics code usually suffices as a good default) to ensure you have covered your bases in the informed consent document your clinic modifies. Typically, only a few sentences of clarification are needed in total.

> *What information should be provided to patients to ensure they understand the nature and benefits of PCBH?*

Let's be honest. 0 to 1% of patients read these things. So, we recommend putting only the basics in a modified primary care informed consent. Put your best energy into training your PCPs, MAs, and BHCs for good verbal introductions to

PCBH services. In the written document, you may want to introduce the following:

- Description of BHC services as a primary care level of behavioral health support
- A statement describing open communication between PCP and BHC, including EHR documentation
- Patient responsibility for any costs associated with scheduled or same-day services

3. *Stigma and Discrimination: How will the clinic address the potential stigma of seeking behavioral health services within a primary care setting?*

The good news is that PCBH, by nature, is destigmatizing. For example, the patient is often seen in the same exam room they see their PCP in. The key is to decrease any differentiation between the PCP and BHC visits; this is why we recommend using exam rooms, not office spaces, for BHC visits. We also recommend using the same procedures for calling patients back to the clinical area from the waiting room and mimicking all registration and other administrative processes. The goal is that only the patient knows they are seeing a behavioral health provider during their visit. To this end, the clinic should also promote the concept of a care team, including behavioral health support, in advertising, written materials, and their website to normalize accessing PCBH services. Finally, the most crucial step a clinic can take to destigmatize behavioral health services is simply teaching its staff to introduce services with consistent, destigmatizing language; this should be a recurring training, not a one-and-done.

What steps will be taken to prevent discrimination against patients with mental health or substance use issues?

This question is particularly salient for patients with substance abuse conditions. Far too often, patients with substance abuse issues are treated differently by care team members or staff. Training on a harm reduction model and trauma-informed care are crucial here. All staff, including registration staff, medical assistants, and other clinical staff, should be culturally on board with an understanding of substance abuse as a chronic disease and trauma-informed communication skills. Along with this training, staff should know policies and procedures for dealing with intoxicated, otherwise incapacitated patients and patients in crisis. This training gives staff tools to understand patient behavior and steps to assist patients who need de-escalation and empowers staff to protect themselves.

4. *Provider Competency and Training: How will primary care providers be trained to address behavioral health concerns effectively and ethically?*

It would be best if you had a plan for provider training that is sustainable and replicable. In other words, think of provider training as you would think of continuing education - it never ends. Far too many clinics think one training will level-set their PCPs. That is not high-functioning team behavior. Here are some topics you may want to include in such recurring training:

• How to introduce the PCBH service

- High-functioning teammate behaviors for the PCP leader
- Working with the BHCs with mental health issues
- Working with the BHCs with physical health issues
- Huddle basics
- Curbside consult basics
- How to access the BHC team

> *What mechanisms will be in place to ensure ongoing professional development for providers in both primary care and behavioral health?*

Well, most of that is up to you, but they should be in place, and where possible, they should cross over both groups. In other words, design as many trainings as feasible involving PCPs and BHCs to foster a shared learning environment. I have had many experiences where PCPs were ecstatic about participating in our PCBH training because they learned so much. We teach and train well in the behavioral sciences, so it's a novel experience for PCPs. As noted in other chapters, at Access, various team communication and training methods exist, including an annual PCBH team in-service experience for all staff and trainees.

5. *Patient Autonomy: To what extent should primary care providers involve patients in decisions regarding their behavioral health treatment?*

Patient autonomy is a critical principle in healthcare. In practice, I rarely see a patient prefer less integrated care, so this concern is not commonplace. That said, it deserves attention due to its importance. The key competing principles here are the nature of the service the clinic is providing and patient autonomy/ preference. No patient should be forced to see a BHC or other care team member. However, the PCP should be clear with the patient that services at the clinic are arrayed in a specific fashion (as per the informed consent) and that, in some cases, the care they provide might be hampered or, in some cases, not be possible due to that structure. For example, a patient seeking psychostimulant treatment for ADHD may not be able to receive medication intervention with the PCP if, per protocol, the BHC must be involved in the care. In that case, with care and respect, the PCP would encourage the patient to seek care elsewhere or help the patient see the wisdom of working with the BHC. Exceptions to team-based care should be few and far between in a high-functioning clinic with PCBH.

6. *Referral and Access: How will the clinic ensure that patients have equitable access to behavioral health services, especially considering potential disparities in access to care?*

Here is where data will help you. PCBH services should evaluate their data, particularly data that enables you to see the penetration into the clinic population. This data should not only tell you how much penetration is occurring (typically, high-performing clinics are around 20% of unique users) but with whom. At a minimum, you should break this data into payer categories, ethnic/racial categories, gender identification, and ages. You can identify disparities if you have local population data or the clinic's general population data. If you want to get fancier, some clinics are working on particular condition categories and seeing if there are access or outcome differences between groups (e.g., depression screening). It can be helpful to coordinate these efforts with the larger quality improvement efforts that the clinic undertakes so that this does not occur in isolation.

> *What criteria will determine when to refer a patient to a behavioral health consultant versus managing their care without PCBH support?*

PCBH, by definition, does not impose criteria. However, this could lead to differential referral patterns from PCPs and different care involvement across groups for the PCBH service. Here, the PCP penetration metric is useful. You should track panel penetration rates across your providers and target an underperforming PCP with positive messaging to support their PCBH referral behaviors. It may be helpful to break down how portions of their panel, for example, Hispanic patients with English as their second language, are being under-treated compared to others in the population. Of course, tact and good messaging are essential here to ensure that PCPs are not accused of discrimination but are encouraged to self-evaluate their PCBH referral behavior.

That said, some clinics have developed protocols for automatically including PCBH for conditions such as MAT, ADHD, triage for specialty MH referral, pre-bariatric surgery referral, and others.

7. *Dual Relationships: Can BHCs see staff and their relatives in clinical care?*

This is a controversial issue. If we adopt our golden rule, then in most cases, the answer will be yes since primary care providers see each other and staff and their relatives for the most part. In most instances, PCBH programs select a "Yes, and" approach where there are limits to the extent and kinds of situations where BHCs see clinic staff. Since we cannot cover all the possible scenarios here, it is most instructive to cover the fundamental principles in negotiating this ethical dilemma.

- **Ethics codes do not prohibit dual relationships.** This is a common misconception for behavioral health professionals. What is prohibited are dual relationships where power differentials are likely to lead to abuse or harm or situations where confidentiality cannot be maintained. You will have to think through how the PCBH service can provide care without introducing harmful dual relationships or violate confidentiality. For example, it does not make sense for a BHC to work with their direct supervisor or family, for instance, due to the power dynamics in the relationship.
- **Staff deserve equal care to patients.** By avoiding serving staff through rigid prohibitions, PCBH services can inadvertently create two levels of care, one for patients and one for staff who are patients. We should not tolerate sub-standard care for staff who have elected to have their care at their clinic; this does not mean that reasonable limits cannot be imposed or options provided such as an EAP service. The one criterion for staff to formally receive services from the PCBH service is that they are legitimately an enrolled clinic patient and, therefore, the care team's responsibility.

- **BHCs need training and supervision to know how to work with staff who are patients.** The key to working with co-workers clinically is to have training and processes in place to ensure that BHCs have supervisors they can go to to discuss ethical and logistical aspects of care. Policies and procedures should also be in place to guide the service in resolving situations. These should be developed with input from Human Resources and the Chief Medical Officer.
- **Informal consultation is acceptable, but BHCs should exercise good boundaries.** It is common for PCPs to consult one another informally for personal health issues; thus, reaching out to their BHC colleague will feel natural. In most cases, this will work well if the BHC is clear when specific consultation questions are outside their area of expertise or ability to comment. A certain amount of wisdom is needed to discern situations where no comment is better than offering an opinion.

8. *Cultural Humility: How will the clinic address the cultural and linguistic needs of diverse patient populations in the context of behavioral health care?*

Here is a list of the routine activities that should become a part of your care team culture at a minimum:

- Training on cultural humility
- Training related to populations, especially vulnerable populations, such as LGBTQ+, ethnic/racial minorities in your area, and persons with disabilities (centered on health equity implications)
- Training on the use of interpreters

- Workforce development plans, including career ladders within your organization that increase your chances to hire persons that reflect the patient population you serve (e.g., peer support specialist, care manager, internships, etc.)

What data elements are being tracked with a health equity lens in mind?

Health equity is fundamentally about your knowledge of the population you serve and identifying gaps in care. Your efforts to provide equitable care will hinge on your ability to gather data that tells you how care is distributed and utilized by important groups within your population; this will be unique for each clinic and requires a strong relationship between your health quality director and the PCBH service. A good start is to align first with the existing equity goals of your organization and consider how PCBH services can contribute to bridging the gaps. Then, as you become adept with data and successfully bridge gaps, you can turn your attention to other gaps unique to behavioral health that need to be encompassed in your clinic's existing quality plan. Here are some exemplars of this latter category:

Is PCBH utilization equivalent amongst ethnic/ racial categories, including key indicators such as English as a second language?
Are members of important sub-populations screened for behavioral conditions at roughly equivalent rates?
Are there important trends among markers such as age, gender, or race/ethnicity that show differential utilization of PCBH services?

Since PCBH is centered on solving the access problem in behavioral healthcare, your equity metrics should center on ensuring that access is measurably equivalent, where possible, across important sub-populations.

9. *Resource Allocation: How will the clinic allocate resources for behavioral health services, and how will these decisions align with ethical principles of equity and patient need?*

One of the more worrisome trends in some PCBH service implementations is the apparent disregard that the organization can have in allocating resources to the service; this leads to negative signaling, which impacts staff morale and patient perception of the service, including amplifying feelings of stigma. For example, suppose a PCBH provider has to fight for room space and is allocated a sub-standard space to work in, like a closet. In that case, this will create a bifurcation between the medical and behavioral health services. Clinics must allocate resources to the PCBH service like they would to a new nurse team or medical pod area. The good news is that the PCBH service is not resource-intensive by nature.

> *What mechanisms will be in place to address resource constraints and ensure that patients receive adequate care?*

Some of the most difficult ethical challenges in running a PCBH service involve interacting with clinic financial policies and the payer background of the patient. Resolving these ethical dilemmas, or more helpfully, averting these situations, includes developing a good relationship between the PCBH director and the CFO. For example, you want to avoid creating different levels of care team support based on patient insurance status. If your clinic has prohibitive copays that they charge for warm handoffs, you will dissuade patients who cannot afford extra copays from accepting the standard of care in the clinic. You will also place your medical providers in a bind as they seek to care for some patients independently and others with BHC support. Every clinic with solid relationships between CFOs and the PCBH service has found ways to resolve these situations. Creativity is often needed, such as lower sliding fee scale for behavioral health visits for uninsured patients to decreasing aggressive collection policies. Ultimately, our ethics tell us to do what is right by the patient, adhere to insurance laws in our region, and provide equivalent care across patient groups.

10. *Patient Feedback and Grievances: How will the clinic solicit and respond to patient feedback and grievances related to their experience with the PCBH model?*

Patient surveys are the usual answer to this question when looking at it from a global patient satisfaction approach. The problem is that patient surveys tend to be almost universally positive about PCBH services, so much so that the feedback, while encouraging, is not practical. I still recommend using existing survey data (nearly all primary care clinics collect patient feedback) to rate BHC providers but be prepared that it will not provide actionable intelligence. For patient grievances, the standard grievance procedure used by the clinic should suffice for specific patient complaints. Likely, the most actionable patient feedback might come from focus groups, though health systems rarely utilize this.

11. *Regulatory Oversight: Do we operate as an independent service and thus adhere to regulations as such?*

This is an essential and nuanced issue. All licensed providers are subject to the state laws governing their profession and the ethical mandates of their guild. These are non-negotiable, and they rarely come into conflict with PCBH service parameters. For example, in certain states, specific master's level providers must provide patients with specific statements in their informed consent procedures - that would require some workarounds in the PCBH service procedure to avoid having patients sign separate informed consent.

There is rarely legislation or regulatory language that specifies distinctions between a PCBH model and specialty care regulations, although this is becoming more commonplace. Thus, in theory, a PCBH service must adhere to all the specialty regulations for their region/ state. The good news is that in most instances, the language and requirements are broad enough that standard primary care procedures for patient enrollment, handling of patient records, and other key regulatory mandates are manageable within the normal scope of primary care; this is why we recommend against duplicative procedures such as dual informed consent procedures, separate records, lengthy notes or other non-patient-centered policies.

Where inconsistencies exist, work with your compliance team and C-suite to arrive at reasonable accommodation. Remember that compliance is not about receiving 100% on the compliance scale - it should be about doing what is best for the patient and improving their access to high-quality, timely care.

Over time, PCBH will become more of a norm in regulatory language, and it will become easier to maneuver the distinction between PCBH and specialty mental health. For now, your job as an implementer is to create a service wholly dependent on and integrated into the primary care service while meeting minimum criteria for the licenses of your staff. This approach can feel foreign to many mental health professionals who tend to be high on conscientiousness and rule-following. Just remember that laws and regulations have a spirit and that real human beings administer these rules. I would rather defend my approach to a specific rule based on a patient-centered rationale than work extra hard to adhere to a rule to ensure we get a perfect score on an audit that reduces the quality of care to our patients.

Addressing these ethical issues and questions is essential for successfully implementing a PCBH model while ensuring the well-being and rights of patients receiving care in this integrated setting. Ultimately, the ethical health and readiness of the overall clinic will determine the context for the PCBH service. Where gaps exist, they likely do not just exist for the PCBH service but the entire operation. An implementer can use this reality to alert the clinic to the need and arrive at a workable solution. Rarely will you be working on ethics and legal issues as an independent service because that is not what you are.

Chapter 31: One More Thing... The Community Health of Central Washington Story

By David Bauman, PsyD & Bridget Beachy, PsyD

Just as ripples spread out when a single pebble is dropped into water, the actions of individuals can have far-reaching effects - Dalai Lama

If a small to medium-sized community health center (CHC) in the central, rural part of the state of Washington can build a leading PCBH service, there is no reason other organizations cannot grow successful services. Just as the Dalai Lama described above, we believe the pebble of PCBH can ripple out in health centers (and communities) through healing, humanity, and compassion. These ripples start with a Behavioral Health Consultant (BHC) being curious about what a patient thinks is feasible via collaborative treatment planning; it is done by a BHC talking with a medical provider about the importance of understanding context and how Adverse Childhood

Experiences (ACEs) could shape someone's worldview; it is done by a BHC partnering with a medical assistant to deliver a presentation on motivational interviewing to the nursing team; it is done by a BHC leading a discussion with the senior leaders on trauma-informed care and the importance of approaching healthcare from a place of cultural humility. Each of these moments carries potential energy to make health care more contextual and compassionate. We know it is vital to examine our past to help shape where we are going, and we hope some of our stories help support you in the ripples being created within your organization.

Additionally, we wanted to point out that we are well aware of the limits of our perspectives, including but not limited to our fickle human memories and perceptions; thus, we know this chapter will not only be incomplete, but there may also be some unintended inaccuracies; this is a story mainly told through our eyes. Regardless of how hard we have worked to ensure the timelines and reflections are as accurate as possible, we know we could never accurately document what happened and what "made things work." Thus, your grace in any unintended errors of commission and omission is appreciated as we tell the story of PCBH at CHCW.

Our journey throughout this chapter will begin with a history of CHCW's PCBH efforts, from its conception as an organization in the early 1990s to where we currently stand in 2023. We will then focus on two primary stories, 1) efforts and lessons learned in BHC clinical care and workforce development (core BHCs and trainees) and 2) influencing our organization's leadership and administration.

Lastly, please take a moment as you read this to pause and reflect on your current moment. Place the book aside, and ask yourself, "What is a moment lately that reflects my values as a healthcare professional?" "What values do I live out in my work?" One of the many reasons we cherish sharing Stories of PCBH is that it reminds us regularly of the "why" of what we do in assisting healthcare in answering the call for high-quality primary care put forth by the National Academies of Science, Engineering, and Medicine (NASEM, 2021).

Implementing high-quality primary care can be draining and, sometimes, even demoralizing. While we will highlight the "wins" at CHCW, we also do not want to leave out the ubiquitous challenges and struggles. We have a saying, "To be on the cutting edge means you will get cut." We are here with you and the tireless efforts you have made and are currently making. Take a moment to be kind, compassionate, and above all, take a moment to be loving to yourself. And let's have that moment of love ripple out throughout these incredible Stories of PCBH at CHCW.

Community Health of Central Washington: A History

Community Health of Central Washington (CHCW) is a CHC in central Washington (the rural, dry part of the state that uses irrigation to sustain its crops). Serving the cities of Ellensburg, Naches, Tieton, and Yakima, CHCW provides comprehensive care (i.e., full-spectrum family medicine, obstetrics, pediatrics, dental, nutrition, pharmacy, senior and residential care, medically assisted treatment, women, infants, and children's nutrition, and integrated behavioral health) to approximately 30,000 patients. CHCW is a CHC that values providing healthcare to those overlooked in the healthcare conversation. Their primary focus is on underserved, uninsured, and underrepresented individuals.

CHCW also houses two formal training programs, including a family medicine residency that dates back to the early 1990s and a primary care behavioral health training program consisting of a predoctoral psychology internship accredited by the American Psychological Association (APA) and a post-graduate fellowship. CHCW's "mothership" clinic is Central Washington Family Medicine (CWFM), which houses most of the outpatient medicine done by residents, faculty, and other core providers. Due to being one of the original Teaching Health Centers (THC), CHCW strives to reach patients through direct service and educate future generations of primary care providers. Dr. Mike Maples, CHCW's founding CEO who served for close to 30 years until 2019, often quipped, "CHCW is the only CHC in the country that has both service and education within its mission statement." While we have yet to verify this claim, written into CHCW's DNA is providing services to underserved populations and ensuring that future generations of primary care providers are trained in settings that offer such services.

As we describe CHCW's integrated behavioral health efforts and history, we must define the goals and philosophy that have guided the organization since 2007. We acknowledge diverse opinions on integration models and whether organizations should adhere to a particular model of integration. Unapologetically, we embrace the Primary Care Behavioral Health (PCBH) model's principles and philosophy. We wish to acknowledge Christopher Neumann, Ph.D., who was so instrumental in first exposing many of us at Forest Institute to this idea of PCBH and primary care psychology. Further, our mentors, who included Jeff Reiter, Ph.D., Kirk Strosahl, Ph.D., and Patti Robinson, Ph.D., are the grandfathers and grandmother of PCBH. We often joke that Kirk and Patti are the six degrees of Kevin Bacon related to PCBH; essentially, if you trace anyone's lineage of training/trainers in PCBH, it would eventually come back to Kirk and Patti. Having them serve as mentors and guiding forces in our careers shaped our relational frames of what integration could and should be.

And, even with these contextual factors, the guiding force that prompts our implementation of and fidelity to PCBH is genuinely believing in the philosophy of primary care. One of our favorite interview questions for our post-doctoral fellowship is, "If a friend of a family member came up to you and said, 'Hey, you work in primary care. Just what is primary care all about? What are the goals of primary care?'" As you are reading this, pause for a moment and reflect on those questions. Where does your mind go? What definitions, guiding principles, and core components come to mind?

If you were like us in the early part of our careers, even after all the education and training, we failed to fully grasp the importance of the body of literature demonstrating the enormous value of primary care; this is one of the main reasons we believe integrated care within primary care fails and falters. Many behavioral health efforts within primary care often try to make primary care something it is not and demands that it assimilate to a specialty approach rather than embracing the vision of primary care. In these cases, integrated care can actually hinder versus help primary care.

For us, it is paramount that individuals understand the goals of primary care to ensure the successful uptake of integration. Although it is not the focus of this chapter, we recommend that individuals visit the Robert Graham Center (https://www.graham-center.org) and read about the Four Cs of primary care, as outlined in the writings of O'Malley et al. (2015). Primary care's values, such as continuity of services over a patient's lifetime, comprehensive care that addresses community members' needs, being the first point of contact for a significant portion of the community, and coordinating care with community partners, have remained unchanged despite the addition of more Cs since the original paper. Lastly, we encourage readers to review the inspiring and enlightening report put out by the National Academies of Sciences, Engineering, and Medicine (NASEM) detailing a vision of primary care that would be healing and build communities of engagement and health (https://www.ncbi.nlm.nih.gov/books/NBK571810/).

With this vision and understanding of primary care, our integrated care efforts began to adapt to the values of the system. Rather than seeing integrated care as a behavioral health intervention focused solely on behavioral health-related concerns (e.g., mental health and substance use), we see our efforts as a health care intervention to assist primary care in reaching its values inherent in those Four C's; this, ultimately, is why we adhere to the philosophy and guiding principles of the PCBH model.

PCBH has always kept primary care at the forefront. For example, a few years ago, we wrote an article for the Washington Academy of Family Physicians journal on our integrated care efforts (Bauman & Beachy, 2020). As we discussed our model's philosophy and explained PCBH through the GATHER acronym (Table 5) described by Reiter et al. (2018), one of the reviewers commented, "Isn't GATHER just the primary care philosophy?" That parsimony and synergy are what we are hoping for BHCs at CHCW. We do not see our BHCs as behavioral health providers; instead, we see them as primary care providers (PCPs), something that our current CEO, Angela Gonzalez, promotes regularly and often, even to our doctorate internship applicants during our annual interview days. That shift in focus and philosophy has been, without a doubt, one of the main reasons we have seen such an exponential growth of integrated care within CHCW.

Table 5. PCBH GATHER Acronym (Reiter et al., 2018)	
Generalist	BHCs working within PCBH strive to see all ages and conditions served by the primary care clinic. Conditions could include traditional mental health concerns (e.g., depression, anxiety, trauma, etc.), as well as medical conditions (e.g., diabetes, hypertension, migraines, etc.) and behavioral concerns (e.g., poor diet, lack of exercise, lack of treatment adherence, etc.)

Accessibility	BHCs working within PCBH strive to provide see patients the same-day the primary care clinic requests services. Via warm-handoffs, BHCs strive to complete meaningful clinical encounters when requested, as well as are available for curbside consultations with the primary care team.
Team-Based	BHCs working within PCBH strive to be a member of the primary care team. This includes working in the same shared clinical space, using the same terminology as the primary care team, and utilizing current clinic operations. Further, BHCs strive to maximize the efforts of the primary care team in all aspects of healthcare delivery.
High Productivity	BHCs working with PCBH strive to apply a population-based approach to serving a high proportion of the primary care patient population. Productivity mirrors PCPs and while emphasis is placed on achieving a high number of meaningful clinical encounters, equal amount of emphasis is placed on serving a high number of unique patients.
Educator	BHCs working within PCBH strive to ensure all members of the primary care team are more confident, comfortable, and competent in behavioral health techniques and philosophies. Through informal conversations and formal trainings, BHCs strive to ensure each member of the primary care team is educated on the biopsychosocial model, contextual, and compassionate model of care.

| Routine | BHCs working within PCBH strive to ensure BHCs are a routine part of healthcare and the involvement of BHCs is so uptaken it resembles involvement of traditional team members, such as nurses, pharmacists, etc. BHCs strive to ensure that their involvement and inclusion in the care for the clinic population reflects less of a rarity and more an expectation. |

CHCW 1992-2014: The Early Years

Community Health of Central Washington (CHCW) is unique for a health center, particularly a CHC. CHCW started as a family medicine residency, which the two local hospitals in Yakima supported at the time. It was not until years later that it became a CHC, an organization comprising multiple clinics and providing services across multiple counties in central Washington state. The humble beginnings of a small family medicine residency clinic still permeate our existence today, including our integrated behavioral health efforts.

According to our founding CEO, Dr. Maples, early in the residency's development, it was clear there needed to be a behavioral health education component. This realization was primarily due to multiple faculty members being graduates of the University of Washington's School of Family Medicine, which has consistently been at the forefront of training future family medicine physicians to understand the importance of a biopsychosocial approach to caring for patients and a community. Additionally, the idea of having a Behavioral Scientist faculty member of all family medicine residency programs was solidified by the Accrediting Council for Graduate Medical Education (ACGME) program requirements.

At CWFM, the initial integration was carried out by Dr. Eugenia English, an OB/GYN physician. During her part-time work with the residency, Dr. Maples noted her significant influence, reflecting her exceptional ability to connect and communicate with others. "She possessed a keen ability to connect and communicate with other humans, and people were quickly drawn to her for the comfort and peace that they found in her company," Dr. Maples remarked. "She was an invaluable resource not just to patients and residents but to this forming/storming/norming group of newbie faculty." Interestingly and remarkably, one could argue that the first signs of PCBH and the current philosophy driving the integrated care movement were ever-present in the program's early days.

In 1997, Dr. English retired, and as CHCW began to form and grow, so did the idea of integrated care. Dr. Dahna Berkson, a psychologist, joined the faculty in 1998 and served in the program until 2005. During this period, CHCW saw its efforts grow exponentially related to its psychosocial medicine within the residency and organization. Also during this time, CHCW became a CHC, acquired a large local pediatric clinic in Yakima, and began to evolve beyond a single residency clinic to a larger healthcare organization with a mission to provide holistic care to the underserved. The work Dr. Berkson engaged in during her time at CHCW helped set the stage for a new view of what integrated behavioral health could be within its primary care offices.

One of our favorite sayings is, "Life is a bunch of accidents," meaning random events in the universe ripple out exponentially and powerfully. When looking back, we like to make connections with these random events and often assign erroneous purposes to them. Maybe our minds do this to provide comfort in the idea that the universe is intentional. Regardless, in 2007, CHCW's PCBH program had one of the most extraordinary accidents, in the form of psychologist Dr. Kirk Strosahl coming on board as the third behavioral scientist in the residency's history.

As most know, Kirk is not only one of the founding figures of PCBH, but he is also a co-founder of Acceptance and Commitment Therapy (ACT) and Focused Acceptance Commitment Therapy (fACT). His influence on the field of psychology and healthcare cannot be understated. The accident that brought Kirk to CHCW was his progress towards semi-retirement status after a long career in academia and consulting and Kirk's move to his childhood home in the Yakima Valley. Another "accident" that this led to was Kirk's partner in life, Dr. Patti Robinson, being connected to CHCW. She was responsible for most of what can be witnessed in CHCW's modern-day PCBH services. Patti's knowledge and wisdom permeated CHCW's infrastructure as she worked intimately with CHCW's leadership regarding its integration efforts. She additionally worked with the early crew of BHCs (including us). It is difficult to fully describe Patti's impact on CHCW's leadership, infrastructure, and PCBH services.

In the early 2000s and into the 2010s, the opportunities were ripe for CHCW as it quickly expanded, including establishing a full-spectrum family medicine clinic in Ellensburg and a rural clinic in Naches in 2007 and 2009, respectively. Continuing the expansion trend, CHCW's leadership saw behavioral health integration as more than just a family medicine residency requirement but something that could genuinely transform an organization's delivery of clinical services across all sites.

Each of these influences started to set up the context for PCBH to be successful at CHCW. CHCW had dynamic physician leaders, including Russell Maier, MD, and Deborah Gould, MD, who were both instrumental in the growth of behavioral health integration at CWFM and the clinical service delivery realms. Soon after Kirk's arrival, more BHCs joined the effort, including Mary Virginia "MV" Maxwell at CHCW's pediatric clinic (now known as Yakima Pediatrics) and Regan Eberhart at the newly established clinic in Ellensburg, WA (CHCW Ellensburg). These two were contracted employees from community mental health agencies in the region, with Ms. Maxwell's position eventually moving from a contract position to a full-time CHCW position.

CHCW implemented new PCBH principles, including having BHCs as part of the primary care team, collaborating with PCPs, completing handoffs, and seeing patients for any behavior-related issues, not just mental health and substance use. This was a first for CHCW. At the same time, patients and PCPs were beginning to appreciate the value of PCBH as they adapted to the new system.

Dr. Maples loves recalling a story of when he first presented the idea of having a BHC at Yakima Pediatrics; the pediatricians at the clinic were not overly enthused about the idea of this new team member. Dr. Maples persisted, saying, "Let's give it some time and see how it goes." A few months later, Dr. Maples followed up with the clinic regarding the efforts, and a pediatrician stood up in the meeting and, while pointing at the BHC (MV Maxwell), proclaimed, "I will NEVER practice again without her, don't EVER take her away from us." Hearing Dr. Maples tell that story never gets old and is a nugget for both BHCs and administrators reading this chapter, in that the beginning of a PCBH program may be rocky, but one should always lean in and carry on. That same pediatrician (now PCBH enthusiast) who was initially apprehensive currently presents at our PCBH trainees' group supervision and even promotes the idea of the medical provider being the consultant to the BHC.

A few additional individuals are worth mentioning for their contributions to the initial growth of PCBH at CHCW. In 2014, CHCW invested in hiring another BHC, Michael Aquilino, to provide clinical services and faculty duties at CWFM. Additionally, Tyra Villifan, a care coordinator, earned her master's degree in social work. She then moved to a BHC role at CWFM and Yakima Pediatrics, marking only the second BHC ever to work at our pediatric clinic.

While all of the individuals mentioned played considerable roles in building and evolving the PCBH efforts at CHCW, undoubtedly, having physician leaders such as Drs. Maples, Maier, and Gould were paramount. We have a philosophy that we regularly promote in that while BHCs can and should advocate and promote their services regularly, integration often takes off when medical providers advocate for the continued expansion and inclusion of BHCs. Drs. Maples, Maier, and Gould were the earliest physician champions who truly advocated and promoted PCBH throughout the organization–further, Drs. Maier and Gould ensured residents were constantly thinking about involving BHCs; this influenced other faculty attendings to create a whole generation of family medicine physicians who were taught to include BHCs in their approach to patient care.

Undoubtedly though, the most significant ripple during this time was Kirk and Patti. Their presence ensured the establishment and fortification of PCBH logistics: 1. charting in the same medical record to BHC documentation, always including a section of "Recommendations to PCPs," 2. BHCs cannot schedule their patients, requiring the operations of the clinics to manage such processes similar to PCPs, and 3. ensuring an easy and seamless handoff process. The skeleton and context were established to make sure PCBH was successful. Further, Kirk's overall prestige and demeanor allowed BHCs to be regarded as true providers, genuine team members, and authentic parts of the system.

Kirk's most powerful impact, at least in our minds, was his continued conviction and devotion to seeing humans as reflections of their greater context. Whether working with residents, patients, or new BHCs, Kirk and Patti ensured that the ideas of functional contextualism, ACT, and fACT were at the forefront. This shift from a symptom and diagnostic focus to a functioning and humanistic focus was ahead of its time. We find great joy in reading articles about trauma-informed care (TIC), person-centered care, and reports like NASEM' Implementing High-Quality Primary

Care that discusses the importance of health care looking beyond disorders and pathologies to acknowledging the patient's context and the need to approach communities and individuals from a stance of curiosity and compassion. Kirk's and Patti's influence went beyond the overt structure of PCBH; it was the philosophy of caring for humans from a contextual lens that indelibly changed the course of PCBH at CHCW.

Not surprisingly, due to Kirk's reputation and popularity, individuals worldwide began flocking to CHCW, wanting to shadow and learn from the guru. These individuals also included two young doctoral students completing their internship in PCBH at HealthPoint Community Health Center in Seattle, WA. With the encouragement of our mentors, Jeff Reiter, and Melissa Baker, we enthusiastically accepted post-doctoral fellowships to learn and train under Kirk at CHCW in the late summer of 2014; this was our most extraordinary professional accident, as the chance to work and learn from Kirk and Patti had been our dream since we first learned about PCBH and ACT in our graduate studies. Little did we know the ensuing ripples that would extend into the coming decade.

CHCW 2014 - 2016: A BHC Metamorphosis

We almost quit our post-doctoral fellowship after the first four months at CHCW. When we arrived at the clinic, we were bright-eyed, enthusiastic, and, probably more than we like to admit, overconfident in our clinical skill set and knowledge of PCBH. As alluded to at the beginning of this chapter, we both were able to complete a primary care psychology concentration at our doctorate program, have multiple practicum rotations in medical settings, have dissertations on topics related to PCBH and ACT, and, in 2014, had just completed our predoctoral internship at HealthPoint CHC where we received robust training in all things related to PCBH.

Indeed, despite recognizing we were going to learn a lot from Kirk and being new to the role of working as a behavioral scientist within a family medicine residency, we largely felt prepared. A few months into our first year, we were left wondering if we had made the right decision to come to CHCW and questioned every aspect of our clinical abilities when working with patients; this, certainly, was related to Kirk's feedback and guidance.

We can both remember when we realized what we knew about psychology and behavioral health was far from complete; and, it was typically after Kirk shadowed us and during our supervision debriefs. Not surprisingly, this is a common experience for those trained under Kirk. As Dave likes to say, "Kirk is just a different dude. He sees things others do not and can articulate it in a way that makes it so obvious that you question how you ever didn't see it that way!" As with most novice professionals, we did not appreciate all of this at the time, and seeing things in a "different way" was one of our greatest struggles.

Throughout our training, our interpretation of PCBH was that it was more about seeing mild to moderate concerns in primary care in brief formats, maybe one to four visits, and the visits lasting a preset 30 minutes. We approached the BHC visits mainly from a medical model perspective; when in the room, you asked questions about symptoms to render a diagnosis and then implement the evidence-based algorithm. Information about the patient's family and living situation was only considered vital if it was related to the issue they were currently facing.

Dave can still remember Kirk shadowing him when he took a warm handoff for a patient with type 2 diabetes. Asking specific questions about diet and exercise, it was clear, or so Dave thought, that the poor management of the diabetes was due to the patient drinking numerous sodas throughout the day. Like a good BHC and informed by the evidence, Dave suggested the patient reduce his soda intake. Twenty or so minutes later, the patient left the room with a plan of reducing his soda intake that everyone in the room, the patient, Dave, and Kirk, knew was never going to happen.

After the debrief, Kirk asked, "Dave, do you even know this guy? Do you remember what he does for work?" Dave responded, "He drives a truck across the country," which was only known because the patient randomly offered that information. Kirk continued, "Correct, and what did he say at the end was most important for him?" Dave responded, "His family." "Exactly!" Kirk proclaimed and went on to detail that perhaps the soda intake was perceived as allowing him to successfully drive and complete long hauls across the country to provide for his family.

Kirk said, "There is always a cost; maybe his is that to provide for his family, his health may suffer. Regardless, helping him to see that connection can give him a more informed choice with his behaviors."

Bridget remembers a debriefing after working with a patient who spent most of the visit crying. She remembers thinking how "patient-centered" and compassionate she was during the visit and was ready for Kirk to praise her presence in the room. During the debriefing, Kirk says with a straight face, "So, what do you know about the patient?" After it was apparent how little she knew from that almost 45-minute visit, he remarked that we have a moral imperative to "learn about the patient's context...because how else will we help them? Regardless of tears, the 'show must go on... that's what we get paid the big bucks for." Kirk would point out early and often, "Do you know what makes that patient tick?" In the beginning, we did not know how to answer that. What is now clear that was not then - we need to *really* know the patient.

Remembering these moments brings up the same emotions for us it did almost ten years ago, as we were beginning to realize what ACT and fACT, as well as PCBH, were and could be all about. It was not about exercising techniques to get people to make the changes "we believed" they should make; instead, it was about functional contextualism, in that all behaviors serve a function and purpose in the individual's life. Rather than focus and try to intervene solely on a weed (i.e., diabetes) that was growing, Kirk instructed us to focus on the soil (i.e., the context) the weed was growing from. This was a complete and often confounding philosophical shift for us as what Kirk was asking for appeared to be more reflective of traditional mental health and not possible within PCBH, or at least what we believed PCBH was.

Asking about an individual's context sounded good, but the idea seemed unrealistic in primary care; this caused us to be unsure of how we could even approach our visits, what questions to ask, and when to follow up on specific answers. We felt a loss of confidence when approaching patients; this is akin to changing your shooting form as a basketball player (we actually both played in college). While it is needed and ultimately will produce benefits down the line, the process can be exhausting and unsettling. Everything in you wants to return to what felt comfortable versus what is best in the long run.

While Kirk educated us on the Contextual Interview (CI; Robinson et al., 2010; Bauman et al., 2018; Table 6), we did not understand how to do it in a manner that did not unnecessarily lengthen a visit nor know which questions to follow up with. As we tell our trainees and new BHCs during orientation, "we hated the CI at first." We remember telling some fellow PCBH colleagues how clunky it felt and how it took us away from the "problem" and how we were not sure how it fit within PCBH.

We laugh (or cry) at these memories now because we may be the greatest promoters of the CI in PCBH outside of Kirk and Patti, but it was a true challenge for those first few months. A challenge that has ultimately changed everything. The ripples of those first few months will be felt by every new BHC or learner who enters our system at CHCW. We will not settle for simple, indiscriminately algorithmic, clinician-centric approaches to patient care. In the words of Kirk, "Do something a handout can't do; do something that no one else on the team can deliver... that's what you get paid the big bucks for."

Table 6. Contextual Interview Domains
❖ **Love (Identify the patient's social relationships)** ➢ Living situation ➢ Relationship status ➢ Family ➢ Friends ➢ Spiritual life
❖ **Work (Identify the patient's work and financial situation)** ➢ Work ➢ Source of income
❖ **Play (Identify meaningful activities to patient)** ➢ Hobbies ➢ Fun activities
❖ Health Risk & Behaviors ➢ Caffeine use ➢ Tobacco use ➢ Alcohol use ➢ Marijuana use ➢ Street drugs use ➢ Diet/supplements ➢ Exercise ➢ Sleep

Key Take-A-Ways

We tell these stories for a few reasons. First, one of our takeaways from those early months was the importance of embracing the same things we were trying to convince patients to do, particularly willingness and psychological flexibility. The discomfort was sometimes tough to bear, and there were moments of actively avoiding Kirk, hoping we could limit the time he shadowed us. Gratefully, there was a moment where Dave decided to apply radical acceptance and throw himself into his feedback, to the point where Kirk began declining to shadow and would quip, "You can't have me in every visit."

Showing ourselves kindness and grace, as well as sharing it, was paramount. We often would talk about how difficult those moments were, give each other encouragement, and intentionally build ourselves up when not in the clinic. It is crucial to not only accept feedback and question assumptions but also establish connections with others and prioritize time for healing during off periods. Doing what we encourage our patients to do, surprise, surprise, was very much what we needed.

Second, we tell the story to highlight the importance of building a training context where challenging assumptions is acceptable. Although Kirk's feedback was occasionally direct, we understood that he genuinely cared about our success and was committed to helping us achieve it. Flexibility, challenging assumptions, and leaning in would not make sense without a context. It is important to create an environment for these actions to have meaning. As we will discuss later, creating this context to onboard and retain BHCs successfully is paramount.

Third, the story also highlights the importance of "reps" and giving BHCs time to adjust to new roles and expectations. One of the main reasons we struggled during those early months was that we could not see what Kirk saw. Moreover, a main reason for this was that we did not have the "reps" or "touches" to do so. After one debriefing with Bridget, Kirk could likely sense she was beating herself up for not "seeing it." She still remembers him telling her that he had a lifetime of these "reps" and that she had just begun. That reassurance meant the world to her and gave her the confidence to "march on."

Bridget recalls how often she tells current trainees that "time is slow" in visits but quickly follows up with the importance of reps to experiencing this phenomenon. She remembers Kirk telling her this very same thing and her thinking, "How could a visit ever feel that slow to where you can see all of that!?" Much like learning a new way to hit a golf shot, deliberate practice is paramount. However, during those initial reps and practice, BHCs will most likely struggle. Reminding new BHCs to "trust the process" and checking in regularly on how they are doing and progressing is essential.

Furthermore, it is a reminder that even if new BHCs or trainees come in with previous PCBH or other integrated care experience, as we did, going through the same reps and process is most likely needed. For BHCs to learn their role and gain a new perspective on human struggles and resilience, it is necessary to establish a context for reps and deliberate practice.

Finally, this story emphasizes the importance of promoting and pushing the boundaries of what can be achieved within PCBH. From our perspective, the philosophy of functional contextualism can greatly aid in successfully implementing PCBH. The most powerful reinforcement for PCBH is the BHC doing good clinical work. Functional contextualism, as this curious, compassionate, and contextual approach, not only produces "good clinical work" from our perspective but also grows a value of serving patients and the community.

Dave was having a recent conversation with the BHC trainees during group supervision regarding striving to see as many patients as possible; Dave's mind remarked that this value began when he truly understood functional contextualism during those initial years with Kirk. Being a BHC who strives to understand the humans we serve and building up kindness and love within our communities was a ripple of this perspective. Functional contextualism had allowed us to practice in a way we had always wanted (and, as Bridget often says, may have saved our career before it even started). Moreover, as we will discuss later, the philosophy has rippled out to how we see patients and interact with the team, clinical staff, and administrators. Indeed, context matters in everything we strive to do.

Context Matters: The Primary Care Context

As mentioned earlier, through our first two years, we became more familiar with primary care and the philosophy and goals of the system; this was an important contextual factor for our evolution. One of the main reasons integration efforts often fail within primary care is the need for BHCs to more clearly understand primary care and embrace its philosophy.

When we began at CHCW as fellows, each week, we would be assigned to shadow a family medicine resident within their clinics to give them feedback on person-centered communication (PCC). Without question, being on faculty provided us with a platform to encourage the uptake of PCBH amongst residents. We were able to imprint early and often, and since CWFM has a history of retaining its graduates, this further provided fertile ground for PCBH to proliferate.

While shadowing residents to give feedback on agenda setting, gathering and sharing information, building engagement with patients, and other skills, we also began to understand more about the context and culture of primary care. Whenever we consult or have a new BHC start at CHCW, we always recommend that the BHC spend some time with medical providers and observe them in the clinic. This exposure not only begins to show the philosophy of primary care but also begins to shape the BHCs' relational frames on how to be helpful to the medical team.

For example, when we began shadowing residents, we realized they had much to do and manage throughout the day. To this day, we still cannot fathom how PCPs manage it all. This awareness then rippled out to us, realizing that for handoffs to occur, it had to be a simple process to get to BHCs; this could not be a cumbersome process filled with multiple steps and, heaven forbid, the PCP having to search for the BHC.

The process needed to be straightforward, standardized, and easily accessible. As Bridget will often say, for any function in primary care to be successful, there cannot be more than three steps (not sure of the veracity of this claim, but we try to think this way); this also made us realize the importance of BHCs striving to get every handoff initiated, as each handoff missed would ripple out to PCPs being less and less likely to give a handoff (remember those extinction principles).

While we know this can be unpopular, we often talk to our trainees about the need to complete every handoff requested and just how improbable handoffs can be. There is a tremendous amount of error within the handoff process in the best scenarios. First, the PCP has to be aware that the patient is presenting with a concern that the BHC could help with and believe the BHC will be helpful. They then need to explain to the patient who the BHC is and get buy-in from the patient, who likely feels stigma related to behavioral health beliefs. If the patient buys into the idea, the PCP must initiate the handoff to get a hold of the BHC. Then, finally, the BHC must be available for said handoff. When you begin to break down all of the steps for a handoff to occur and be successful, there is a significant amount of room for failure. Our shadowings of PCPs brought this subtlety to light.

Realizing the importance of smooth processes and how to ensure we were making collaboration with the PCPs as easy as possible, we began to shape our behavior to create a context that promoted what we were hoping, regular engagement from PCPs and plentiful handoffs. With the help of Kirk, Patti, and Michael Aquilino, we began rounding and scrubbing PCPs' schedules before each morning and afternoon clinic. Scrubbing a PCP's schedule refers to the BHC reviewing the PCP's schedule and identifying potential patients that may benefit from a BHC visit. Not only would we discuss likely patients that could utilize "BHC" (our services have taken on a life of their own in which BHC services and providers are referred to simply as "BHC"), but this scrubbing and rounding also allowed us to do cross-training, and create opportunities for curbside consultations with PCPs.

Maybe the patient did not need a visit with the BHC but would still benefit from a handout on the Anti-Inflammatory Diet or pacing activities for persistent pain. Perhaps, instead of the BHC seeing the patient, we talked to the PCP about how to phrase a difficult conversation; this increased the PCPs' competence, comfort, and confidence in working with behaviorally influenced concerns and subtly reinforced BHCs being helpful to the entire team.

Lastly, it was a stimulus control to constantly remind PCPs what we can help with. As one would expect, most PCPs know quite well their limitations with working with mental health and substance use concerns and will, generally, be incredibly open to having BHCs help with those concerns. However, PCPs may not be as inclined and knowledgeable about how BHCs can help patients with diabetes, hypertension, headaches, sleep concerns, tobacco cessation, adherence to treatment recommendations, and other problem areas. Each rounding and scrubbing reminded the PCP, "Hey, we not only can help, but we also WANT to help - and we can surely help with a lot of things!"

These shadowings also prompted us to rethink the logistics and workflows of handoffs. While we do not have specific data on this, our memories convey that we typically had eight to nine PCPs simultaneously with two BHCs. Not a terrible ratio and one that made it very important that our schedules allowed us to get handoffs when they occurred. We needed to be easily accessible even if we were not visibly present in the respective medical pod, as there were four medical pods in the clinic and only two BHCs typically.

Eventually we developed a system of having whiteboards in shared areas that identified which BHCs were in the clinic that day. The whiteboard system was something medical assistants (MAs) were already using to help track which PCPs were on that day and which MAs were working with each PCP. Whenever a handoff was needed, the PCP could easily check the whiteboard instead of trying to remember who was available.

Additionally, we developed a system in which MAs could send a message to our cell phones with the handoff request, and we made it a requirement that BHCs had to respond with their estimated arrival time within three minutes of receiving the message. This workflow assured rapid communication with the medical team and BHCs. It made sure the BHCs working together in the clinic collaborated and strove to ensure each handoff requested was completed.

Interestingly, in some form, all of the above still exists within our current 2023 structure. BHCs are still required to huddle and scrub schedules before each clinic, whiteboards are still utilized to indicate which BHCs are on, and while we utilize Microsoft Teams instead of messages to our cell phones, we still aim to respond within three minutes. These interventions, again, were not by accident; they were a result of shadowing medical providers regularly and often, learning their system, seeing firsthand what they had to do, and understanding how to ensure BHCs were helpful to them.

Beyond shadowing residents, we began to learn more about family medicine and primary care by attending weekly faculty meetings, all-staff meetings, and casual conversations with our fellow medical attendings and staff. Quickly, our minds began to understand that we may have been looking at PCBH completely wrong, as we had typically seen it as just taking BHCs and placing them in primary care for a brief form of traditional therapy. During this immersion, we began to see how much we could learn from primary care.

Bridget often quips with BHC learners, "We always talk about what primary care can learn from BHC; let's talk about what the psychology and counseling fields can learn from medicine, especially primary care." From learning how to establish rapport rapidly and agenda set with patients to embracing the power of a continuous relationship throughout someone's life, we began to break from our traditional mental health mindset and become more versed on the copious worldwide literature on the power of primary care. We began to regularly utilize point-of-care resources, such as *UpToDate*, to help inform us of the most evidence-based interventions possible, albeit within the context of the human we were working with.

We also began attending family medicine conferences and learning about the different medical specialties. In 2015, with the support and encouragement of our residency program director, Dr. Maier, Dave applied and was awarded a scholarship through the Society of Teachers of Family Medicine and attended the American Academy of Family Physicians Congressional Conference. During this conference, we finally learned how to describe primary care's philosophy as a representative from the Robert Graham Center gave a presentation on the Four C's of primary care. While a simple, one-hour presentation, this rippled out exponentially within us as it began to give a framework for how we should be as BHCs within this primary care system.

Simultaneously, Bridget completed the Behavioral Science/ Family Systems Educator Fellowship through STFM and was mentored by Larry Mauksch, a pioneer and innovator within integrated care. Bridget learned the basics of family medicine and primary care, like Dave did while attending the Congressional Conference. These two experiences, while seemingly just routine professional activities, had profound impacts on us, truly igniting the fire within us for PCBH and, maybe for the first time in our career, we began to truly understand what the founders of PCBH meant when they intentionally placed primary care before behavioral health in the name.

In retrospect, the clarity for us that was unlocked by these key points made all the difference in our PCBH efforts. We now realize what philosophers and researchers have known for years, the key to expertise is a deep understanding of core principles and not memorizing superficial protocols and procedures.

Delving Into Leadership

One last contextual influence to discuss during this time period was our understanding of the importance of advocating for BHCs within the organization and the significant gaps in knowledge and skills we had related to leadership. At the end of 2015, the BHC team was rocking and rolling; Kirk was approaching retirement, and CHCW was at a crossroads with its integration efforts. The team that just four years ago had only three BHCs, two of whom were not CHCW employees and another part-time, had quickly grown to a team of seven BHCs.

PCPs were happy with the service, as shown by our annual PCP satisfaction survey, which we started formally tracking, and many patients were being seen; yet, uncertainty remained. As most organizations have faced with their integration efforts, CHCW was ahead of the curve at times, resulting in ambivalence about the next steps for a program that was not even an official department within the organization. The team had doubled in four years, yet there appeared to be more need than ever. Patients were requesting more access to BHCs, as were PCPs; this does not include the equally growing call for more BHC involvement in the residency and training aspects of the organization.

Many questions began to come to our minds. If CHCW did expand its efforts, could it do so via the same avenues and means it currently was doing? Or did it need the more formal structure of a department to ensure standardization and oversight? While people liked the service, the growing narrative was that BHCs needed to bring money to the organization (emphasis here on the word narrative). How could a program expand in personnel if it was a drain on finances?

Additionally, Drs. Maples and Maier began advocating for their long-held dream, bringing an APA-accredited doctoral internship to CHCW to run alongside its family medicine residency. If pursued, would there be openness from the staff, medical providers, and residents to this new program that could take away resources from the established training program? With BHCs already spread thin and working well beyond the 40-hour work week, where would the resources come from for this initiative?

Bridget remembers keenly thinking we needed a division of labor and certain BHCs to "own" certain aspects (e.g., clinical vs. educational), as it was all becoming overwhelming.

All these questions began to surface, and while there were moments of trepidation, we both knew we needed to apply the same approach we did when we started at CHCW. Armed with what Kirk had taught us, we had to advocate for ourselves, lean in, and figure it out. While we continued to focus on our clinical skills, we began to see the importance of building our knowledge regarding finances, reimbursement, billing, coding, electronic health record (EHR) template design, operations of clinics, marketing, and multiple other areas not related to the traditional role of a behavioral health clinician. We began to understand even more the importance of relationships, not only with PCPs and medical staff but administrators and departments we rarely interfaced with, such as billing, finances, IT, and our EHR support team.

When Dr. Maples decided in late 2015 to formalize two departments, a clinical PCBH department, which Bridget would oversee, and a training PCBH department, which Dave would oversee, we had no idea and still are not sure if it was the right decision and were worried it could lead to us being less integrated. On a side note, you might think it was well thought out regarding who played what role; however, it largely worked out this way because Bridget admittedly was overwhelmed with the prospect of a training program and said if Dave wanted it, he could oversee that aspect. Bridget often jokes that although she shares the credit for the training programs, it might not have happened if it was not for Dave insisting on it!

One thing was clear, we would need to apply the same effort and learning that was required to get to this point as clinical psychologists working in primary care if we had any chance of success with influencing the organization and ensuring the growth and expansion of the two newly formed PCBH departments, clinical and training. Yes, leaning in again became our mantra, and we read religiously and relentlessly to learn as much as possible about leadership.

CHCW 2016-2020: Growing Up

From formalizing departments to building EHR templates (and the umpteen iterations of these templates), to developing reports and dashboards for metrics, to officially starting our PCBH training programs, to the team growing from a team that translated to 4.3 FTE of clinical coverage in 2016 to a team that translated to 8.0 FTE of clinical coverage at the end of 2020, the evolutions and iterations were many; and occurred, what seemed like, daily. While it would be impractical to discuss all the iterations and efforts made during this incredibly dynamic five-year stretch, we feel it is important to highlight the progressions, including but not limited to clinic layouts, leadership development, recruitment and retention strategies, EHR template developments, and data reporting.

Remodels

A lot happened at CHCW in 2016; the organization had just opened its latest rural clinic in Tieton, WA, to serve a predominately Latinx, farm-working community. Additionally, CHCW's previously mentioned "mother ship" clinic, CWFM, was about to have a dramatic facelift to its clinical space. While a relatively large clinical operation, typically housing 8 - 10 medical providers at a time, CWFM was about to double its clinical space, make the clinical layout more conducive to team-based primary care (ironically, we were initially very concerned about some of the changes that ended up being huge positives such as increased proximity to MAs and nursing), and prompt more engagement from patients with aesthetic changes.

As young leaders and recently promoted directors, we look back on this transformation and are surprised at how well it went! We owe a great deal of gratitude to Dr. Maples, as he was instrumental in helping ensure BHCs would have a place to see patients and sit within shared medical spaces and pods. One of the contextual pieces we always struggled with at CWFM was the BHCs largely seeing patients in "counseling rooms" rather than exam rooms. For sure, during handoffs, there was often a chance that we could stay in the exam room after the patient had completed their visit with the PCP; however, due to exam rooms being a high commodity, we often found ourselves striving to balance staying in exam rooms and not wanting to upset MAs and nurses who were trying to "turnover" exam rooms.

BHC/Ps As Providers In Primary Care

As discussed throughout this chapter, BHCS need to see themselves more as PCPs than behavioral health providers. The question then arises, what contextual changes and factors would prompt BHCs to see themselves as more like PCPs? During this time, we frequently addressed this question and tried to be perceived more as PCPs by adapting to contextual changes. We prioritized using language and terminology aligned with the primary care system to achieve this. As we detailed in a PCBH Corner, examples of this included requiring BHCs to use a lexicon that was reflective of primary care, including using "patient" instead of "client," "treatment or intervention" instead of "therapy," "visit or encounter" instead of "session," among others.

Each year when we onboard our new BHC trainees, we inform them of these lexicon realities and let them know that if and when we hear them use language more reflective of traditional mental health, we will provide a stimulus-controlled prompt of "Lexi." If a new trainee says "client," a supervisor will respond with compassion and kindness, saying, "Lexi."

Further, we strove to make sure our processes were reflective of PCPs, and while this was ever present at CWFM due to Kirk's influence, as BHCs expanded into all of

CHCW's clinics, we made sure patients had the same check-in and check-out process for BHCs as they did with PCPs. We also ensured that contacting the BHC was the same as contacting the PCP, which resulted in nursing teams routing and triaging patients calling in to talk with BHCs, as they would for PCPs. Furthermore, we strongly advocated for BHCs to see patients in exam rooms.

We are influenced by functional contextualism and Relational Frame Theory (RFT; Barnes-Holmes et al., 2001), supported by extensive research. An easy way to describe the concepts of RFT is to do an exercise we like to call the "peanut butter and jelly metaphor." We often will use this with patients and new BHCs; the goal of the exercise is to give a glimpse of how automatic our thinking can be. We can even do this exercise now as you are reading this. To complete the exercise, we will say or type a word or a phrase, and we want you to notice what your mind automatically responds with. As we tell patients, this is not a psychological trick dating back to the psychoanalytic days of free association; rather, it is more of an exercise of the plentiful relational frames in our minds. Ready, okay, what does your mind automatically say when you read or hear:

Twinkle, twinkle, little...
Mary had a little...
Up...
Good?

We predict your mind automatically responds with star, lamb, down, and bad. Moreover, even if your mind did not respond with those words, it responded with something. Furthermore, even more interestingly, no matter how hard you worked to stop your mind from saying lamb after Mary had a little, it will say or think it; this is because we learned these combinations, and the words have a relational frame with each other.

Amazingly, this happens so regularly throughout the day that we have no idea they even occur. Moreover, it does not have to be overt language to prompt them. Walking into a doctor's office sets off a cascade of relational frames that prompts the patient to adjust and adapt to the context of a doctor's office. What causes this simple example of RFT to be paramount in the discussion of exam rooms is the reality that if we truly desire to have BHCs be providers and truly be a part of the medical team, having a room that resembles a traditional therapy room will, unintentionally, ignite relational frames of therapy, not of primary care.

While potentially subtle, it is important to have the BHCs igniting as many possible relational frames of primary care and not siloed traditional therapy; this is one of the reasons that Bridget has almost a cringy response to BHC services at CHCW being referred to as "behavioral health" instead of phrasing such as "BHC." People's relational frames with "behavioral health" generally are NOT an integrated primary care service. Across the whole system, including in writing and documents, we push for it to say either "PCBH" or "BHC" versus "BH" or "behavioral health."

A quick sidenote about this, often, when we have shadowers to CHCW, they comment that our exam rooms look "sterile." We could not agree more with this, and we often have pondered, "Why do exam rooms look the way they do? Sterile, uninviting, and, dare we say, scary at times. Does it have to be that way?" Moreover, these are all completely relevant questions and ones that should be explored not for the BHC exam rooms but for ALL exam rooms in the medical system. Luckily one of our providers donated artwork to each exam room to help improve the aesthetics. The question, to us, is not how do we make BHC exam rooms more inviting and engaging; rather, how do we make all of our clinical spaces more inviting and engaging, which is part of what initiatives such as Trauma-Informed Care are trying to accomplish.

Getting back to the story about the remodel, Dr. Maples approached us early in the process and informed us that the four medical pods would have a designated "BHC room" that would resemble a traditional office rather than an exam room. Dave can still remember Dr. Maples' face when we said, "Oh, that is great, but let's not make it an office; let's make it an exam room and just know that it is the one for the BHC." We explained that we did not want differences between where patients saw PCPs and BHCs.

Further, we told Dr. Maples that allowing the BHC exam room to be fully functional would allow us to complete reverse warm-handoffs to PCPs, where the patient, would not need to leave the room they were originally in if handed off to a PCP from a BHC. Lastly, it allowed the medical team to use the exam room if there was no assigned BHC in that medical pod that day.

Now, while many "wins" occurred this time, including the remodeled clinics being more conducive to team-based care, there were hard-fought battles and contentious conversations. We both remember Bridget's meeting where two clinic leaders asked, "Can't your BHCs just stay in the exam rooms? Do they need to be out in the medical pods?" Trying to contain her frustration, Bridget objected and advocated that BHCs must be in these medical pods, explaining the research on bumpability (Gunn et al., 2015). One of the medical leaders asked, "Well, Bridget, you have to decide which hills you are willing to die on," which, Bridget responded confidently, "this is a hill I will die on."

This previous story is just one of many that produced numerous scars for us as early leaders and directors. There were multiple days and nights when we left work feeling demoralized and asking ourselves regularly, "Are we still having this conversation?" From trying to have BHCs seen as a regular part of primary care to medical staff and providers understanding that BHCs could help with more than mental health and substance use concerns, it felt like we were constantly going against the grain and swimming upstream.

Gratefully, we had tremendous mentors, including Dr. Maier and the Chief Medical Officer at CHCW at the time, Michael Schaffrinna, MD. There were many times Drs. Maier and Schaffrinna had to provide words of wisdom and calm our frustration. We both look back with a chuckle and hold our actions and mentors' actions with grace and lightness, as many of the heated frustrations, and rumbles were directly with them!

We predict some of our frustrations and subsequent reactions were due to us being green when it came to the realm of leadership, and we also know now that this is what most, if not all, directors will go through when striving to achieve the highest level of integration possible. As we approach our tenth year at CHCW, we still regularly see how difficult it is to have BHCs recognized as "core business" within primary care.

There are several reasons why this is the case, some of which are due to the field's failure to effectively communicate its potential impact and a medical culture that has historically disregarded behavioral health and integrated care due to a rigid power dynamic. During these initial years and subsequent battles, we had to constantly remind ourselves of sayings such as the one mentioned earlier in this chapter, "If you are on the cutting edge, you will get cut," as well as other sayings, including "If you say something once, you said it once;" and "It would not hurt if it was not important." We highlight this reality for two reasons. First, for directors, leaders, and even new BHCs: be kind towards yourself.

Additionally, be intentional with celebrating wins regularly and often and finding healing outside of work (more on this later). Furthermore, be intentional in building up your skills related to leadership. As mentioned, consider the time, effort, and devotion you put into learning your clinical skills. That same time, effort, and devotion must be applied to gaining leadership skills to build a service successfully.

Leaders Are Not Born

We have many pet peeves, and one of our least favorites is the idea that "leaders are born" and the often erroneous adage, "You either have it, or you do not." Both sayings are decontextualized and create a context of leaning out rather than leaning in. As we were beginning to engage in many conversations and, at times, "battles," we began to realize that we were neither skilled nor had the abilities to advocate for our needs and support our growing team. In 2017 CHCW entered a consulting contract with the *Studer Group*, a healthcare consulting firm dedicated to developing leaders within systems and helping achieve the ever-elusive concept of employee engagement. Dave was not initially included in the group of leaders, which was difficult to deal with in those early times. Bridget was adamant and unwavering in her urging for Dave to advocate for himself, and he eventually was granted access into the group of leaders to receive the trainings.

On the other hand, Bridget was immediately immersed into the trainings, thus she was able to immerse herself in this knowledge and skills requisition. We will discuss lessons learned throughout this chapter and provide suggested readings. Recognizing limitations in skill sets and striving to address those deficits was paramount for our sanity, our department's growth, and, most importantly, our recruiting and retention efforts.

Workforce Realities

As most directors and health organizations know, there need to be more well-trained and available BHCs. Not only is there a shortage of mental health providers in general (HRSA, 2016), but potentially even more problematic is the lack of training behavioral health providers receive regarding integrated care, let alone the mission and purpose of primary care. As we have evolved in our efforts with our training programs, we have realized that the way we train mental health providers, in general, is the exact opposite of how we want our BHCs to be. We need a shift in focus towards a functional contextualist approach to clinical work.

Traditionally, mental health providers are taught that having enough time indicates treatment quality. Whether it be not being interrupted during visits or that visits should be 50 minutes long and for a specified number of visits, the traditional approach to mental health trains and sets providers up to fail in the primary care setting. Compounding these training realities, as organizations add additional BHCs, the need for BHCs grows linearly. This results in the need to be constantly recruiting, training, and retaining BHCs in health systems. It should be noted that all three (i.e., recruiting, training, and retaining) are difficult in their unique ways. When directors do not have the skill sets to manage this reality, each can prove quite damning for program development.

When we look at our current team, which now includes 20 plus BHCs (in the fall of 2024, we will have at least 16 core BHCs and five trainees), we often think, "How the hell did we get here?" The beginnings of 2016 and 2017 were fundamental in creating a foundation to expand personnel. Before discussing recruiting, training, and retaining efforts, we thought it important to discuss our experience advocating for new BHCs. In our experience, we have found that BHCs are quite adverse to understanding the realities of health care and what allows for the expansion of programs. As we will discuss in coming sections, we have a great deal of data related to PCP satisfaction with the PCBH services, as well as a treasure trove of data related to patients' love of the service; while impressive and inspiring, this data is often not collected and, even more, not what necessarily will lead to programs growing.

Advocating For BHC Expansion

During the five years from 2016 to 2020, there was persistent pushback when attempting to add more BHC positions to CHCW. We came to meetings prepared with data to show how much PCPs and patients loved the service. However, despite our efforts, the conversation usually ended with the response that they could not add a position; this was not only demoralizing for us at times, it was confusing. We were left wondering, "What are we doing wrong?"

Gratefully, we continued to apply the lean-in approach and began requesting meetings with our senior leaders in hopes of not only building relationships with them but also seeking to learn and understand the inner-workings of our health centers. As we had these meetings, we started to understand how CHCs were funded and how tight our budgets were. We began to understand that our senior leaders' resistance had little to do with them not seeing or understanding the value of PCBH; it was more that we did not see nor understand the reality of finances and just how CHCs made money.

Further, it became clear we were paying for the sins of previous years where BHCs were not even considered in metrics conversations and never held to productivity expectations. As soon as we type this out, our minds predict that readers may have negative relational frames when talking about productivity and, heaven forbid, expectations. As we will discuss when discussing retention, this is a conversation directors of programs need to embrace. While tracking productivity solely for financial means will never motivate medical providers and BHCs, we have realized that productivity and the subsequent financial realities that measurement reflects are paramount within the conversation of growth.

We both remember feeling disillusioned when we learned about this reality early on. Indeed, we had to work against our relational frames about finances. In healthcare, if being financially stable is necessary to better serve the community, we must accept this reality instead of opposing it. When we did this, we began to see that our leaders were not saying "no" to expansion because of a lack of understanding of the benefits or because they were cold-hearted capitalists who only worried about profits. The "no's" were because they were worried that adding positions that could potentially lose money and the rippling impact on the organization's financial stability.

Additionally, during this time, we began to understand that there was no clear way of measuring what BHCs were doing to the bottom line of CHCW's financial statements. Traditionally, BHCs' reimbursement and expenses were rolled into the BHC's respective clinics, which resulted in being unable to separate what BHCs brought into the organization and the total expense. After realizing the situation, we had to make a tough choice: request a separate BHC budget to better define our financials.

We knew that separating budgets runs contrary to the idea of true integration. Keeping the finances as they were or separating them had numerous pros and cons. Creating a separate budget had the obvious pro of knowing the financial realities of BHCs in the system. While it would be helpful if it showed BHCs brought in money, it could be a death sentence if it clearly showed BHCs lost money for the organization, which many believed was the case at the time. Keeping the BHC finances as part of the larger clinic budget allowed for more clinic ownership and promoted true integration; on the other hand, it would prevent anyone from taking a deep dive into what BHCs did financially, allowing arbitrary narratives to direct expansion or lack thereof.

After many conversations with leadership, we ultimately agreed that separating the BHC-related departments' budgets was the best option. While we still believe this was one of the main reasons we have been able to expand services, it also created those negative consequences, such as clinics having less invested ownership of BHC operations. Indeed, why would a clinic dedicate more support staff to helping BHCs if they do not receive any financial support?

Still, knowing our financial impact, good or bad, was monumental for our program. And it took some time to get it right. Initially, the financial reports we received were nearly impossible to decipher and appeared to include only some of the grants and funding that should be going to our departments. We had to, at times, rumble with leadership to ensure our budgets were right regarding income, especially the grants and our expenses. It took time, and starting in 2018, we began to feel better that our budgets were more a true reflection of what was happening in our departments.

We worked closely with Dr. Maples and our Chief Financial Officer (CFO) at the time, Paul Kashmitter, whom we are grateful for as he showed great patience towards two young directors asking questions about everything related to finances. At times, we were sure our questions did not make sense or were so elementary that they had to be comical. Still, our engagement with Paul rippled out to him regularly consulting and talking with us about what budget line items meant and why certain months, we got specific reimbursements and others we did not. Further, our Controller at the time and now current CFO, Desiree Ashbrooks, as well as personnel related to billing and insurance, including Lana Barnes and Julie Durston, were key to our growing understanding of not only the PCBH departments' finances but the finances of the entire organization.

Starting at the end of 2019, as we began to improve our precision and scope with our budgets, as well as welcomed new payment methods to our Medicaid and Medicare contracts, we started to see that BHCs not only did not lose money, our two PCBH departments were significantly in the black. Moreover, while grants helped support the program, we learned how to sell leadership on the idea of expanding positions even without including any grant or other funding sources. Grants can go away at any time and we wanted to make sure our expansion was secure if they ever did.

In 2019, we saw that goal become a reality. We felt the shift in our fight to expand positions, culminating in an annual senior leadership meeting about the state of the PCBH department. During prior meetings we would have many rumblings about expanding the department. At that specific meeting, we readied ourselves to fight to add a position to the team. At the end of the meeting, senior leadership did not agree with us; they felt that two BHC positions should be added, not just one.

Recruiting A Workforce

With the narrative changing about BHCs losing money for the organization, we were simultaneously focusing on recruiting, training, and retaining BHCs. These efforts began with us working with our provider recruiter, Julie Finley, who is currently our Chief Experience Officer, and educating her on just what we were looking for in a BHC. We knew early on that we would have to face the reality that any new BHC, even if having previous experience as we both did, would take significant onboarding and constant support to be a successful BHC in our system. Thus we began to realize that instead of recruiting solely people with previous experience, we needed to recruit people with meaningful values that would align with what we were hoping to do with PCBH.

To us, values such as serving a community, wanting to reach people not otherwise reached, and working collaboratively on a team were paramount. Further, individuals who were flexible and were okay with being interrupted, as well as stepping outside of their comfort zone, was whom we began to look to hire. Lastly, we coveted individuals from systems and functional contextualist perspectives who held lightly to traditional ways of seeing patients. Working with Julie during our early years was crucial. We communicated our desired provider, and she assisted us in refining our message and dedicated herself to recruiting our BHCs with the same level of effort as she did for medical providers.

From 2016 to 2018, we recruited and hired five BHCs. Our original PCBH crew, including Michael Aquilino, Tyra Villafan, and Kirk all moved on to different chapters in their careers as well as Regan Eberhart, who fulfilled our community contract position. The only BHC who remained from that original crew other than us was our part-time BHC. Those early departures were completely understandable and not personal from our perspective, and at the same time, handling this turnover could not help but feel like a gut punch. It was a disorienting time where we often felt panicked about how we were going to make this work.

In hindsight, Bridget realizes she could have prevented some hardship with more fully developed leadership skills. One of the BHC positions that CHCW had came with strings attached as a contract position. Although both organizations were trying to do the right thing, contracted positions between two organizations involved additional difficulties. We greatly advise against hiring contract positions, especially when there is an expectation of sharing duties between organizations when trying to establish PCBH. There are so many nuances necessary for PCBH to work, as we have detailed already, and adding in other layers of double duties, supervisors, and organizational norms, makes things unsustainable.

Bridget feels that if she had known then what she knows now, she would have been able to advocate to move away from this approach. The contract position eventually was dissolved after the employee moved on from that position, and all hires henceforth were directly CHCW employees. Luckily, so many "wins" during this period provided hope that we could grow the program.

Our first hire came in the late spring of 2016. Sarah Ortner, a licensed marriage and family therapist, had never worked as a BHC. While we were apprehensive, particularly Dave, Julie assured us this was someone we wanted to interview. After the interview, where Sarah completely nailed our interview task of looking at a provider's schedule and identifying patients we could potentially see, it was obvious Sarah was one of us. Eight years later, she still is and was not only pivotal to our growth as a program but a reminder to us of just what we were looking for in a BHC. Soon after Sarah, we recruited psychologist Dr. Arissa Walberg, a contact through a colleague, to join the team in September of 2017.

She was followed by another psychologist and former doctorate school classmate of ours who reached out after seeing Bridget's CHCW BHC open position posting on her Facebook. Dr. Ruth Olmer and her husband, Dr. Steven Olmer (more on Dr. S. Olmer later), moved to Yakima, and she joined the team in February 2017. We also procured and hired a local mental health counselor, Michelle Austin.

All three of them brought incredible experience to the team as Dr. Walberg had significant training in PCBH through her internship and fellowship, Dr. Olmer was additionally licensed as a marriage and therapist and had extensive knowledge of systems and how to work flexibly within a variety of settings, and Michelle was a guru with working with a pediatric population with specialized training in CBT, resulting in all BHCs becoming more confident, competent, and comfortable working with pediatrics. We hired another core BHC, Tasha Hansen, a licensed clinical social worker who had worked previously in an FQHC primary care setting in 2018. The core clinical team was composed of individuals with varying backgrounds. Some had experience in integrated care, while others had not worked in a primary care office before. The team included members with extensive training in systems and functional contextualists and those who identified more with traditional CBT and were strict behaviorists. Regardless, we all had a mission and values that aligned our behaviors with the goals of PCBH.

Making The PCBH Training Programs A Reality

With the additions of Drs. Walberg and Olmer, we unlocked a final piece of the puzzle towards completing Drs. Maple's and Maier's dream of bringing a formal, APA-accredited doctoral psychology internship to CHCW. It also gave life to the idea of "growing our own" PCBH service. Before their arrival, we had taken numerous meetings with programs across the state regarding developing such a training program. The process appeared somewhat impossible for us as a small-to-moderate-sized CHC.

During one meeting with a director of a newly accredited program in a CHC, the director asked, "Wait, have you started this process yet?" When we responded that we were just in the exploration stage, she said, "Don't do it!" It is daunting for anyone who has gone through the development of an APA-accredited internship. It requires much administrative support and oversight to get it off the ground.

The entire process can be overwhelming. From the APA self-study to developing formal processes such as evaluation forms and time-tracking to developing schedules and didactic training. This director explained that developing these aspects could take as much as a .8 full-time equivalent (FTE), essentially removing an entire BHC from our mix. Moreover, at organizations such as CHCW, where the primary mission is direct patient service delivery, it is difficult to support the start-up and subsequent continued costs. At the beginning of exploring the possibilities of bringing an internship to CHCW, it appeared dead on arrival.

During our writings (including earlier in this chapter), consulting, and speaking gigs, we often joke, "90 percent of what we say comes from Kirk." His wisdom not only transformed our clinical skill set and knowledge but also fortified us when faced with situations that appeared daunting and "dead on arrival." We can remember talking to Kirk about consulting efforts and what to do when faced with situations where you were unsure of the answer or if you were not an expert in an area that someone was asking about; his response was once again, "... that is why you get paid the big bucks. Say 'yes' and figure it out." While we are still waiting for those "big bucks," his words inspired us not to accept the premise that we, as a CHC, could not bring a formal training program to CHCW.

As we explored our options, our minds kept returning to the main sticking point, the overall administrative support and cost required to complete such a program. Perhaps with too much confidence, we felt we would be able to organize a training program that provided robust PCBH experience. Furthermore, with the residency approaching its third decade of existence, we knew that we would be borrowing ideas and structure from an already established program. As we wrestled with the administrative support reality, we gratefully felt a cascading ripple that occurred a few years before we ever heard of CHCW!

During our doctorate work at Forest Institute, we took courses from and eventually became Teacher's Assistants (TAs) for one of our professors, Adam Andreassen, PsyD (we also knew each other from fierce pickup basketball games at the local community center, but we digress). Dr. Andreassen wore many hats for our graduate school, one of which was overseeing an internship consortium that included several traditional internship sites throughout the state of Missouri. The consortium, called Heart of America Psychology Training Consortium at the time, provided numerous training spots for future psychologists to complete their internships. The consortium received APA accreditation in 2014 and started a second region in Indiana, officially changing its name to the National Psychology Training Consortium (NPTC).

NPTC's focus was to partner with community-based agencies, many of which were community mental health centers (CMHCs), and provide the logistical and administrative support to alleviate the burden accreditation and subsequent requirements create. The consortium also focused on providing care in rural settings and underserved communities, and, as fate would have it, they were beginning to be interested in training future psychologists to work in integrated primary care.

We both recall Dr. Andreassen asking us to go to dinner before we left Forest Institute for our doctoral internships. We remember him knowing how passionate we were about integrated care and him saying something along the lines of not knowing if or when our paths might meet again. This meeting set the stage for us to reach out to Dr. Andreassen.

When we first reached out to Dr. Andreassen, we were solely looking for advice and guidance on how to start an internship. During the initial conversation, Dr. Andreassen proposed starting a separate NPTC region in the pacific northwest. At that moment, we finally saw a solution to the logistic and administrative burden preventing us from seriously considering a training program at CHCW. We knew we needed to get Dr. Andreassen in the room with Dr. Maples. As predicted, once these two innovators met and discussed the idea of partnering, agreements were signed, and timelines were set to welcome the first cohort of interns for the 2017- 2018 academic year. Dave can still remember meeting with Drs. Maples and Maier during a cold February day when the residency held its winter retreat. The meeting occurred in a rented ski lodge and ended with Drs. Maples and Maier said, "We got ourselves another training program."

While there is much more we can say about this time and the development of the training program, we hope to highlight a few areas. First, it highlights the importance of collaborations and partnerships with community members and individuals. Not only did starting an internship produce a collaboration with NPTC, an organization hundreds of miles away in Springfield, MO, but it also prompted us to look for community partners that may be interested in starting a similar training program. During the initial phase of searching out partners in the region, two fellow Washington state CHCs agreed to join us in the journey. HealthPoint CHC, where we both completed our predoctoral internships, recognized the unfortunate burden and reality of doing an independent training program and saw this collaboration as a way to keep and evolve their training program.

Further, Yakima Neighborhood Health Services (YNHS), a CHC in the Yakima Valley, also expressed interest in growing its integrated behavioral health efforts and agreed to serve as a rotation experience for interns at CHCW from 2016 until 2020. Dr. Steven Olmer led this rotation at YNHS for the interns during this time. Six years later, Yakima Valley Farm Workers, a large CHC throughout the states of Washington and Oregon, also came on board and welcomed its first internship cohort in 2022. Without question, none of these internship programs would exist in their current forms if not for the partnerships with each other and NPTC.

Additionally, while part of starting an internship was undoubtedly to train future psychologists to spread the word about PCBH and create radical ripples throughout the country, we also saw a training program doing the same thing for CHCW and Yakima that the medical residency had shown to do for close to thirty years. Research related to Teaching Health Centers (i.e., residencies designed to operate in community-based agencies, often in rural areas; Davis et al., 2022) has shown that trainees often stay at the organization or, at the very least, in relative proximity to where they train.

Drs. Maples and Maier knew this reality well, as many of the CHCW's family medicine resident graduates stayed at CHCW and filled many medical positions within the Yakima Valley. Dr. Andreassen also knew this reality and discussed it regularly when discussing NPTC's impact within the communities that house the internships.

He often quips, "Bringing interns to your organization is often like a rom-com movie of an individual moving from the big city to a rural community. They struggle and despise it at first, and then, by the end of the movie, they have fallen in love and now call the rural community home." This vision of a training program meshed well with our vision for PCBH at CHCW, at which time we saw an opportunity for rapid growth and expansion. We knew there was a dearth of well-trained BHCs, particularly in rural Washington. We saw this training collaboration as a way to bring people to the communities we hoped to serve and teach them as much as possible regarding PCBH.

PCBH Standardization

As we focused on developing and standardizing our training efforts for our interns and fellows, we also began to structure and standardize onboarding processes for new core BHCs. As we conveyed earlier, one unfortunate reality is that traditional training of mental health providers does not necessarily translate to the primary care setting.

Throughout many experiences, conversations with colleagues, and consulting work, we have come to believe that for BHCs to be successful in implementing the goals and mission of PCBH, directors and onboarding practices should truly mirror a yearlong fellowship program, with an intensive onboarding, yearlong shadowing, and consistent training and upskilling in specific domains. The main reason that integrated care has difficulty being established by a system often has less to do about the system and more to do about the lack of training the BHC had to be successful. As with most places in healthcare, it is a constant battle to have enough time and rest to figure out ways of working smarter and not necessarily harder. Although we have made progress, much work must be done to provide new BHCs with the necessary context to understand and effectively become a part of the PCBH mission and system.

While it has taken years to evolve, our current onboarding process for core BHCs (as well as our trainees) is intensive and extensive. Before we get into more specifics regarding general onboarding for any BHC in our system, it is important to note that the trainees in our system have plentiful additional support via individual supervision, group supervision, precepting, and formal didactics. They have peer support given that they onboard and train with a PCBH and medical resident cohort. The many core values and principles, as well as the strategies discussed in this section and many other initiatives, are also implemented with the PCBH trainees. In Bridget's opinion, there is almost no group of people at CHCW who have more support than the PCBH trainees. For ease of communication, we will describe approaches to onboarding that extend to both our core BHCs and our trainees, with some of the experiences being more geared toward cores and some for trainees.

Our core BHCs are provided an intensive six to eight weeks of onboarding, followed by a continued reduced schedule and productivity requirements. We cannot overstate this point enough; we do not expect full productivity of a new BHC until they have been in our system for one year.

This reality may be difficult at times for administrators to understand and accept. For new PCPs, the generalizability of roles from clinic to clinic is relatively high. If a PCP switches from one organization to another, training would be needed to adjust to clinic workflows and a new EHR system; however, the clinical responsibilities, including presenting concerns, prescriptions and interventions used, and visit content, would remain the same. For BHCs, not only do they need training and time to adjust to new workflows and a new EHR, but clinical work may also look vastly different from previous training and positions. Once established, habits are difficult to change, given that PCBH constantly swims against the current, resulting in a high likelihood of old behaviors returning if not intentionally prevented.

Onboarding materials. During the initial onboarding of BHCs and in the training programs, reading lists and training are provided to help increase their knowledge base. Materials on the Four Cs of primary care, Implementing High-Quality Primary Care, and contextualism and Focused Acceptance and Commitment Therapy (fACT; Strosahl et al., 2012) to name a few, new BHCs are inundated not only with the philosophy of primary care and PCBH but also the philosophy of care we are hoping to promote within our healthcare system. Additionally, we provide several YouTube playlists, including Dr. Beachy's BHC Onboarding Intro and other recorded webinars.

These videos offer examples of BHC introductions, visits, interventions, podcast-like discussions regarding core components of the work, and frequently asked questions about PCBH. While BHCs progress through these assigned readings and videos, they will begin to shadow core BHCs (all BHCs at all sites are included to help distribute the workload and has the simultaneous benefit of exposure to many different styles, skill sets, and clinics) at the CHCW clinics.

Initially, new BHCs are a "fly on the wall," solely observing and then debriefing with the paired BHCs after visits. A helpful feature of Microsoft Teams is doing a screen share so the new BHC can follow along with how the core BHC is managing the EHR and responding to WHOs. After a few days of shadowing, new BHCs will begin to practice concordant charting while the core BHC completes the visit. As the BHC increases their confidence in concordant charting, they will begin to complete visits with patients while the core BHC completes concordant charting. After a few weeks, the new BHC will complete both the visit and concordant charting with patients, allowing the core BHC to observe, shadow, and provide feedback and support after and during visits. This scaffolding approach helps the new BHCs feel confident in their growing abilities. Once comfortable, they will operate as independent BHCs; however, the number of scheduled visits is limited and increase as the BHCs' confidence improves.

Intentional meetings with PCBH leadership. During this process, the core BHC meets regularly and often with Bridget, including but not limited to reviewing 360 peer feedback from the team at the 90-day mark and continuing to answer questions and address any concerns. Further, during these meetings, Bridget also assesses knowledge of specific concepts, such as the GATHER philosophy of PCBH and the Four Cs of primary care. She begins to discuss further aspects related to productivity and other job-related expectations.

While these expectations are detailed in proceeding sections, Bridget strives to imprint the culture and values of the department during these meetings, constantly discussing expectations as reflections of the organization's and department's infinite values. Bridget also intentionally begins to develop a personal and human relationship with the new BHC, allowing discussions of PCBH and conversations about family, personal values, and the BHC's own journey to get to this point in life. More about the purpose and pursuit of these efforts are discussed in the Contextual Leadership section below.

Ensuring Competencies

Bridget meets monthly with new BHCs to complete monthly rounding, more on this later, and check in on how the BHC believes they are progressing and provide constructive and reinforcing feedback from the team. Bridget also strives to shadow the BHC when possible. While we are working on making this process more standardized and structured, when shadowed, BHCs are evaluated based on a combination of Core Competency tools developed by Robinson and Reiter (2016) and the CHCW BHCs' innovations. Additionally and during this year of onboarding, we strive to focus on ensuring operational and clinical competencies.

Operational competencies. Operational competence would include being able to concordant chart when completing a handoff, responding to all handoff requests via teams within three minutes of the requests, developing comfort in running late to a scheduled visit to ensure a handoff occurs when requested, understanding how to effectively communicate with PCPs and other team members, amongst others. Clinical competencies would include a sound introduction, organization of initial and follow-up visits, delivery of context-dependent interventions and goals, ensuring after-visit summaries are completed, determination of needed follow-up visits, and time management within visits, amongst others.

Clinical competencies. Clinical competencies are a high priority as we know the best way to help a BHC succeed is to ensure they can do good clinical work. None of this works if BHCs cannot be helpful to providers or patients.

Clinical Competencies: Introductions

Starting with the introduction, we are intentional about making sure new BHCs not only have their introduction memorized and include core components but understand the why behind having an intentional introduction. One of our favorite humans is well-known Single Session Therapy guru Robert Rosenbaum, Ph.D. Bob regularly talks about the importance of noticing and utilizing moments, free of time, to create a human connection and change potentiality. From a well-timed pause to an intentional curious question regarding internal moments or a shift in body language, Bob regularly talks about how to utilize every moment as one that connects us to another human being.

Introductions are infinite moments that, when done intentionally, can create a context of confidence, love, and compassion. We train our BHCs to follow AIDET principles (Braverman et al., 2015), which include Acknowledging all individuals in the room, Introducing ourselves and our role at the clinic, Duration of the interaction, Explanation of what will occur during the interaction, and a Thank-you at the end of the interaction. Several videos in the onboarding playlist provided earlier give examples of such introductions.

BHCs onboarding in our system review these videos and write out their introduction with the hopes of internalizing it as soon as possible. During their initial weeks of onboarding, trainees are prompted regularly and spontaneously by the BHC team to say their introduction and given feedback. By the time they move to be solo, they have done their introduction many times, resulting in moments of confidence, love, and compassion when introducing themselves to patients.

Clinical Competencies: Functional Contextualism

We strive to ensure new BHCs gain confidence and comfort within the philosophy of functional contextualism; this does not necessarily mean we require all BHCs to come from an Acceptance and Commitment Therapy (ACT; Hayes et al., 2011) or fACT approach. Regardless of their primary theoretical orientation or approach, whether traditional cognitive behavioral therapy (CBT), Solution Focused Brief Therapy (SFBT), family systems, etc., we try to ensure all of these approaches and interventions come from a place of curiosity, humility, and contextualism.

Clinical competencies: The CI

We require all BHCs to complete the CI with each new patient to accomplish this. As discussed earlier, we discuss regularly and often with new BHCs to approach the CI as a procedure. Like a new physician learning a suture technique, the BHCs ask about the patient's living situation, their relationships, and so on. We also discuss early on the importance of allowing the CI and subsequent questions to be an intervention in and of itself. The CI is also a stimulus control for the BHC to prompt them to remain curious about the patient's context.

As we found for ourselves, we are adamant that BHCs get reps doing the CI in the same order and in the same way. We do this to ensure the delivery of the CI becomes natural, purposeful, and intentional. On a side note, we provide all medical residents training on the CI and any interested medical provider in our system.

Clinical Competencies: Mental Representations

Further, we encourage the BHCs to apply deliberate practice with the CI, completing the CI in the same sequence and manner with patients, in role-plays, and with colleagues. By engaging in such deliberate practice, we hope BHCs will begin developing mental representations to help them see the human before them.
As discussed in the phenomenal book Peak (Ericsson & Pool, 2016), these mental representations enable our work in PCBH. In early 2022, Bridget developed a mental representation mnemonic that can be activated when utilizing the CI, specifically, the mental representations of Adverse Childhood Experiences (ACEs; Felitti et al., 1998), Culture Implications, Context (internal; Strosahl et al., 2012), External context (Strosahl et al., 2012), Social Determinants of Health (SDoH: Plamondon et al., 2020, Stages of Change (Miller & Rollnick, 2002; 2013), and Values (Hayes et al., 2011).

This ACCESS-V mental representation allows the CI to be a true intervention in and of itself and uncover many contextual variables that impact human development and behavior. A video on this approach can be found here.

Other mental representations include Kirk and Patti's CARE approach, which includes contextualizing the concern, identifying the avoidance, reframing the problem, and experimenting with a new behavior by expanding their behavioral repertoire. These mental representations allow the CI to become more than just a set of questions and allow the BHC to begin filtering evidence-based interventions through these mental representations. This filtering ensures that any intervention the BHC provides is contextualized and relevant to the patient's context.

Further, via the CI, these mental representations allow common concerns seen in primary care with great complexity to have more parsimony and clarity. Simultaneously, while providing parsimony, it also discourages the BHC from approaching concerns from a decontextualized perspective. For example, the CI and subsequent mental representations may allow the BHC to view a patient with type 2 diabetes as a function of a context that includes ACEs, cultural relevance, an internal context that includes a critical mind, external factors such as lack of social support, SDoH such as lack of healthy food access, the individual being in the contemplative stage of change, and one who holds values of family.

Due to these contextual factors, simply suggesting to the individual to begin the evidenced-based algorithm of diet and exercise to help with lowering the individual's A1C would not make much sense. Instead, the BHC, with the help of the CI igniting the mental representations of ACCESS-V, may work with the individual to build up social support, frame any health behavior improvements as reflections of their values of family, or work with the individual to build up more kindness and compassion, all of which increase the probability of better A1C control.

For new BHCs to be successful, PCBH programs must intentionally train them in ways that prompt parsimony while also not decontextualizing and overly simplifying concerns. The functional contextualism approach, the CI, and the mental representations discussed allow this hope to be realized. To assist with this potentially large shift in philosophy, we have our BHC trainees complete a Relational Frame Theory course that details functional contextualism and the implications of this approach. Further, we have our new BHCs progress through many of our PCBH Corners.

Moreover, during meetings, shadowing opportunities, and case consultations, the concepts promoted here are regularly discussed and reinforced, creating a context where the ideas of functional contextualism radiate through the program.

Other Growth Factors

As our recruitment and onboarding efforts began to reap benefits and our team expanded exponentially during this time, other developments aided the department's growth.

One of these developments happened in late 2016: a Centers for Medicare/Medicare Services (CMS) audit. While discussing the ins and outs of the audit is not necessary for this chapter, a few takeaways occurred during this stressful period. First, the mantra and theme of "lean in" was ever present during this time. While scary and worrisome, as there were definite moments where we were concerned that the results of the audit could be catastrophic and potentially program ending, it was one of the best accidents that ever occurred for our program.

For the first time in the program's history, we were able to sit down with personnel from CMS and ask them questions regarding requirements for billing and documentation for PCBH. To our surprise, much of what we had heard from colleagues and presentations did not match what the auditors were informing us, and, ironically, the proposed changes caused our documentation process to be more straightforward; this also produced an opportunity for us to collaborate and grow close to our billing, coding, and EHR personnel.

As we attended meetings with our billing and coding personnel, we learned more about their roles, and they learned more about ours. We not only got to ask each other questions related to each other's work, but we also got to know about each other's families and lives, resulting in a bond that transcended beyond figuring out how to make it through the CMS audit.

Additionally, once we had a clear direction of what was needed for documentation to receive reimbursement, sometimes down to the literal words that were required, we were able to quickly meet with our EHR personnel to build templates, check-boxes, and "dot" phrases to ensure all billing requirements were included in the documentation, as well as creating a context for BHCs to efficiently complete concordant charting.

Lastly, this allowed us to recognize how our contextual approach blended well with billing guidelines and requirements. Not only did we see parsimony within these two often competing realities (i.e., billing requirements and contextualism), we could structure our templates to utilize stimulus controls and prompts to remind BHCs of our contextual philosophy and the importance of staying open and curious when working with patients.

Data Reporting And Connection To Infinite Values

Until this time, we largely relied on hand counting to show data related to productivity and other metrics of importance, such as handoffs. As we began to reformat our templates based on feedback from CMS and to ensure reimbursement, we also began implementing discrete fields that were mineable and subsequently report-producing. Dave can still remember the glorious moment of being shown the first initial dashboard regarding BHC metrics, which included yearly and monthly breakdowns of each BHC for total visits, handoffs, and initial visits, amongst others.

This data reporting also coincided with us continuing to read as much as possible about leadership and stumbling on a transformative book by Simon Sinek, The Infinite Game (Sinek, 2019). This book began to change our relational frames with data and showed us how to use data to tell incredible, value-congruent stories of PCBH. As we both read this book, we reflected on just what were CHCW's and our PCBH programs' infinite values.

For us, the most basic infinite values that we hoped guided our BHCs were serving our community, reaching populations otherwise left out of health care, and providing contextual, compassionate, and team-based healthcare at the moment when it was needed. As we formed and articulated these infinite values, we also began identifying metrics that could reflect if we were moving closer to those values. For example, visits per day could be a great reflection of us being able to determine if we were reaching and serving our communities. Handoffs per day could be a way of determining if we were providing care when it was requested.

Moreover, patient engagement could determine if compassionate and contextual care was being rendered. As we learned and Sinek's book detailed, no matter how reflective, the metric would never again become our goal. Rather, it was paramount that the metric always be placed in the context of the overarching infinite value and purely used as a reflection point rather than a goal.

KISS

As these infinite values became more defined and our data tracking more refined, we applied a philosophy Bridget's father taught us from his days as a Home Depot district manager: keeping data and metrics simple and to a few key indicators. Specifically, the keep it simple, silly [original version was "stupid"] (KISS) method became our standard for tracking and reporting data, focusing on six primary areas 1) visits per day, 2) handoffs per day, 3) patient engagement, 4) PCP satisfaction with the PCBH program, 5) BHCs' penetration rate within respective clinics, and 6) employee engagement. Table 7 provides an overview of our data from 2018 to the present day within these six domains, and we will discuss in the proceeding sections how we rallied the team around these metrics and shared them regularly with our senior leadership team.

Table 7. Metrics that Reflects CHCW's PCBH's Infinite Values

	Visits/ day*	WHOs/ day**	Penetration ***	Pt Eng.#	PCP Sats.^	BHC EE^*
2018	8.4	3.0	20.0	89.5	4.8	N/A
2019	8.4	3.0	21.5	89.7	4.8	89.4
2020	8.8	2.2	20.6	93.5	4.8	90.2
2021	8.6	2.6	21.2	94.7	4.9	88.3
2022	8.4	2.8	23.5	N/A	4.8	95.0

* Visits per day per BHC; visit defined as a meaningful visit encounter that includes a gathering of context and a delivered intervention; rendering ~95% of visits to meet billing requirements
** Warm-handoffs per day per BHC; WHO follow the same criteria as visits above and occur the same-day that was requested by the primary care team
*** The percent of patients that had a medical visit in the past 12-months that also had a BHC visit; visits follow the same criteria as visits above
# Patient engagement measured by quarterly scores out of a composite of 100. Score is an combination of patient perception for Provider Listening, Provider Time Spent, Provider Explanation of Care, Provider Knowledge of Health History
^ PCP satisfaction measured by annual survey and out of a 5-point Likert-type scale. Specific question is "Overall, rate how satisfied you are with the PCBH service."
^* BHC employee engagement measured by CHCW's annual employee engagement and out of a composite score of 100. PCBH departments have had the highest employee engagement out of any CHCW department since the survey was implemented in 2019.

By the end of 2019, the BHC team had grown to 14 BHCs and expanded to all of CHCW's primary care clinics, including providing services at a new school-based health center at a Yakima high school. In 2016, the BHCs saw 4,143 visits, completed 1,458 handoffs, and provided services to 3,436 unique patients, resulting in a total BHC penetration rate within the CHCW clinics of 13.5%. In 2019 the BHCs saw a total of 10,513 visits, 4,222 handoffs, 5,232 unique patients, with a CHCW-wide BHC penetration rate of 22%, meaning one out of every five patients that saw a medical provider in 2019 also saw a BHC.

Patient engagement scores soared, and PCP satisfaction surveys produced not only quantitative responses from highly satisfied PCPs but also qualitative responses such as, *"In the future, I will never practice without a BHC partner on* the team" and "*I have come to believe this brings more value to the care I can offer patients than any other service in our clinic.*"

Furthermore, beginning in 2019, more changes were on the way! After the start-up years, which often involved working ungodly hours, we finally received administrative support due to a BHC expansion grant; this resulted in us hiring a BHC coordinator position to support all things related to PCBH programmatic growth.

There were also new challenges, as many of the senior leaders who had been our champions began to retire. From 2019 to early 2022, almost every senior leadership team member turned over, including organizational pillars, Drs. Maples, Maier, Schaffrinna, and CFO Paul Kaschmitter. These departures prompted a new challenge, namely selling the idea of PCBH to a new group of senior leaders. Little did we know that a devastating global pandemic and unsettling social unrest would, ironically, aid us in this process.

CHCW 2020: Beyond A Context Realized

We can still remember our excitement at the start of 2020. In January, we returned from a healing trip to the east coast to visit family, and the team began the months of January and February by posting records of total visits and handoffs. Dave can recall the energy from the team and the enthusiasm that permeated the PCBH team and the entire organization. As we welcomed our new CEO, Angela Gonzalez, meetings were occurring where BHCs were genuinely seen as primary medical team members who provided core business.

During one of CHCW's quarterly leadership summits, where all leaders within the organization met to discuss various activities and initiatives, leaders were voting on programs that should be considered for expansion or implementation. Expanding the PCBH services was discussed, and while receiving universal support, Angela paused and questioned, "Do we really need to vote on this one?" While our hearts began to sink, Angela went on to clarify, "Should we not approach this like we do expanding PCPs? Meaning, if we expand a clinic or a service line, just like it is standard to add PCPs, MAs, nurses, should we not just also add BHCs?" Remembering this moment prompts much emotion, as we both remember thinking, "We finally made it; we are finally seen as primary care."

COVID Times

Little did we know the world we knew would change drastically in just a few short weeks due to the COVID-19 pandemic. At times, it is still difficult to remember all that transpired during those early months of the pandemic, as workflows changed daily, new concerns were constant, and keeping our heads above water was challenging. During our evening walks, a COVID-era staple due to pandemic-related restrictions, we often talked about BHCs' role during this time. We regularly heard from our colleagues around the country about BHCs beginning to be furloughed or sent home to complete virtual work. Both options did not appeal to or feel right to us, the latter only making sense if that was what medical providers were asked to do. Dave remembers Bridget being steadfast and unapologetic with her approach during the early stages of the pandemic that rippled out for the pandemic's entirety; quite simply, her approach was, "BHCs are primary care, we do as primary care does." If PCPs were in the clinic seeing patients, so were BHCs. If PCPs were completing virtual and telephone visits, so were BHCs. If PCPs were striving to serve their community, so were BHCs.

In addition to Bridget's fierce leadership and determination to ensure the status of BHCs, something we had been working towards for five years, our leadership welcomed this call to action. Dr. Schaffrinna, who was a little over a year away from retiring, was adamant about supporting our efforts and joked with us later into the pandemic, "Could you imagine if I even tried to tell the BHCs to go home?" Further, the BHC team followed Bridget's lead and never questioned their purpose or place within the primary care team. Not only did the BHCs lead the charge to say, "We MUST reach our patients," but they also provided monthly, weekly, and sometimes daily support for staff struggling with the reality of the world. Often during organization-wide calls, a BHC would be asked to provide perspective and complete grounding activities to help create a calming context in these turbulent times.

Covid Times: PCBH Stories. During the pandemic, Dave became more intentional in writing Stories of PCBH, our blog (https://www.beachybauman.com/blog). The pandemic provided an opportunity to showcase the healing, restorative, and grounding power of love, connection, and storytelling. By intentionally producing genuine reflections, particularly about the team's and patients' successes, the PCBH team created a calming presence that helped alleviate fear, uncertainty, and worry.

This approach resulted in a more flexible way of dealing with the pandemic, as we shared wins and moments of gratitude with the PCBH team and clinic leadership. Despite the exhaustion and constant worry about the community and family members, the team's reflections, storytelling, and sharing of kudos provided a mild balm to the events around us. Although we never asked the leadership team directly, we received emails and spoken words of gratitude from them, particularly when we shared patient care wins. Leaders often remarked that the stories fortified their resiliency, especially since they were removed from the clinical space.

Covid Times: JEDI. This time also included the murders of unarmed black members of communities and greater awareness of the ongoing effects of centuries of discrimination and racism in the United States (and healthcare, too, was forced to address its role in institutional racism and discrimination). Again, the BHCs within CHCW helped craft messaging, sat on committees, and often led difficult, yet, needed conversations within our health system. Although a value held by the team, our health center had not been as clear on its stance and involvement in an active anti-racist approach. BHCs regularly held space for difficult conversations with staff members who were curious about the increase in discussion of terms such as institutional and structural racism and unsure why CHCW was talking so actively about them.

Furthermore, this involvement was primarily led less by us (the authors) and more by the PCBH team. Our team consistently supported and educated us as we grappled with our biases and uncertainties. Again, similar to the BHC response to COVID, BHCs responded in a way that showed their value to the organization and healthcare beyond direct patient care.

Covid Times: BHCs Growing Like Weeds. As expected, visits plummeted during the initial days of March 2020, and we were left wondering if we would ever return to the patient volume we had in 2019. We wanted to continue to help our community members and show up for them, which is what we did. Not only did the volume return, but BHCs hit record numbers in total visits in 2020, with 12,003 total visits completed. While handoffs decreased in 2020, over 3,500 handoffs were completed, and BHCs still saw 20% of the population served by the medical team during the year. In the following years of the pandemic, BHCs continued to set records each year for the number of visits, with 12,079 in 2021, 13,488 in 2022, and a staggering 14,880 in 2023.

Further, handoffs rose to over 4,000 yearly and we continued to set records each consecutive year. In 2022 we completed 4,782 handoffs and in 2023 we eclipsed that record as we completed a whopping 5,520 handoffs. And, moreover, by the end of 2022, the team broke records for unique patients served for a year and achieved a penetration rate of 24%. Due to a change in our EHR we do not have the final numbers for 2023's penetration rate, but it will eclipse the 24% record! Each month, we sent emails to the PCBH and leadership teams acknowledging the records and their underlying meaning- the realization of our infinite values, namely providing compassionate, contextual, and team-based care to a large majority of our communities that are often left out of the healthcare conversation many of whom were devastated by the impact of a global pandemic.

The BHC team grew again in 2022 with 17 total BHCs, four of whom were alumnae of our PCBH training programs. As the team grew, our focus remained on recruitment with a focus on retention and implementing leadership strategies that we have begun to refer to as Contextual Leadership.

Our View Of Contextual Leadership

Functional contextualism is a healing, grounding, and unique philosophy for working with patients and approaching all that life brings. When applied, functional contextualism naturally promotes kindness, love, and self-compassion. The idea of every behavior serving a purpose, and context producing all psychological events, prompts us to stay more curious, intentional, and gracious when faced with unwanted or challenging behaviors. This philosophy and perspective is difficult to apply as a leader. Playing out the philosophy would mean that employees' behaviors are not solely representative of personality traits or flaws but an accumulation of the individual's past and current context.

In a sense, if a BHC is not engaged or producing desired behaviors, a leader from a functional contextualist perspective would not automatically assume that this is due to a character deficit; instead, the behavior must be evaluated in the context of the individual. The leader's style and abilities significantly influence that context and produce behaviors that may frustrate the leader. If you are a director, pause, and reread that sentence to understand its significance.

This approach we take is the result of reading dozens of leadership books and Kirk's influence on us. Essentially we began to approach our team with less interest in problematic behaviors and more in the context we created for the team's operations. If we were concerned about a BHC's productivity, we would ask ourselves what contextual factors were preventing the BHC from being productive. If we were disappointed that more BHCs did not understand the philosophy of primary care, we would become curious about what factors were present to create this lack of uptake.

While this is challenging, this contextual approach, we believe, has been the most significant influence for what has produced our BHCs achieving the highest departmental employee engagement scores for four straight years. Outside of that initial 2016 year, we have achieved high retention rates, even through the Great Resignation and even as the team was tasked with more responsibilities and increased productivity.

Is there a simple or catchy way of practicing Contextual Leadership? While we will provide a definition below, we also want to acknowledge the reality of what we discussed earlier in this chapter. Specifically, leadership, similar to working with patients, should not be reduced and simplified into a few steps that leaders must take to engage their teams. In our opinion, doing so produces the unintended error of making it seem "easy" or something devoid of "complexity."

Thus, while we will discuss a few suggestions and present an overly simplified definition of Contextual Leadership, please, do not mistake the explanation as the totality of the reality. To us, Contextual Leadership is a three-step process for us: 1) Seeing them, 2) Celebrating them, and 3) Expecting them.

Contextual Leadership: See Them. Seeing them involves a genuine desire to get to know your team; this starts from the initial recruiting process, mainly asking questions regarding their values, what got them into healthcare, and what drives their mission and purpose. Not only does this allow us to assess any potential incongruences of our mission as an organization and theirs, but it also allows us to begin to know them as a professional, and, potentially more importantly, as a human being. Additionally, when people arrive at CHCW, they are introduced to our not-so-subtle efforts to encourage people to bring their whole selves to work.

We recognize the potential dangers of blurring boundaries with employees with this approach. If done indiscriminately and unintentionally, this could be harmful and disastrous. At CHCW, we hope that through specific strategies we can support staff bringing their values, being, and humanity to work. Getting to know our team is paramount, from understanding how they like to be recognized, to their mission and values, to who makes up the folks in their inner circle.

Contextual leadership: See them - get to know your employees. We get to know our team through many formats and means. Monthly, each of us offers to meet with our direct reports and completes a Studer concept of rounding (Studer, 2013). Refer to Table 8 for questions we ask during these monthly meetings, which vary in length and can be as short as five to 10 minutes or up to an hour. Before starting these meetings, Dave begins each by asking a simple question that he took from the book The Trillion Dollar Coach (Schmidt et al., 2019). The Trillion Dollar Coach details the life of Bill Campbell, who provided coaching and mentorship to many executives in Silicon Valley, including Steve Jobs, Larry Page, and Eric Schmidt. As the book details, one of Bill's starting questions to every meeting and coaching session, after his initial hug, was, "How is your family?" Even in the often-described cold and ruthless world of the tech industry, the individual mentoring the CEOs of major companies started his interactions with them by seeking to get to know them as individuals and humans, particularly about their social relationships. Reading this aligned perfectly with our values and the desired context we hoped to shape.

Table 8. Monthly PCBH Rounding Questions Examples
What is working well for you?
Is there a care provider or colleague I can recognize and thank for living our mission and going above and beyond?
Do you have the tools, training, and equipment to do your job safely and effectively?
What "tough questions" can I address for you today?

Table 8. Monthly PCBH Rounding Questions Examples
What systems, processes, or safety/quality concerns can be improved for our department/organization?
Tell me about a meaningful connection you made with a patient, family, or co-worker.
What is at least one thing I can start, stop, or continue to do to help improve your experience as an employee?
What can I support you with to benefit your "5 years from today's self?"
What do we need to listen to more?

Contextual leadership: See them - Create moments. After reading another inspiring book called The Power of Moments (Heath & Heath, 2017), we sought to intentionally onboard and celebrate anniversary moments with our team. As The Power of Moments poses to the reader, think back to the first day of your onboarding. Did you feel seen this day? Undoubtedly, a moment was created; was it one of engagement or disengagement? After reading this book, we revamped what we do when folks start at CHCW. Specifically, our coordinator, Maria Ortiz, will have all the BHCs sign a card welcoming them to the organization. Further, before the individual starts, our coordinator will reach out to them, asking about their favorite snacks and drink. When the new BHC shows up to the administration offices for their first day of onboarding, Maria meets them there with the card and a gift basket filled with their favorite snacks and drink. While subtle, this creates engagement and reflects our desire to see them as employees.

During annual evaluations, we ensure the annual evaluation is a way of not only providing performance feedback and reemphasizing expectations (more on this soon) but also seeking to create a context where we celebrate the past year's successes and help them within their careers and personal lives. In fact, in 2023 we renamed the annual evaluations to the "annual recruitment meetings" or "ARRMs" (it is pretty fun to say, give it a try if you'd like). Our ARRM form includes prompts and questions such as, "List your three why's/values related to your role at CHCW," "What are three professional goals you have for the next year?" "What are three personal goals you have for next year?" "What can we do to help you reach your goals?" These meetings have turned from sterile and, often, disengaging meetings, to ones that are filled with life and purpose and allow us, again, to "see them."

Contextual leadership: See them - workspaces. We also have worked hard to create a context of seeing our team by ensuring they have productive and healing workspaces. Over the nine years, we have been at CHCW, the team has not only grown, we have grown to the point where we did not have enough space for people to complete paperwork, work on projects, and rest. We advocated for BHCs to have a dedicated space in the clinic where they can do non-clinical tasks in a nurturing environment. In 2021, CHCW received grant money, and senior leadership allowed us to use some of the monies to renovate our office space. This office space is purposed for BHC use when they are not in the clinic and working on projects or paperwork.

As we worked with the interior designer and she asked us what our vision was for the space, we said, "A healing space that prompts productivity." Our office includes many subtleties that remind our team that we see you: we added signage in early 2023 to the shared spaces that include slogans such as "WHO or die" (thanks to Ruth Olmer for this one), "context matters," "stay curious," "GSD (get shit done; thanks to Bridget)," "Service. Education.,"; a snack station filled with the team's favorite snacks and drinks, nameplates with their hometowns listed (thanks to Dave)- all of these are subtle ways of reminding everyone of the journey they have been on and their context, current and past, that they bring on this journey.

Contextual leadership: See them - Compensation. Without question, one of the most potent ways of demonstrating or seeing someone is to ensure they are compensated based on their value to the organization. Dave often says, not jokingly, that BHCs can be some of the most influential people in healthcare if they hone their ability to bring a contextual and compassionate lens to healthcare. As anyone in the behavioral health field can attest, salaries, for various reasons, have not matched our medical counterparts.

Not surprisingly, we found early conversations about compensation frustrating, invalidating, and simply disengaging. Even multiple years into our program, and after numerous successes, conversations about salary increases for the team regularly ended with "the market does not support it."

While the overall conversation has evolved from "the PCBH budgets lose money," to being in the black, the current state of the salary market continues to be a problematic context to navigate. During one of our State of the PCBH department presentations to senior leadership, we asked for salary increases for the team and ended by saying, "We do not care what the market is, as we are not doing market things." One of the senior leaders, quite appropriately, asked, "How do you know you are unique?"

After we got through our initial frustration, we realized it was a fair question, as most people probably think they are unique and, yet, how does one know they are? One answer is to track data on how productive the team is beyond just the clinical realm, showing how influential the team is across organizational priorities; from the committees, education, and training initiatives to projects, groups, and non-clinical activities, we can delineate all of our team's activities. At that meeting, while we very much knew salary increases would primarily come down to how the overall organization's budget looked and the current state of the market, our efforts to illuminate the full spectrum of BHC contributions to the organization has allowed us to create a compelling argument for continuing to push compensation upwards.

As we write this chapter, we are currently in another pivotal moment for salaries for our teams. While we were able to receive sizeable increases across the board regarding compensation, BHCs (and medical providers) are still pushing for better compensation. While the outcome of the current talks is unknown, especially given the tough economic times organizations find themselves in, one thing is clear, CHCW is dedicated to fairly compensating our BHCs (and medical providers). We do not think this would have been possible without us seeing our team and making sure the totality of the organization, especially senior leadership, sees our team.

Contextual leadership: See them - engineering the BHC position. One last point we would like to highlight regarding *seeing* our team is structuring weekly schedules and activities that allow our team to succeed. As we discussed earlier, our belief in functional contextualism means that a BHC being productive and engaged at work reflects the BHC and their context at work. We constantly ask ourselves, "What makes a BHC engaged? What makes them productive?" Freeing providers of extraneous responsibilities and tasks and supporting their autonomy within passion projects has been paramount. We want BHCs to focus solely on seeing patients and supporting the primary care team during the clinic.

As discussed earlier, this means ensuring documentation requirements are as efficient as possible, having tasks such as resources and care coordination handled by other staff members, and ensuring processes involving patient care (e.g., completing handoffs, scheduling patients, etc.) are seamless. The latter point has prompted us to ensure clinic schedules produce enough flexibility for BHCs to have scheduled follow-up visits and buffer time to take handoffs and catch up throughout the clinic. As Table 9 shows, a BHC that has been in our system for over a year will have five scheduled slots per four half-day, which are set at 30-minute intervals. After each scheduled slot, a 15-minute buffer follows, allowing the BHC to work flexibly throughout their day to see scheduled and in-the-moment handoffs.

For example, as Table 9 shows, a scheduled visit may occur at 9 AM; however, let us imagine a handoff occurs at 8:59 AM. With the way we have engineered the schedule, we want the handoff to be completed before the scheduled visit at 9 AM. Let us imagine the handoff occurs, lasts 20 minutes, and then the BHC sees their 9 AM at 9:19 AM. Let us continue to imagine the visit lasts 25 minutes, taking us to 9:44 AM, allowing them to be on time to see their 9:45 AM, barring any other handoffs before then. This scheduled flexibility throughout the clinic day allows for the BHC to produce the very behaviors we are hoping for, dedication to patient care and giving preference for in-the-moment connection with patients.

Table 9. Example of CHCW PCBH Schedule Template
8:00 AM
Buffer (BHCs huddling with and scrubbing PCPs' schedules)
8:15 AM
BHC Scheduled Visit
8:30 AM
8:45 AM
Buffer
9:00 AM
BHC Scheduled Visit
9:15 AM
9:30 AM
Buffer

Table 9. Example of CHCW PCBH Schedule Template
9:45 AM
BHC Scheduled Visit
10:00 AM
10:15 AM
Buffer
10:30 AM
BHC Scheduled Visit
10:45 AM
11:00 AM
Buffer
11:15 AM
BHC Scheduled Visit
11:30 AM
11:45 AM
Buffer

Contextual leadership: See them - approach to weekly scheduling. Seeing our BHCs also means engineering a weekly schedule with respite moments for paperwork and predictable project time, only changing for rare occasions due to coverage needs; this was a concept we realized after reading this book's first edition. As Neftali discussed his comparison of BHCs that work five days of full clinical activities versus BHCs working four days and how the two groups saw the same number of patients, we knew we needed to do that for our team. As Neftali has described, the basic theory is that if BHCs are provided time to heal, do charts, do deep work, and work on projects, their clinical time will be more productive. Rather than having a BHC who works 100% clinical, actively not take handoffs due to knowing they have no time to do their charts or are tired from a lack of respite, BHCs who have time to recharge will be more willing to actively seek out patients when they are in the clinic.

We have applied this theory to our team, and the results have been profound. Not only has productivity continued to increase and grow for each BHC, even as we add more, the projects and initiatives the BHCs have produced during their respite time have been nothing short of inspiring. From creating a community walking group that patients and staff members attend on weekends (developed by Sarah Ortner), to developing training modules for family medicine residents on topics related to contextualism and compassionate care (developed by Emily Faust), to focusing on making charting more efficient for the entire team (contributed by Ruth Olmer, Heather Harris, and Amelia McClelland), to a weekly PiYo exercise class (developed by Ruth Olmer), our talented group of BHCs has used their abilities in incredible ways.

We ensure that the weekly schedule, which usually includes a breakdown of 70% clinical work, 10% charting, 10% faculty/rendering training activities, and 10% project time, is set and only changes when clinical coverage needs are apparent. (Another considerable benefit of having training programs, including the medical residency and the PCBH training programs, is the ability to offer our core BHCs more time out of the clinic to engage in education activities. Education and training work is also a massive recruitment and retention strategy.) A predictable schedule allows our BHCs to prepare for their upcoming weeks and months, ensuring they are most productive during each assigned task. At a recent PCBH retreat, multiple BHCs commented that the predictable schedule has been beneficial as it eases their mind about what is coming in the future and assures that the schedule reflects an understanding of the demanding job that is PCBH.

One consequence of expanding the BHC coverage to all of our clinics is that the clinics began to adjust to a more standard ratio of clinical coverage. In our early days, our mothership clinic averaged a PCP to BHC ratio of 4.5:1; however, due to the uptake of PCBH, now it can be very busy even with a ratio of 3:1. Thus, we have developed an Excel sheet algorithm for our schedule templates to alert us whenever coverage at a specific clinic dips below our desired ratio of PCPs to BHCs. We move around coverage, project, and charting time when alerted to ensure acceptable coverage. If unavoidable, we begin adjusting BHCs schedules to allow for more buffer zones in anticipation of high warm handoffs at a particular clinic. A few years back, we partnered with our human resources to develop per diem contracts for all interested in BHCs. Thus, if low on coverage, we will offer per diem clinic opportunities where we will pay our BHCs for any additional clinics they work beyond their regular schedule. Previously, if we needed BHCs to provide extra coverage, there was no formal compensation, which is not conducive to work-life integration. Our efforts in ensure consistent coverage is a way for us to show BHCs we not only *See* the challenges of the job, it also reinforces to them how vital their jobs are. Similar to hospitals needing to have so many medical providers on to cover patients, so too must we have BHCs on due to the invaluable and life saving work they do.

Contextual leadership: Celebrate them. We often joke during leadership training, "Yes, even adults who are professionals need positive reinforcement." One of the common themes discussed in leadership books is how much time and energy is focused on things not going right as opposed to what is going right in an organization. When a team celebrates wins, a context is developed that engenders team members' feelings of value.

Contextual leadership: Celebrate them - BHC monthly meetings. At the beginning of every BHC monthly meeting, the BHC team shares wins, kudos, and moments of gratitude/reflection for the greater CHCW team and each other as BHCs. This space is free of time and has no limit on how long the moment lasts. Dave can remember during a BHC meeting where the sharing of wins and kudos was entering its 40+ minute. At this time, Dave texted Bridge, "We need to move on; we have a lot of important things to go over." Bridget responded, "This is the important stuff." Bridget, as she usually is, was right. Creating a space where the team shares appreciation, gratitude, and basks in recent wins is not only healing for each member of the team, it brings the team together as a unit.

Sarah Ortner leads this section of our meeting. She brings many themes and prompts, including what things are rejuvenating folks, what PTO they have coming up or were able to enjoy this past month, and other outside-of-work milestones such as anniversaries, birthdays, and momentous family events. Our previous CEO, Dr. Maples, made it a point to attend the BHC monthly meetings even with the 7 AM start time. He regularly commented to other leaders in the organization, "If you want to feel positive and energized after a meeting, even at 7 AM, go to this meeting!"

We send weekly emails to team members highlighting moments of appreciation and gratitude. These emails include celebrating a BHC hitting a daily visit record, a team of BHCs covering many handoffs during the clinic, or a patient story that reflected healing and engagement. Of course, keeping these to ourselves would not be a functional contextualist approach. We regularly share wins and kudos with care team members. A formal version is done monthly during the clinics' All-Staff meetings, where we give out the monthly Warm-Handoff trophy. Each clinic's respective BHCs will provide nominations of staff members, including PCPs, MAs, nurses, and front desk staff members, who have done an incredible job with handoffs in the past month. The team will gather nominations and vote on a winner announced at the All-Staff meetings. To say the Warm-Handoff trophy is a coveted award is an understatement. It has been humbling and awe-inspiring to see its impact on some employees, as one employee became tearful when winning, expressing, "This is the first time I have ever won anything at work."

Contextual leadership: Celebrate them - sharing with senior leadership. Additionally, we share regular emails and comments about our team's successes with clinic management, leadership, and our senior leadership team; this is another strategy Kirk introduced to us in those early months of starting at CHCW. He explained that we must demonstrate our contributions overtly and often. This sharing has cultivated a culture from upper management that views the BHCs as talented and inspiring individuals; it also has solidified the reality of the BHC team being value-driven and high-performers.

In meetings with leadership and management, everyone knows the wins and successes the team has accomplished and achieved, resulting in more engagement from our senior and clinic leaders. The BHC team gets it done whenever something needs to be executed, such as mandatory training, peer chart audits, closing charts, etc. As Bridget regularly shares with the team, this engenders positivity amongst the senior leaders and allows us to "earn chips," as Kirk used to say. As you will hear Bridget tell the team, a contract exists between employer and employee. If we expect high leadership standards, then we need to execute high standards, plain and simple.

Notably, focusing on kudos, gratitude, excellence, and GSD does not mean we support a culture of toxic positivity. Part of celebrating the team is also to celebrate vulnerability and struggles. As regularly seen by members of the PCBH team, BHCs will share moments of losing patients, complex clinical interactions, and struggles. When Bridget had a devastating loss in her family and friend group, she emailed the team about the vulnerability and how it impacted her. The team responded by celebrating the vulnerability and an appreciation for allowing them to be with Bridget during the difficult time. When Dave lost a patient unexpectedly, he emailed the team, letting them know how it impacted him, resulting in the team surrounding and lifting him through the next few days of clinic. Celebrating them means celebrating each moment and experience BHCs endure, including the difficult and uncomfortable ones.

Contextual leadership: Celebrate them - The Award Show. Formal celebrations occur during the monthly PCBH meetings and annual evaluations. At each monthly meeting, we complete the famous CHCW PCBH Award Show. During this part of the meeting, Dave walks the team through a PowerPoint slide deck highlighting the team's wins and accomplishments in the past month. Maybe a record was set for the number of visits or handoffs, or a BHC completed an important project; moments that reflect the infinite values of the PCBH department are highlighted. Then, we begin passing out awards through the monthly club and award winners. Table 10 details each of the monthly clubs and awards handed out. The Award Show usually elicits a lot of laughter and engagement.

A year ago, we asked the BHCs what their favorite parts of the monthly meetings were, and they responded, almost universally, "the sharing of wins and kudos, and the monthly Award Show." It is important to note that Award Shows can sometimes prompt discomfort for team members, both for winning and not winning awards. Similar to indiscriminately applying a behavioral intervention without knowing the context of the individual, we believe it is paramount to ensure that leadership provides a context of celebrating wins and kudos before introducing the idea of the Award Show.

Table 10. CHCW PCBH Monthly Award Show Clubs and Awards

Benjamin Club

BHCs who completed at least 100 visits in the month

All-State Club

BHCs who averaged at least 1.5 warm-handoffs per clinic

Sharp-Shooter Club

BHCs who averaged at least 4.2 visits per clinic

Task Destroyer Club

BHCs who completed all charting and submitted clinic counts on time with no reminders

Be a Friend Club

BHCs who completed all peer reviews in the month

Consistency Club (quarterly)

BHCs who had zero call-outs during the past quarter

Producer Award

BHC who completed the most visits in the month

All-State Award

BHC averaged the highest number of warm handoffs per clinic in the month

Marathon Award

BHC who completed the most clinics in the month

New Heights Award

Table 10. CHCW PCBH Monthly Award Show Clubs and Awards
BHC averaged the highest number of visits per clinic in the month
Culture Shaper (quarterly)
BHC has profoundly shaped CHCW's culture. Voted on by the PCBH team
Shining Star Award (quarterly)
BHCs with the highest quarterly and rolling 12-month patient engagement scores
BHC of the Month
BHC with the highest BHCr score, an algorithm that includes visits/clinic, warm-handoffs/clinic, and initial/clinic.

The Award Show is a place for our team to celebrate each other and individuals who had incredible months. If the context is lacking, the Award Show could produce an air of resentment and disengagement. At the end of every Award Show, our program coordinator (Maria Ortiz) creates slides with pictures of the team completing fun activities outside work. Essentially, every month she sends an email with a request for BHCs to send in pictures showing their families, pets, accomplishments, and them engaging in other meaningful activities. And, although it is 100% optional, the vast majority of the team participates in sending in photos the vast majority of the months. It is truly amazing to see how this "photo dump" activity has evolved. There are so many special moments that we share in at the end of the award show as our coordinator prompts the team to say a few comments about the photos' significance. It truly gives the team an opportunity to both see and celebrate each other.

Additionally, we intentionally celebrate the team members taking paid time off (PTO). We have dedicated ourselves to working against the glorification of overwork (something we both struggle with) and to model taking PTO and not working on CHCW tasks during PTO. Having our BHCs take their PTO is good for all parties - it allows us to plan and have appropriate budgets and allows BHCs to come back rejuvenated; this is something we overlooked in the early years but now have brought to the forefront as a critical strategy in employee engagement. In recent years, we have worked diligently to eradicate sending emails on weekends or holidays. We are, again, attempting to model a more sustainable approach to this work.

Contextual Leadership: Expect of them. Each club and award from the Award Show ensures that we, as a program, are reinforcing metrics or data points that reflect our infinite values of providing contextual, compassionate, and team-based healthcare to our population; this translates into us creating a context of expectations for our team.

Simply seeing and celebrating employees will only produce satisfaction, not engagement. Expecting of them allows for the final piece of engagement to be realized. As we learned through our Studer training, having clearly defined expectations for employees that are understood and universal for the team creates more engagement. We rumble about this regularly when consulting and talking with colleagues, as unquestionably, expectations of employees can sometimes create tension and resentment, both from leaders and direct reports.

We strive to create a culture and context of *expecting* in the following ways:

Contextual leadership, Expect of them: Metrics. First, we have worked hard to ascertain our infinite values and what metrics and data points reflect those values. Six data points best reflect our infinite values:
1. visits per day per BHC,
2. handoffs per day per BHC,
3. penetration rate of BHCs into the clinic's population,
4. patient engagement,
5. PCP satisfaction with the PCBH program, and
6. BHC's overall employee engagement

Each month, the first three data points are shared regularly during the Award Show, with the first two data points (i.e., visits per day and handoffs per day) shared for each BHC's numbers. Patient engagement data and an award for that metric are shared quarterly. Penetration rates, PCP satisfaction, and employee engagement are shared annually.

We analyzed years of data to gather information on daily visits and handoffs. We determined the minimum expectation for a core BHC would be 4.2 visits per clinic (or 8.4 visits per day), with 1.5 handoffs per clinic (or 3.0 handoffs per day) occurring. As a reminder, a visit for us is a meaningful clinical encounter, including gathering context and providing intervention, rendering ~95% of these visits billable. During each monthly meeting, not only are each individual's metrics shared with the entire team, each BHC receives a PCBH Scorecard after the meeting that details their past three month's metrics related to visits and handoffs, along with a comparison to the team average. If BHCs have three consecutive months of not meeting these minimum requirements, they will meet with Bridget or Dave to troubleshoot their productivity.

As you read this last passage, we ask you to pause and notice your body's response and where your mind is going. Does this prompt discomfort? Does your mind wonder how your team will respond? Does it say, "Absolutely not?" At the start, our team faced similar challenges, and we often disagreed on establishing a culture that prioritized recognizing and appreciating our staff while holding them accountable.

Reading several books such as A Culture of High Performance (Studer, 2013), Dare to Lead (Brown, 2018), and Radical Candor (Scott, 2017), we began to realize that creating a context of candor and expecting was potentially the most potent contextual factor possible. It created clear expectations for the team and allowed us to ensure that it was reasonable and realistic to expect what we were expecting of them. As discussed in the *Seeing* them section, if we were to expect them, we had to ensure the context was conducive to the behaviors we hoped to see.

Contextual leadership, Expect of them: Radical candor. This encouraged us to strive to create a context of radical candor amongst the team. Dave likes to reflect and share books he has read about Google and Apple, not as an endorsement but as an example of what a candid context can produce. Google and Apple have been known to have meetings of fierce debate and radical candor, rippling out to challenging assumptions and regular evolution. In the context of PCBH, we need to adapt continually, asking ourselves, "How do we reach our communities in more efficient ways?" However, as Scott's book (2017) discussed, candor and rumbling make sense only when there is a context of love, connection, and engagement.

Dave recalls never believing the stories about Google and Apple meetings, as his mind often said, "No one would be able to do that truly." Years into this program, we can say it happens regularly and often at our program. If people attended our monthly meetings or other individual meetings, they would observe a significant amount of celebrating and connecting and a great deal of rumbling, debate and expecting of one another. Assumptions are regularly challenged, and statements such as "with all the grace, love, and compassion" (that one is a favorite of Emily Faust) alert everyone that a rumbling is about to begin; this has led the team to not only embrace each other, it has prompted us to expect of each other.

Further, this continual discussion of expectations, rumbling, and radical candor paves the way for more engagement. For example our annual evaluations (renamed ARRMs as mentioned earlier) are largely a time for celebration versus a negative and nerve-wracking experience. BHCs enter the space fully knowing the expectations, if or if they are not meeting those expectations, and this allows for more genuine conversations about performance, their goals, and their future. We have a saying that there should not be any new information shared at the ARRMS, as that should have been done in the moment there was a concern.

Without question, this context of expecting has influenced some individuals to recognize that the work of PCBH may not be for them. Rather than responding with resentment and demoralization, the context of expecting allows these candid conversations to be handled with more kindness and compassion, allowing us to celebrate folks moving on even when they realize that maybe PCBH at CHCW is not their career.

Radical candor works the opposite way as well. CHCW PCBH leadership asks BHCs directly what it will take for us to retain them. There have been times when it was clear CHCW would not be able to help the employee reach their professional or personal goals. Thus, they needed to move on. Instead of resentment or negative feelings when BHCs decide to move on, these employees' next adventures can be shared and celebrated. Expecting each other and being candid creates engagement for current members and can also prompt a movement towards a more value-congruent professional path, within or not within PCBH.

CHCW PCBH: Next steps

Transitioning to the end of this journey, we reflect on areas we see coming down the road. Unquestionably, we have continued to advocate for more representation at all levels of leadership within the organization. Over the past year, Bridget was asked to serve on Senior Leadership and invited to participate in all Senior Leadership functions. We have also had conversations regarding BHCs serving and chairing committees, accepting positions historically reserved for physicians, such as one of our BHCs, Ruth Olmer, PsyD, serving as the EHR Provider Champion and leading us through an EHR transition. We hope this continues to grow the status of BHCs as essential team members and as dynamic leaders within the organization.

CHCW PCBH: Justice, Equity, Diversity & Inclusion

Further, we know our efforts to embrace diversity, equity, and inclusion must be improved and evolve. Recruiting and hiring BHCs who are representative of our patients' demographics is essential. Additionally, we must ensure that we have more bilingual BHCs on staff. We continue to highlight and require that all BHCs at CHCW share a value of cultural curiosity and humility, which is paramount for our program to evolve. We are looking into offering internships for high school students and current employees to provide exposure to the role of a BHC and help individuals further their careers within the organization. We are currently investigating opportunities to collaborate with nearby graduate education programs that have a track record of recruiting and training a diverse range of students who share a commitment to serving underserved communities.

The Evolution Of Primary Care

Rethinking how primary care could work and be delivered continues to be an iterative endeavor. Our goals include:

- Reducing barriers to care, such as having a mobile unit that not only includes medical and dental but also includes BHCs
- Expanding hours of service and locations to schools and other community venues
- Exploring having a ratio of one BHC to one PCP
- Developing better data tracking and clear outcomes for integrating BHCs into primary care
- Research what happens when a health system embraces a contextual and compassionate approach delivered by all team members (not just BHCs).

Lastly, we wonder, "What would it look like if a BHC was truly a PCP?" We hope to answer this in the coming decade at CHCW.

Gratitude

We want to thank you for taking this journey with us; we at CHCW could talk for days about PCBH and the efforts of CHCW. We want to again acknowledge the limiting context of this story being told through our eyes. We have, unquestionably, not acknowledged everyone in this story. We also acknowledge the bias (and error) inherent in us being the ones to tell this story, and yet offer ourselves grace as it is impossible to recollect every pebble over these past few decades.

Further, we hope you do not walk away with misconceptions. First and after reading this, you could conclude that everything is perfect at CHCW and it is a PCBH nirvana. Again, we hope it was clear that it took an iterative process over decades to get a well-functioning

PCBH service. Moreover, we hope there is no implication that CHCW's success is solely due to us being the leaders of these efforts. We can talk for days about the mistakes we have made along the way. We created a PCBH Corner regarding <u>Instagram vs. Reality</u>, discussing the importance of directors and BHCs in programs being kind, showing grace towards yourself and your program, and applying what can be applied realistically.

While we take great pride and ownership of what has been accomplished at CHCW, we are acutely aware of the many contextual accidents and randomness that facilitated this story.

We also know that all of the BHCs, past and present are responsible for where we are today. These include Ruth Olmer, Amelia McClelland, Steven Olmer, Carrah James, Emily Faust, Julie Aubrey, Heather Harris, Sarah Ortner, Graciela Ortiz, Mayra Correa Barada, Ryan Boggess, Lacey Sheppard, Hilary Richardson, our coordinator, Maria Ortiz, and all of our trainees past and present. Further, our Senior Leadership team, consisting of Angela Gonzalez, Christopher Reed, Gray Dawson, Stephanie Macias, Desiree Ashbrooks, Caitlin Hill, Vanessa Krantz, Julie Finley, and Laura McClintock, as well as past senior leaders, have created a context where PCBH can flourish. Our governing board, as well as every employee at CHCW, contributes to the context of being able to produce radical ripples of PCBH. Without question, our patients and community continue to embrace the idea of PCBH- they are also crucial to this story.

We would also like to end with a few themes we hope pulsated throughout the chapter. First, we hope you, as the reader, have taken away the importance of understanding the context you are striving to integrate within. For us, this context is primary care, and regardless if that is your context or not, strive to understand the setting's purpose, mission, and values. And, while undoubtedly work to evolve the setting's mission and values, strive to not only understand but believe in the mission. Understand that context reigns supreme and whether it is working with a patient, striving to integrate into a system, gaining buy-in from an organization, or obtaining engagement from your BHCs, approach these behaviors from a functional contextualist perspective, asking regularly, "what context would produce the very psychological events I am hoping to see?"

Second, embracing and understanding accidents can be turned into opportunities with intentionality and a will to lean in. Even when the world appears to be crumbling around you, and you have to tell the same nurse for the millionth time you can help with diabetes, lean in and keep fighting. One of our previous trainees, Will Summers, alerted us to a Buddhist story of the farmer that details a series of events in which there appeared to be a positive outcome or a negative outcome, only to have the proceeding event change the positive outcome to a negative one and the negative one to a positive one. Will would often impressively say, "good, bad, or too soon to tell," and as we have learned, life has an interesting way of making everything "too soon to tell." Lean in, be kind, and embrace accidents (even difficult ones) as opportunities.

Lastly, be intentional on creating a context for yourself to be successful. Whether you are a student interested in PCBH, a new BHC to a PCBH system, a leader of a growing PCBH program, an administrator looking to learn, whatever your role and place in the universe, cultivate a context of kindness, compassion, and love. Find someone to share wins with, as well as vulnerability when needed. Find meaning and purpose not only in your clinical and administrative work, but outside of work. Find time to reflect on moments that happen so regularly that we have habituated to their awe-ness. Find your values and connect regularly with them. And, find behaviors that cultivate a context of those three healing and life producing contextual factors, kindness, compassion, and love.

One final request of you as a reader, reach out to us. When we share regularly on listservs and through social media about PCBH Corners or Stories of PCBH, we love receiving emails from people about their own stories. For sure, we love answering questions, and more so we love hearing the passion and values from people doing this work. It, literally, is healing for us. So, reach out regularly and often to let us know what was helpful about this chapter and what was confusing (we assume much)! Also, if our paths cross at a conference or workshop, please, engage with us as connecting and knowing others are carrying the same conviction as us only fuels our spirit and desires.

Our gratitude again for reading about the radical ripples PCBH has created at CHCW. Be kind, be compassion, and, above all, be love. Our gratitude for you and this journey.

References

Barnes-Holmes, Y., Hayes, S. C., Barnes-Holmes, D., & Roche, B. (2001). Relational frame theory: a post-Skinnerian account of human language and cognition. *Advances in child development and behavior*, 28, 101-138. https://doi.org/10.1016/s0065-2407(02)80063-5

Bauman, D., & Beachy, B. (2020). Integrated behavioral health in primary care: A look at Community Health of Central Washington. *Washington Family Physician: The Journal of the WAFP*, 20-21.

Bauman, D., Beachy, B, & Ogbeide, S. A. (2018). Stepped care and behavioral approaches for diabetes management in integrated primary care. In W. O'Donahue & A. Maragakis (Eds), *Principle-based stepped care and brief psychotherapy for integrated care settings*. New York, NY: Springer Science, Business Media, LLC.

Braverman, A. M., Kunkel, E. J., Katz, L., Katona, A., Heavens, T., Miller, A., & Arfaa, J. J. (2015). Do I Buy It? How AIDET™ Training Changes Residents' Values about Patient Care. *Journal of patient experience*, 2(1), 13-20. https://doi.org/10.1177/237437431500200104

Brown, B. (2018). *Dare to lead: Brave work. Tough conversations. Whole hearts.* New York, NY: Random House.

Davis, C. S., Roy, T., Peterson, L. E., & Bazemore, A. W. (2022). Evaluating the Teaching Health Center Graduate Medical Education Model at 10 Years: Practice-Based Outcomes and Opportunities. *Journal of graduate medical education*, 14(5), 599–605. https://doi.org/10.4300/JGME-D-22-00187.1

Deao, C. (2016). *The E-Factor: How engaged patients, clinician, leaders, and employees will transform healthcare.* Pensacola, FL: Fire Starter Publishing.

Ericsson, A., & Pool, R. (2016). *Peak: Secrets from the new science of expertise.* Houghton Mifflin Harcourt.

Felitti, V. J., Anda, R. F., Nordenberg, D., Williamson, D. F., Spitz, A. M., Edwards, V., Koss, M. P., & Marks, J. S. (1998). Relationship of childhood abuse and household dysfunction to many of the leading causes of death in adults: The Adverse Childhood Experiences (ACE) study. *American Journal of Preventive Medicine,* 14, 245-258.

Gunn, R., Davis, M. M., Hall, J., Heintzman, J., Muench, J., Smeds, B., Miller, B. F., Miller, W. L., Gilchrist, E., Brown Levey, S., Brown, J., Wise Romero, P., & Cohen, D. J. (2015). Designing Clinical Space for the Delivery of Integrated Behavioral Health and Primary Care. *Journal of the American Board of Family Medicine : JABFM,* 28 Suppl 1(Suppl 1), S52-S62. https://doi.org/10.3122/jabfm.2015.S1.150053

Hayes, L. J., & Fryling, M. J. (2019). Functional and descriptive contextualism. *Journal of Contextual Behavioral Science,* 14, 119-126. https://doi.org/10.1016/j.jcbs.2019.09.002

Hayes, S. C., Strosahl, K. D., & Wilson, K. G. (2011). *Acceptance and commitment therapy: The process and practice of mindful change.* Guilford press.

Heath, C., & Heath, D. (2017). *The Power of Moments.* New York, NY: Simon & Schuster.

HRSA. (2016). *National projections of supply and demand for selected behavioral health practicioners: 2013-2024.* : Department of Health & Human Serivices. https://bhw.hrsa.gov/sites/default/files/bureau-health-workforce/data-research/behavioral-health-2013-2025.pdf

National Academies of Sciences, Engineering, and Medicine; Health and Medicine Division; Board on Health Care Services; Committee on Implementing High-Quality Primary Care, Robinson, S. K., Meisnere, M., Phillips, R. L., Jr., & McCauley, L. (Eds.). (2021). *Implementing High-Quality Primary Care: Rebuilding the Foundation of Health Care.* National Academies Press (US).

O'Malley, A. S., Rich, E. C., Maccarone, A., DesRoches, C. M., & Reid, R. J. (2015). Disentangling the Linkage of Primary Care Features to Patient Outcomes: A Review of Current Literature, Data Sources, and Measurement Needs. *Journal of General Internal Medicine,* 30 Suppl 3, S576-585. https://doi.org/10.1007/s11606-015-3311-9

Miller, W. R., & Rollnick, S. (2002). *Motivational interviewing: Preparing people for change (2nd ed.).* New York, NY: The Guilford Press.

Miller, W. R., & Rollnick, S. (2013). *Motivational interviewing: Helping people change (3rd ed.)*. New York, NY: Guilford Press.

Plamondon, K. M., Bottorff, J. L., Caxaj, C. S., & Graham, I. D. (2020). The integration of evidence from the Commission on Social Determinants of Health in the field of health equity: a scoping review. *Critical Public Health*, 30(4), 415-428. https://doi.org/10.1080/09581596.2018.1551613

Reiter, J. T., Dobmeyer, A. C., & Hunter, C. L. (2018). The Primary Care Behavioral Health (PCBH) Model: An Overview and Operational Definition. *Journal of Clinical Psychology in Medical Settings*, 25(2), 109-126. https://doi.org/10.1007/s10880-017-9531-x

Robinson, P. J., Gould, D. A., & Strosahl, K. D. (2010). *Real behavioral change in primary care: Improving patient outcomes & increasing job satisfaction*. Oakland, CA: New Harbinger Publications, Inc.

Robinson, P. J. (2015). *Contextual Behavioral Science: Primary Care. Current Opinions in Psychology*, Elsevier.

Robinson, P. J., & Reiter, J. T. (2016). *Behavioral consultation and primary care: A guide to integrating services (2nd ed.)*. Springer International Publishing. https://doi.org/10.1007/978-3-319-13954-8

Schmidt, E., Rosenberg, J., & Eagle, A. (2019). *Trillion Dollar Coach: The Leadership Playbook of Silicon Valley's Bill Campbell*. New York, NY: HarperCollins Publishers.

Scott, K. (2017). *Radical Candor.* New York, NY: St. Martin's Press.

Sinek, S. (2019). *The Infinite Game.* New York, NY: Penguin Random House, LLC.

Strosahl, K., Robinson, P., & Gustavsson, T. (2012). *Brief interventions for radical change: Principles & practice of focused acceptance and commitment therapy.* Oakland, CA: New Harbinger Publications, Inc.

Studer, Q. (2013). *A culture of high performance: Achieving higher at a lower cost.* Gulf Breeze, FL: Fire Starter Publishing.

About the Authors

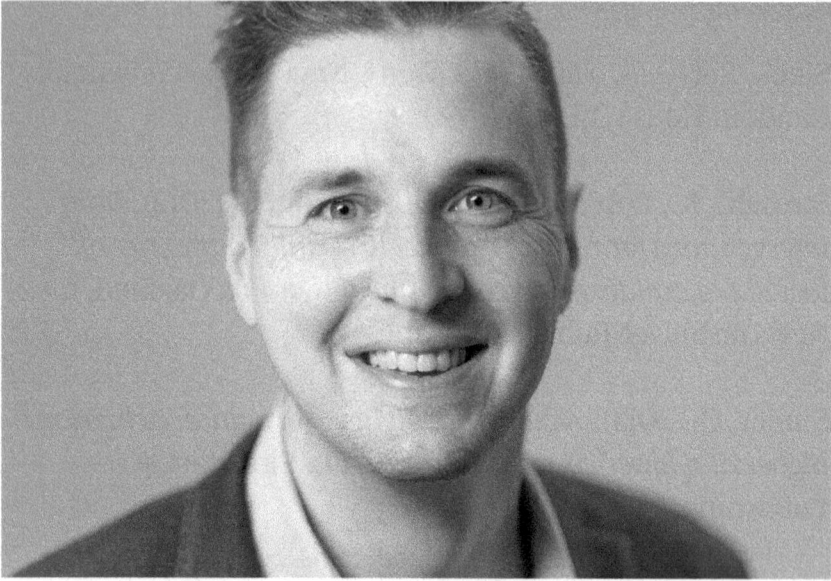

David Bauman, PsyD is a licensed psychologist and the Primary Care Behavioral Health Education Director at Community Health of Central Washington, where he oversees a variety of behavioral health training programs (i.e., predoctoral psychology internship, post-doctoral psychology fellowship, and psychosocial medicine curriculum within the family medicine residency). He also is the principal member of Beachy Bauman Consulting, where he is able to consult with health systems around the globe regarding the integration of behavioral health into primary care, as well as helping providers and systems provide contextual and compassionate healthcare. Dr. Bauman can be found on X at @PCBHlife.

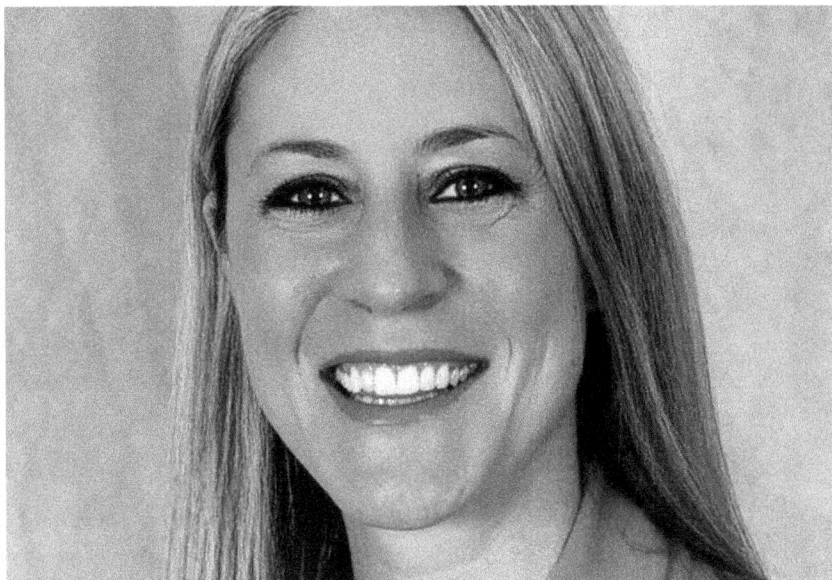

Bridget Beachy, PsyD, is a licensed psychologist who's passionate about all things integrated care! During her day job, Dr. Beachy is the Director of Primary Care Behavioral Health at Community Health of Central Washington (CHCW) in Washington state where she serves on CHCW's executive team, oversees the PCBH service, supervises and trains learners, and still loves delivering clinical services to patients of all ages. In other pursuits, she's Co-Principal for Beachy Bauman Consulting where she and her partner, David Bauman, help other organizations and individuals around the globe pursue integrated care efforts. Dr. Beachy is an author as well as an avid speaker and presenter, and can additionally be found on Beachy Bauman Consulting's YouTube Channel as well as CFHA's Integrated Care Podcast.

For more training opportunities, <u>consultation support</u> &
networking opportunities visit
<u>integratedcareassocation.com</u> or <u>cfha.net</u>.

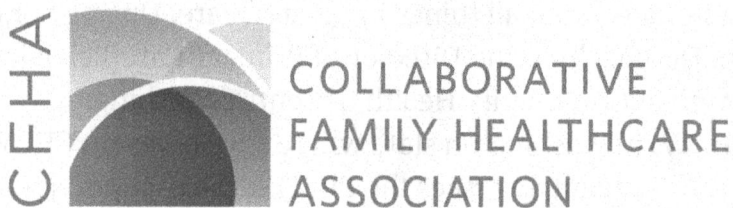

COLLABORATIVE
FAMILY HEALTHCARE
ASSOCIATION

www.ingramcontent.com/pod-product-compliance
Lightning Source LLC
Chambersburg PA
CBHW072037020426
42334CB00017B/1305